Making Medical Decisions

How to Make Difficult Medical and Ethical Choices for Yourself and Your Family

Thomas Scully, M.D., and Celia Scully

Formerly published as Playing God

A FIRESIDE BOOK
Published by Simon & Schuster Inc.
New York   London   Toronto   Sydney   Tokyo

THOMAS SCULLY, M.D., and CELIA SCULLY

New York London Toronto Sydney Tokyo

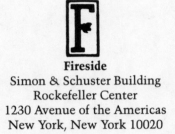

Fireside
Simon & Schuster Building
Rockefeller Center
1230 Avenue of the Americas
New York, New York 10020

Copyright © 1987 by Thomas Scully, M.D., and Celia Scully

First Fireside Edition, 1989

FIRESIDE and colophon are registered trademarks
of Simon & Schuster Inc.

Designed by Irving Perkins Associates
Manufactured in the United States of America

1   3   5   7   9   10   8   6   4   2
1   3   5   7   9   10   8   6   4   2   (Pbk.)

Library of Congress Cataloging in Publication Data
Scully, Thomas J., date.
Playing God / Thomas Scully and Celia Scully.

p.cm.
Bibliography: p.
Includes index.
1. Medical ethics.   I. Scully, Celia G., date.   II. Title.
R724.S396 1987   87-20610
174'.2—dc19   CIP

ISBN 0-671-60144-X
ISBN 0-671-68731-X (Pbk.)

for
Leslie, Marty, Geary
Chris, Michelle, Cathy
Peter and Barbara

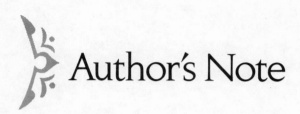 Author's Note

MY wife and I collaborated in writing this book because of the experiences we have shared and our mutual interest in health care ethics. However, we have chosen to use the first-person singular form throughout this book because the clinical and professional experiences described are mine.

Thomas Scully, M.D.

Contents

Acknowledgments   *11*

1. Making Hard Choices You Can
   Live With   15

2. Taking the Lead in Building a
   Healthier Doctor-Patient
   Relationship   34

3. Knowing and Exercising Your
   Rights as a Patient   59

4. The Living Will, the Durable
   Power of Attorney, and Naming
   a Proxy—the Pluses of Thinking
   Ahead   92

5. Transplanting Human Organs
   and Tissues—a New Lease on
   Life   124

6. Making Babies—Conflicting
   Rights *in Utero* and Beyond   152

7. The Baby Doe Dilemma—to
   Treat or Not to Treat   194

8. Who Speaks for the Child with
   a Disabling, Life-Threatening, or
   Terminal Illness?   230

9. Making Life-and-Death
   Decisions for Another Adult   272
10. From Malpractice to Billing
    Fraud—Getting Action When
    You've Been Wronged   306

   Appendices   341
   A A Patient's Bill of Rights   342
   B A Medical Research Patient's
      Bill of Rights   345
   C A Pregnant Patient's Bill of
      Rights   347
   D An Institutionalized Person's
      Bill of Rights   350
   E A Nursing Home Patient's
      Bill of Rights   354
   F Living Will and Durable
      Power of Attorney for Health
      Care (sample forms)   356
   G Uniform Anatomical Gift
      Act; Donor Card and
      Consent by Next of Kin for
      Removal of Organs (sample
      forms)   364
   H Withholding or Withdrawing
      of Life-Prolonging Medical
      Treatment: AMA Statement   370
   I Pointers on Working with
      the Media   372
   J National and Regional
      Centers for Medical Ethics   375

   Notes and Sources   383
   Selected Bibliography   411
   Index   417

Acknowledgments

THIS book could not have been written without the help of many people who shared their experiences, information and, sometimes, their tears with us. While some case histories are the result of professional and personal experience, many came from colleagues, friends, and students who suggested we interview still others with important stories to tell. In a few instances we have changed names, locations, and occupations to protect the privacy of the person and his or her family.

We are grateful to University of Nevada School of Medicine Dean Robert M. Daugherty, former dean Ernest L. Mazzaferri, and former pediatric department chairmen Burton A. Dudding and Robert Bonar—all of whom supported our studying medical ethics at the Hastings Center and encouraged us to write this book.

Special appreciation goes to Daniel Callahan, director, and Willard Gaylin, President, of the Hastings Center, and to Arthur L. Caplan, Ronald Bayer, Thomas H. Murray, Ruth Macklin, and Carol Levine for their encouragement, stimulating ideas, thoughtful discussions, and sound advice.

A generous gift from Claude I. Howard and assistance from

Hastings Center librarian Marna Howarth enabled us to collect many books, journals, and other materials needed in researching this project. Invaluable, too, was the help of reference librarians at Washoe County Library and at the University of Nevada–Reno Getchell and Savitt libraries.

We are indebted to all who reviewed chapters in their areas of expertise, giving second opinions and making suggestions which have been incorporated in this book:

Judges William N. Forman, Procter Hug, Jr., and Charles E. Springer; attorneys David B. Clarke, Jr., Mary M. Devlin, and Larry D. Lessly; physicians Robert J. Barnet, John M. Davis, Sandra A. Daugherty, Burton A. Dudding, Barry S. Frank, Richard C. Inskip, Paul Jensen, Roy F. MacKintosh, Jeffrey Millman, Larry M. Noble, John Peacock, Michael V. Pokroy, Chris J. Scully, Peter A. Scully, Stewart Shankel, Geoffrey Sher, and Sandra Wilborn; nurses Linda Hicks, Barbara Juergens, Virginia Marriage, Sylvia Smith, and Patricia Rutherford; health care administrators Louise Bayard-de-Volo, Dale G. Breaden, Ann A. Dailey, Michael J. Hoover, Kathleen Lewis, and Thomas Morton; medical ethicists Arthur L. Caplan, James F. Drane, John J. Paris, S.J., and David C. Thomasma; pastoral counselors the Rev. Richard Engeseth, Sister Maureen, O.P., and Rabbi Myra Soifer; psychologist Georgia S. Dudding; health communicator Barbara C. Thornton; political scientist Richard L. Siegel; and patient advocate Virginia Turk.

We wish to thank Edna and Robert Brigham, Evangeline Fernandez, and Leslie Scully, who critiqued chapters from a layperson's viewpoint; Roni Cooley, Derek Newman, and Bill Chau for typing and research assistance; and editorial consultants Connie Emerson and Myrick and Barbara Land.

Special thanks go to our agent, Jacques de Spoelberch, and to our friends at Simon and Schuster, former editor Don Hutter, senior editor Bob Bender, and copy editor Ted Johnson. We are grateful for their confidence in the project and for their help.

This book is not intended as a substitute for legal or medical advice. Readers should consult an attorney regarding personal legal affairs and see a physician about questions related to their health—especially with respect to any symptoms that may require diagnosis or medical attention.

Making Hard Choices You Can Live With

IT'S been more than twenty-five years, but I still clearly remember a U.S. Air Force Hospital maternity ward in Spain where a young mother had just given birth to her first child—a beautiful little girl with no arms.

"Why?" she asked. "What did I do wrong?"

I was stationed in that hospital as a pediatrician, and I had no answer for that distraught young mother. Seemingly there was no explanation until three months later, early in February 1962, when the child's father came to my office with a copy of *Time* opened to a picture of a "flipper" child. A related article suggested a link between his daughter's birth defect and Thalidomide, a drug effective in treating nausea of pregnancy. Tearfully, he showed me a vial containing seventeen pills.[1]

When just six weeks pregnant, his wife, he said, had suffered a bout of morning sickness in Germany, where they were vacationing. A pharmacist provided her with twenty pills, and in the five days that followed, she took only three. But she was not the only one. During the early 1960s, scores of women throughout Europe took Thalidomide for morning sickness and gave birth to an estimated eight thousand deformed babies.[2]

The Thalidomide disaster was the beginning of an ethics revolution in medicine—a broad rethinking of traditional medical values in the light of ethical problems posed by rapid advances in high-tech medicine and research.

Further fueling the interest in medical ethics, both in America and Great Britain, was Sherri Finkbine's flight from Arizona to Sweden in 1962 for the abortion of a Thalidomide-affected infant, an event which focused world-wide attention on the issues of therapeutic abortion.[3] Back home, the nation's first patient selection committee formed in 1962 to choose patients for artificial kidney treatment in Seattle agonized over the difficult task of allocating scarce medical resources.

New technology, new problems— but age-old issues

Physicians, of course, have always been challenged by diffi-cult cases. In making tough decisions, they have been guided by professional codes of ethics based on moral principles to care for the sick, ease suffering, and not abuse the vulnerabil-ity of the sufferer. For example, the Hippocratic Oath with its noted dictum "first, do no harm" has been the cornerstone of Western medicine for centuries.

But now, for the first time in history, physicians have the ability, know-how and sophisticated technology to sustain the physical life of patients beyond any reasonable quality of life they might want to endure. What does that mean?

"Our great tradition of medicine has always had a bias to-ward saving life," explains Daniel Callahan, director of the Hastings Center, a New York facility he cofounded in 1969 to study issues in medical ethics.[4] "It made a great deal of sense until we had the kind of medicine that keeps people alive longer than is good for them, treating them beyond anything good for their benefit."[5]

And that is the *key* issue: what will be of most benefit to you or the person for whom you are making a decision?

Remember, you don't have to sit back and passively let a doctor or a nurse or a hospital do things *to* you or your loved one. You don't have to say (unless it's your choice), "Well, that's how it is and I'm stuck with this treatment," or "What's the use of battling the system—patients can't win because doctors protect each other."

When I was a member of the Nevada State Board of Medical Examiners (the group which licenses and disciplines physicians), I frequently received calls from people who felt wronged, frustrated, angry about their health care—or lack of it. "I don't know how to handle this," they'd tell me. "I don't know where to go, or who to ask—or even what to ask."

As a health care consumer, you have more clout than you realize. But to participate fully in decision-making with your doctor, the hospital, and the "system," you've got to know what your health needs are, what the best way to meet those needs is, and how to get information. You also need to know what your rights are, how to obtain them, and where to go for help and support when you can't do this by yourself.

What you may not realize, however, is that never before have you had so many factors going *for* you.

These range from the so-called doctor glut, resulting in increased competition among doctors for *your* business, to a new focus on encouraging patients to become more responsible for their own health and a growing awareness of patients' rights—backed up by numerous court rulings, federal laws, and the reports of the congressionally mandated President's Commission for the Study of Ethical Problems in Medicine and Biomedical and Behavioral Research.* (You'll find these documents in many hospital and medical school libraries. They can also be purchased directly from the Superintendent of Documents, U.S. Government Printing Office, Washington, D.C. 20402.)

But depending on the nature of your dilemma, one or more

---

*In chapters which follow, this group will be referred to simply as the President's Commission.

ethical principles will determine the choices you make either for yourself or—as a proxy—for someone else. You should be familiar with these principles because ethical dilemmas often arise from a conflict between two or more of them and the underlying values at stake.

Guiding principles

To protect yourself and those you love, you need to be aware of these four principles:

Autonomy is your right to determine what is done to you, to make decisions for yourself, to be told the truth and be sufficiently informed that you can make those decisions. Your rights to personal liberty, privacy, and confidentiality, to be left alone and to be respected as a person, all flow from this principle, and your physician has an obligation to promote and respect your rights, values, preferences, and choices.

Do no harm (nonmaleficence) includes your right not to be injured or hurt in any way. It is the basis for risk-benefit analysis, as well as the notion of "ordinary" and "extraordinary" treatment, a concept explained in Chapter 9. Your doctor has the duty not to harm you or expose you to a risk which is out of proportion to its potential benefit.

Doing good for others (beneficence) obliges us to act in the best interests of others and to help them further their own welfare and well-being. This principle is the basis for treating one another with compassion, respect, and kindness. Beneficence imposes on your doctor the duty to promote your health and welfare and foster your autonomy.

Justice in health care stems from the concept of fairness and the sharing of resources in an equitable way. As citizens, we each have a stake in equal access to health care and the sharing of both benefits and burdens in providing adequate care to everyone. Hospitals and governments should be guided by this principle in establishing policies, guidelines, and legislation.

When it comes to the care of an individual patient, however, experts disagree on the extent to which the principle of justice should influence medical decisions. For example, most ethicists agree that doctors should not deny a patient a treatment, solely based on its cost, if that treatment would greatly benefit the person. However, through its laws and reimbursement policies, society can deny a treatment, based on cost or availability, to *all* patients in a given category—as the government of England has done in refusing to pay for kidney dialysis for all patients over 55 years of age.

Other principles, such as *rationality* (you have a reason or justification for what you're doing) and *universalizability* (you act the way you'd expect all others to act in similar circumstances), also come into play in decision-making. But the first four principles described above are the chief ones which are balanced against one another in most bioethical dilemmas involving patients and their families.

What is bioethics?

Bioethics, explains Arthur Caplan, director of the University of Minnesota's Biomedical Ethics Center, is the examination of policy questions and clinical decisions that have to be made because of advances in medical technology. "Or to put it another way," he says, "bioethics is the attempt to decide what values will govern the practice of health care, what values *ought* to govern what people do."

What would *you* do?

What if *today* you were faced with a life-and-death decision you hoped you'd never have to make—either for yourself or for someone you love. Would you want to have some "say"—

or would you rather leave the choice to someone else? Whom would you go to for support, advice, solace, information?

You can answer in many ways.

You can say yes, you'd want to have a say in the decision, and tell me you'd turn to your minister or priest or rabbi for advice. Your faith would provide a spiritual basis for your choice.

You could describe how you'd consult your doctor or your child's doctor about risks and benefits of treatment or no treatment, and take it from there—a medical basis for your decision.

You might call your attorney after talking to your doctor, adding legal input to your choice.

You could couch your reply in terms of autonomy, best interests, justice, rights, or a heady concept like personhood—calling on philosophy to point you in the right direction.

If time allowed, you'd probably talk it over with your family and, possibly, your friends, even the people you work with or socialize with. One of these people might be a counselor, a hospital social worker, or a university professor who could suggest other experts you could call for advice.

But if you resented my question and felt the adrenaline pumping, if you told me, "Doctors have no business playing God—and neither does anyone else," or "No, I don't think we should make life-and-death decisions for ourselves or others," I would say this book is especially for you.

First of all, there's no such thing as *not making a decision* when it comes to your health. (Suppose, for example, you have a sore throat and fever. You're debating whether or not to call your doctor and you put it off for three days. At first glance, it seems as though you made no decision. But in fact, during the time you waffled back and forth, you made a decision *not* to call but to wait out the symptoms.)

Second, all of us are under increasing pressure today from doctors, insurance companies, the government, and hospitals —to name but a few sources of pressure—to take a greater responsibility for our own health and to share in making decisions that affect ourselves and our families.

Tough decisions when health care dilemmas hit home

In making hard choices involving health care, each of us must come to grips with two questions: "What are my options?" and "Which ones are in my best interests and the best interests of my family?" What would you do if:

- You've taken a new job and will be driving a U-Haul truck across the country. You'd feel safer having your medical records with you, but your doctor won't give them to you.
- You recently underwent amniocentesis, which has revealed that your child will be born with a severe birth defect and probably will be mentally retarded.
- Your 12-year-old child has Hodgkin's disease and a cancer expert has advised chemotherapy and radiation treatment, but you want to try new diet and herbal treatments.
- Your 75-year-old mother has lived alone for years, but she fell recently and is still confused, and her doctor says she shouldn't live by herself any longer. She says she's fine.
- Your 8-year-old daughter is terminally ill and is being treated with experimental drugs at a large medical center. She says she's had enough and wants to go home.
- When you go to renew your driver's license, the clerk asks if you want to sign an organ donor card which can be attached to the back of your license.
- Your son, his wife, and their new baby have come to visit during the holidays. Before they leave, your son surprises you by asking if you've given thought to what you'd want him to do if you ever were in a serious accident or very ill and unable to make decisions for yourself.
- Your doctor makes overt sexual advances.
- You've just given birth to an infant with Down syndrome.[6]

Doctors say the baby's intestines are blocked and he'll die without emergency surgery, but you're worried about the quality of his life if he *does* live.

· Your 85-year-old father, who's in a nursing home, is senile and no longer recognizes you or anyone else. He refuses to eat and his doctor has written orders to start intravenous fluids and stomach-tube feeding.

· Your 37-year-old fiancé, who has no living relatives, had a stroke during surgery and has yet to regain consciousness. His doctors say it's unlikely he ever will, and recommend withdrawing all treatment, including the respirator.

· Your child, who is mentally retarded, has lived at home for sixteen years. Her doctor thinks it's time to place her in a state facility, but the nearest one is two hundred miles away.

· You're hospitalized at a university medical center with advanced cancer of the pancreas, for which there is no cure. Your doctor suggests an experimental new drug.

· You and your wife dearly want children, but are infertile. You've read about sperm banks, frozen embryos, and surrogate mothers, but you don't like the idea of paying someone to have your baby or having "orphan embryos" left in the laboratory if something happens to both of you.

What should you do?

From one end of the lifespan to the other, these examples illustrate some of the most troubling bioethical dilemmas patients and their families face today. How do you, either as a patient or family member, choose the best course of action in situations like those just described?

Good decision-making begins with good communication between you and your doctor and, in many cases, among the members of your family as well.

But you may find yourself at a loss unless you're familiar with the "language" of ethical decision-making in health care matters. That's where this chapter can help by stating these moral principles in plain English, describing the process by which medical dilemmas are resolved—sometimes by doctor and patient alone, other times with the help of others.

What it boils down to is this: you don't have to make hard choices alone—but you must be involved.

If you're in the middle of a health-related dilemma, you need information: you need to know what your options are, how to protect yourself and those you love, and how to ensure that your wishes are respected—whether you want treatment or don't want it.

Media headlines and news broadcasts so often focus on dramatic "pulling the plug" and Baby Doe stories in which the issue is withholding or forgoing treatment that it's easy to forget that many people want every effort made to save them or a family member. "Do all you can"; "Leave no stone unturned"; "If there's a chance, go for it"—such pleas are heard every day by doctors from coast to coast.

Dr. Sandra Wilborn, for example, heard this loud and clear from one of her patients, a 78-year-old man who was incapacitated with chronic heart disease. He had already been resuscitated several times when, one day, she felt she should talk to him about his impending death and these dramatic efforts to stave it off. Did he want them to continue?

"You know," she told him as gently as she could, "you are very ill, and if we try to resuscitate you again, I don't think you've got one chance in a thousand of surviving." But her patient gingerly responded, "If you don't try, I don't even have *that* chance."

"He wanted it all—everything medicine could offer to the very end," says Wilborn. "Some people do, no matter what it takes; others don't."

What's important to you?

According to the Declaration of Independence, all men (women, too) are created equal and are endowed by their creator with the inalienable rights to life, liberty, and the pursuit of happiness. Nowhere, however, is a right to health mentioned.

Yet in terms of what Americans value, a 1982 Gallup poll showed that good health ranked second only to having a good family life. And, says Daniel Callahan, "some minimal level of health is necessary if there is to be any possibility of human happiness."[7]

If you are being asked to make a health-related choice that's difficult, one of the first things you must be clear about is what's important to you. In part, this stems from your *personal values.*

Values are items to which you assign high worth and esteem. They are standards by which you test and judge yourself, people around you, society—and things seen and unseen. In a complex world, your values can help you set priorities and give your life meaning, structure, and direction. Your values reflect your attitudes and, consciously or unconsciously, become the basis for your actions as well as what you're willing to spend money on.

Most of us, however, can't come up with a list of our values on short notice. And it's even more difficult to rank them in order of priority. Yet this is important when you realize that an ethical dilemma stems from a conflict of values, loyalties, and obligations—in which every choice has both good and bad elements.

Values you hold dear may come in conflict with the values of other people, including the doctors and nurses caring for you.

Even if you and your doctor see eye to eye on everything from sports and politics to *nouvelle cuisine,* it may not be enough to ensure you'll be given all the medical information you want if your doctor thinks it's your job to "trust" him and his task to do what's right and "protect" you from worrisome news.

You value being able to make decisions for yourself; he values being able to do what he believes is best for you.

This isn't simply a personality clash. As Georgetown University Medical Center physician-philosopher Edmund D. Pellegrino says, "The growing conflict between patient autonomy and physician authority is the central crisis in medical relationships today."[8]

Look over the values in the accompanying list. There's no right or wrong way to rank them, and the list is far from complete. But they may trigger your own thinking—and suggest other values that would be important to you in making health decisions for yourself or for someone you love. Inherent in the way you identify and line them up are your feelings about quality of life, a meaningful life, and what you consider a life worth living.[9]

Keep in mind, however, that sorting out your values is not a once-in-a-lifetime task, but an ongoing process.

What's important to you may change with new information, new situations, new events—good or bad. The birth of a handicapped infant, a cancer-revealing biopsy, the need for an organ transplant, and having to place a parent in a nursing home are but a few of the events which can change your viewpoint overnight.

Happiness then and now

Former Chicago Bears wide receiver Dan Plater once had his hopes set on the Super Bowl. Now the 26-year-old University of Southern California medical student says the simpler things of life have taken on new meaning for him. "Three years ago, happiness was getting a good workout, catching a

How Important are These Values to You?
The following list of values* is by no means complete. Only you
know which *other* values would be important in making a personal
health-related decision for yourself or someone you love.

Independence (not to be dependent)
Freedom to make one's own choices (self-determination)
Freedom to be left alone (privacy)
Self-respect (sense of self-esteem)
Freedom from pain and suffering
Love (sexual and spiritual intimacy)
True friendship (close companionship)
Freedom from anxiety and fear
Happiness (contentedness)
Pleasure (enjoyable experiences, fun, leisure, travel)
Salvation (to be saved/eternal life)
Health (freedom from illness, disability)
Sense of control over one's life
Wisdom (a mature understanding of life)
Family life
Sense of accomplishment or fulfillment
Peaceful death
Faithful to one's beliefs (personal philosophy or religion)
Opportunity to earn a living
Sense of belonging (community with others)
Others _____

great pass," he explains. "Now, if my lawn is watered and my
boys are tucked in bed for the night, that's what peace of
mind—contentment—means to me now."

What changed Plater's outlook a few years ago was failing
eyesight caused by a tumor doctors discovered in his pituitary gland as he was preparing to open the 1983 season with
the Bears. Seemingly overnight, the star player headed for the
Super Bowl was instead on his way to brain surgery—not
once, but twice.

*Adapted from Milton Rokeach, *Understanding Human Values* (New York: Free
Press, 1979).[10]

Denial, he says, was his first reaction. "Why me? I had the whole world in my hand, I was where I'd always wanted to be, and then all of a sudden, doctors are telling me, 'You've got a tumor in your cranial vault.'" With tremendous support from his wife and fellow teammates, especially his good friend Bears quarterback Jim McMahon, Plater says he got hold of himself and decided, "I wasn't going to let it affect my life."

Plater today speaks candidly about the nonmalignant tumor, which was partially removed—and about his concerns for the portion that remains. Doctors say he has received all the radiation treatment his body can tolerate, and all they can do now is hope that the tumor won't continue to grow. "This tumor is going to be part of my life," Plater says, "and I've got to get on with it. But it's hard. I watch the Super Bowl and think, 'I should be there.'"

Hard choices—thinking it through

Whether you must make a decision for yourself or for someone you love who is unconscious or mentally incompetent, the following questions, adapted from a publication of the North Memorial Medical Center, Robbinsdale, Minnesota, may help you think through the problem and reach a workable solution to your dilemma.[11]

Even though answers to some of these questions may seem obvious, just putting the problem in writing helps to clarify what you're thinking and feeling. It also helps to say the unsayable and think the unthinkable. You're not a bad person if you're angry at what's happening or thinking it's time to stop all treatment and let your loved one die in peace.

Remember, there is *no* dilemma when everyone *agrees* on the best course of action to take. Problems surface when there are good arguments on both sides, or some evidence suggests that an action may be wrong, but equally good evidence indicates it may be right—yet neither position is strong enough to be conclusive.[12]

To resolve a dilemma, you must first weigh the conflicting loyalties, values, obligations, and then try to balance the pros and cons of all possible alternatives—so that you can do what seems best, even if it's the lesser of two unappealing choices. And that's when you or perhaps someone very dear to you is caught between the proverbial rock and hard place.

Working through these questions can help you in making a choice or, at least, knowing where you need additional input before you reach a decision.

Questions to ask yourself

1. What is the problem as you see it? In your own words, what is the dilemma you are trying to resolve?

2. What has the doctor or nurse told you about the situation?

3. Do you have all the facts you need? (If not, list any questions that you still have.)

4. Whom else do you want to talk with? (Chaplain, lawyer, another doctor, relatives, a counselor, a member of a bioethics committee?) It's important to gather all the information you can.

5. What are your available options?

6. Given those options, what in your opinion is the best that could happen to you?

7. Given the same options, what in your opinion is the worst that could happen to you?

8. Have you talked to your family about your options? If not, would it be helpful to do so?

9. What possible solutions to your dilemma do you see now?

10. What do you think you should do?

11. Why do you think this? That is, upon what belief or value do you base this decision? (Again, now may be the time you need to talk things over with a counselor, spiritual adviser, or friend whose opinion you respect.)

(If you are making a choice for someone else, here are additional questions you will need to consider.)

11a. Is this, as far as you know, in accord with the beliefs or values of others in your family?

11b. Did the patient leave any written instructions, such as a Living Will, Durable Power of Attorney, or letter to relatives expressing his or her wishes?

11c. What do you think your loved one would do if competent and able to decide for himself or herself?

11d. What do you think your loved one would want you to do? (Did you ever talk with him or her about this type of situation in the past? What do you remember about that conversation? Questions 11c and 11d help you to realize that a patient may have often talked about what he or she would have liked done.)

11e. What would you want for yourself in a similar situation?

11f. What, given the available options, is the best that could happen to your loved one?

11g. What, given the available options, is the worst that could happen to your loved one?

12. What is your next step? (Will you sit down and discuss your feelings and beliefs, along with the medical information you've gathered, with family? with your physician? your attorney? clergy? a hospital ethics committee or consultant in bioethics?)

How can experts in bioethics help?

"Who or what, pray tell, is an ethicist?" asks Harvard University Health Service physician Graham B. Blaine in a recent letter to the editor of the *New England Journal of Medicine.*[13] Referring to an earlier *Journal* article written by a medical "ethicist," he wants spelled out exactly what makes someone an expert in the field and on the basis of what credentials. Blaine is not the only one—many a lay person wants to know, too.

As advances in medical technology have changed the way doctors and patients deal with life and death, many hospitals have formed ethics committees to help clarify issues and make recommendations in complex and controversial cases. Committee members usually include one or more physicians, a nurse, a social worker, sometimes clergy, a nun, a lay person, and, often, the hospital attorney.

But these days, a new face is showing up on more and more ethics committees—that of the professional "ethicist" whose role is to advise, consult, and help clarify any ethical issues which have arisen.[14] (Many times, for example, the problem is poor communication or confusing medical facts rather than conflicting ethical principles.)

Although many ethicists hold degrees in philosophy, theology, humanities, sociology, medicine, nursing, or law, the academic degree (M.D., R.N., Ph.D., or D.D.) alone is not the key to who is called an ethicist. The role evolves as an individual specializes in research and study of ethical issues in health care and gains experience in dealing with the practical problems which arise in patient care.

Dr. Ruth Macklin, for example, is a pioneer in the field of professional bioethics. A member of three New York hospital ethics committees, she holds a Ph.D. in philosophy, has collaborated in developing a model curriculum on bioethics, and since 1980 has been a full-time faculty member at New York's Albert Einstein College of Medicine.

"It used to be thought that life was sacred and that not treating a patient meant you were playing God," Macklin is quoted as saying in a March 1985 *Esquire* article. "Now it is sometimes thought that by prolonging life with vigorous treatment you are playing God. The lines aren't as clear-cut."[15]

Quality of life versus the sanctity of life, what treatment is "ordinary" as opposed to what's "heroic" in a specific case, are typical of conflicting issues that ethicists can help doctors and family members come to grips with. Most often, this will take place in an ethics committee session.

But frequently, I get calls at my office or at home from patients and their families who just want to clear up one or two points that are troubling them. Consulting with a specialist in medical ethics can save you a great deal of worry, time, and energy—especially if you're in the midst of a crisis or feeling overwhelmed by what's happening in your life.

Today more and more hospitals are forming ethics committees. Names and telephone numbers of committee members are usually available upon request, and often are posted in the hospital as well. Any doctor, patient, or family member can request a committee meeting, though usually the patient's request is forwarded by his or her doctor or the hospital social worker to the committee chairperson. Most medical schools and many universities have faculty members who specialize in medical ethics, and there are several major research institutes of bioethics in the United States. (See Appendix J.)

"Stay out of court if you can"

Just as there are few "atheists" in foxholes, there are few absolutists at the bedside—and no magic formulas for resolving bioethical dilemmas. Even if you feel the best choice is to do nothing and let nature take its course, that in itself is a decision. The role of physicians, nurses, attorneys, clergy, ethicists, and others involved is to help you come to the best decision for yourself or for someone else for whom you must make a choice if you're a parent, guardian, or proxy.

In almost all cases, you, your doctor, and your family will be the decision-makers. Occasionally, a dilemma cannot be resolved without an appeal to the courts.[16] Before going this route, however, take a tip from Nevada Supreme Court Justice Charles E. Springer, who says, "Stay out of court if you can. Courts make decisions because people who *should* be making them aren't...but often, by the time the court reaches a decision, the patient is already dead."

Knowing you did your best

In trying to resolve a health care dilemma, it's important to follow through in a way that's caring and sensitive, and takes into account the feelings of everyone involved.

"Sometimes, you can play by all the rules and still not feel good about the outcome," says Georgia Dudding, a registered nurse and psychologist. "Hard choices are stressful—and the choice you make and have to live with may be as painful as the one you forgo. Because of that, you may be tempted to let someone else make the choice for you, but that can add to your stress if you end up feeling helpless or victimized. What's important is to be willing to engage in an honest struggle to find an answer. Then you know you did your best —even if the outcome is less than perfect."

Each chapter that follows suggests where to turn for help, how to get the best deal in a health care system that is becoming increasingly impersonal and cost-oriented, and what the medical, legal, and moral issues are that may affect your options.

Certainly, what you believe in, what the law allows, and what medicine can offer all enter into health care decision-making. Yet often, these hard choices pose dilemmas which cross fine legal-medical-moral lines that leave you frustrated, confused, and angry at the "system" that invites decision-making and then seemingly thwarts it.

In dealing with health care professionals, facilities, and third-party payers such as insurance companies, the first and great commandment is: don't let the "system" *intimidate* you.

The purpose of this book is to help you avoid intimidation and to enhance the dialogue which *must* take place if you are going to protect yourself and your loved ones, get the best medical treatment available, and become an equal partner in bioethical negotiations in which, traditionally, health care professionals have had the upper hand.

If you have a problem and must make your choice right away, you may want to turn immediately to the chapter which deals with your specific dilemma. There you'll find discussed the medical and ethical issues related to the particular situation at hand, a brief description of the landmark legal cases which may affect your decision, examples of how other people have coped with similar problems, and, most important, questions you will need answers to *before* you can make the choice that's right for you.

Unfortunately, no simple formula exists for dealing with medical and moral dilemmas. All of us are heirs to conflicting and often confusing lines of ethical thinking. The rule book has yet to be written. Nor is one very likely to be written which covers all health care situations now or in the future.

"Life," poet Carl Sandburg once said, "is like an onion; you peel it off one layer at a time, and sometimes you weep." Bioethical dilemmas bring you to the heart of life, your values, your innermost resources. Nearly always, resolving such dilemmas calls for making a hard choice—and sometimes, you weep.

We believe that once you have balanced information, the medical facts you need, and an awareness of bioethical issues and how health-related dilemmas can be resolved, you'll be better able to make the choice that's *right* for you and those closest to you.

That certainly is our hope.

2 Taking the Lead in Building a Healthier Doctor-Patient Relationship

GETTING good medical care starts with getting to the right doctor. Sometimes luck plays a role in the match-up. But more often it's a matter of shopping around, checking on a physician's qualifications, talking with friends or relatives *and* acting on your own intuitive sense that a certain doctor is the right one for you. Consider what happened to me.

In 1978, I was the dean of the University of Nevada Medical School—then a two-year institution in the midst of converting to a four-year school which would grant its own M.D. degree. Deadlines to recruit department chairmen, develop a curriculum, and obtain accreditation had to be met month after month. Faculty members and I were working seven days a week to stay on schedule. The workload was enormous; the stress, intense. My colleagues were holding up, but I wasn't.

My blood pressure was elevated and no longer responding to the drugs I had been taking for several years. I was exhausted, not sleeping well, losing weight without trying to. At night, I was gettng up more and more often to urinate; during the day, I felt down and even weepy at times. Some mornings, it was all I could do to go to work. I was 46.

"Midlife crisis," said some associates. "Converting a medical school is stressful business," said others. "If you can't take the heat, get out." Opposition to the changeover to a four-year school was coming from many sides—ranging from legislators who said a medical school would cost the state too much money to doctors who were against training more physicians when a "doctor glut" was on the horizon.

My own doctor was one of those who was vehemently opposed, and I had become increasingly uncomfortable as his patient. About the same time, I hired six clinical department chairmen for the school. One was a nationally renowned endocrinologist, now chairman of medicine at a major medical center.

As we began working together, I told him more about myself. My father had died when he was 51; a brother, who had severe hypertension, at 32. Kidney disease "ran" in the family. For about four years, my doctor had been treating me for what was considered to be essential hypertension with evidence of mild kidney disease. I was taking medications as prescribed, but not feeling any better. Off and on, my blood pressure would be markedly higher, and I was troubled by excruciating headaches.

Although my doctor and I attributed most of these symptoms to the stress of being the medical school dean and all that went with it, I decided to seek a second opinion. I went right to the best doctors I could find—my new department of medicine chairman and his associate. "You look too sick to have just essential hypertension due to stress," they told me. "Let's see what else we can find."

After several tests, a careful review of my past medical records, weekly office visits, and a few months of observing me, my new doctor came to the house one evening and told me he believed I had primary hyperparathyroidism. This is an insidious disease known to cause high blood pressure, signs of kidney disease, and a number of vague symptoms including fatigue, weakness, depression, headache, and stomach and bone pains—all of which I'd had from time to time.

I could have kissed him. I wasn't "crazy," in midlife crisis, or incapable of handling the stress of the job. I was sick, and it was treatable.

In June 1979, tests confirmed his diagnosis and surgery was recommended. After consulting with other doctors, he suggested a surgeon affiliated with the University of California at San Francisco School of Medicine. I talked to this surgeon and read all I could about the disease in medical journals, including articles written by the surgeon himself.

I checked on the hospital where he operates and on his track record for success in such surgery, which consists of removing pea-size glands located on each side of the thyroid. I found out that the risks of such surgery include postoperative recurrence and possible, but rare, vocal cord paralysis.

Both surgeon and hospital inspired confidence.

When I signed the consent form for surgery, I knew as much as any patient could about parathyroid surgery and was convinced that the potential benefits outweighed the risks. The operation to remove three of my four parathyroid glands was successful and I was able to return home a few days later.

That's when I discovered, much to my dismay, that one of my faculty members had called the hospital's laboratory the day I was operated on to find out the results of my surgery and the pathology of the glands removed. Although I certainly had nothing to hide (later I publicly discussed my surgery when I resigned as dean for health reasons), I was surprised and angry that the results of the pathologist's report had been released to physicians other than my own—a clear violation of my right to privacy and the confidentiality of my medical record.

I tell this story because many people think that if you're a doctor you get the red-carpet treatment from your colleagues —more accurate diagnosis, better care, and more respect in the hospital.

But the truth is, there's often breach of confidentiality in the health care system no matter who you are, who your doctor is, or which medical center you're in.

Few people have the opportunity, as I did, to recruit and hire a nationally renowned professor of medicine who later becomes their personal physician. But the *process* is the same—whether you're looking for a second opinion from a surgeon or choosing a family doctor to take care of everything from head colds to your baby's colic.

To get the best care possible—and your money's worth—don't *assume* you'll get it just because you've checked into a hospital, lined up a private physician or signed up with a pre-paid group practice or health plan, such as a health maintenance organization (HMO), preferred provider organization (PPO) or independent practice association (IPA).[1] Regardless of who the third-party payer is, you still need to know the limits of your coverage both in terms of services and who can deliver them.

Where do you start? Today, it's with a new look at the doctor-patient relationship.

A new ethic for the "new" medicine?

Nearly all the ethical debates surrounding medicine today—the right to die, whether to save a severely deformed infant, whether to give a dying patient an artificial heart—arise from technological advances. The result is that there's more to being a patient these days than simply following doctor's orders. And some experts are calling for a new ethic for this new era of high-tech medicine.

At issue are patient autonomy, responsibility, and consumerism.

Speaking at a 1986 conference on medical ethics jointly sponsored by the American Medical Association and the Hastings Center, Morris B. Abram, who chaired the President's Commission on medical ethics, contrasted the old with the "new" medicine, which has spawned an era of health care consumerism. The "old" medicine, he said, was a home-based art with "caring and authority," but it was woefully lacking in relation to modern science.

Today, he explained, the new medicine is very scientific, and that science has created great expectations. But care is institutionalized, delivered by teams of people, heavily influenced by government involvement and paid for mainly by third-party payers. And, he stressed, *"he who pays must be told*—therefore there is always in that arrangement some invasion of what would have been regarded as privacy."

Consumerism is a double-edged sword. "There are a lot of good things about it," Abram says, "but consumerism requires that almost everything paid for and advertised as a service or a system must bear a warranty—and medicine is still too *uncertain* to carry warranties."[2]

As a result, the traditional doctor-patient relationship is changing, and so is the language used to describe it.

For example, Robert M. Veatch of the Kennedy Institute of Ethics in Washington, D.C., sees this relationship as a contract or "covenant." This contract, he says, is the result of a "complex set of understandings" among professionals, patients, and society in general and built upon layers of mutual loyalty, fidelity, respect, and support. Furthermore, says Veatch, "the ethic of patient *benefit* was adequate in the past but it is now outmoded. Today, we need an ethic of patient *responsibility.*"[3]

Other ethicists agree with David Thomasma, director of medical humanities at Chicago's Loyola University School of Medicine, who thinks the patient-autonomy enthusiasts "have beaten beneficence into the ground" and that it's time to bring it back—not in a paternalistic guise, but in the form of *negotiation* based on trust and shared values.[4] And the President's Commission on medical ethics strikes the balance in arguing strongly for "shared decision-making" between patients and their physicians.

Don't wait until you're sick to choose a doctor

Why should you line up a doctor before you need one? "Because," says Dr. Richard Inskip, past president of the American Academy of Family Physicians, "it's important to have a physician who is 'your' doctor—someone who knows you and can help you gain access to the health care system. My bias is that you should have a good family doctor you feel comfortable with who can take care of your needs, and then either refer you to a specialist or obtain additional consultation for your health care needs."

According to Dr. Lloyd H. Smith, Jr., professor of medicine at the University of California at San Francisco, patients expect their doctors to be professionally competent in medical science and technology. But they also want their doctors to listen to them and understand, be interested in them as fellow human beings, keep them reasonably informed, and not abandon them as patients.[5]

In addition, I believe a caring and competent doctor takes seriously the patient's values and encourages a dialogue which enhances the patient's autonomy and ability to make crucial decisions about his or her life.

To avoid the pitfalls of doctor-hunting in an emergency (when decision-making as to the kind of medical care you're willing to accept is altered dramatically because you're desperate), take a tip from Dr. Inskip and choose you doctor *before* you get sick. "Make the decision about what kind of doctor you want," he says, adding that "probably what you want is a doctor of first contact—someone who's reasonably available, whom you can call and discuss your health problem with, and who will see you in a reasonable period of time."

Don't rely on your hospital's emergency room staff to be your "personal" doctor. "In this setting, you're rarely treated by the same physician each time, you don't get what's known as 'continuity of care,' and the episodic care you do get is twice as expensive as that you'd get from your own doctor," says Inskip.

Depending upon your needs or those of your family, you'll most likely want a *primary care* physician—a doctor who can be your first line of health care defense. These doctors include pediatricians for children, gynecologists and obstetricians for women, general internists (specialists in adult medicine involving internal body systems), and family physicians, whose focus is caring for medical needs of family members of all ages.

Secondary care physicians, by way of contrast, deal with special diagnostic or therapeutic needs and usually see patients referred for consultation. Among these physicians are orthopedic surgeons, anesthesiologists, urologists, and neonatologists, to name but a few. (A third group, such as pathologists, radiologists, and public health physicians, are not usually involved in direct patient care and primarily serve as consultants to other doctors.)

Put together a list of doctors and check them out. Now's the time to ask friends and neighbors which doctors they'd recommend and why.[6] Don't overlook nurses, who are excellent sources of information about doctors they work closely with and see in action with patients. According to a survey done for the American Board of Family Practice, most people give less thought to selecting a doctor than they do to finding inexpensive supermarkets and bargain-price clothing.

So do your doctor-shopping with care. Simply put, it's vital to your health.

Call two or three doctors' offices and make some initial inquiries. Ask about the first visit—how much time will be devoted to taking your medical history, doing a physical examination, and answering your questions? What's the usual fee for the first visit? Who covers the doctor's practice when he or she is gone?

Before you schedule an appointment, however, give yourself time to check on the doctor's credentials. Although they're no guarantee a physician will be competent throughout his or her professional life, diplomas, licenses, certificates, and faculty appointments are an important first step.

Checking on a doctor's qualifications

When physicians choose a doctor for themselves, the first questions they ask are about his professional experience and competency—where he went to medical school and where he did his specialty training. The best residency and fellowship training programs generally are based in university or community hospitals and clinics which are affiliated with medical schools or research centers and accredited by national organizations.

Three other criteria are very important. Is the doctor *fully* licensed to practice in your state? (Some physicians may legitimately practice with a limited or restricted license—and you can find out what these limits are by calling your state medical licensing and/or disciplinary board.) Is he or she a member of a hospital staff, and of a county or state medical society? Is he or she board-certified (or eligible) in a recognized specialty and a member or fellow of a national specialty society?

You want a doctor who has passed, or is eligible to take, the certification examinations given by the professional board which supervises that specialty. Remember that so-called generalists—family physicians and internists—are also medical specialists who must meet certification requirements.

Many physicians also hold faculty appointments at medical and nursing schools and regularly teach students and residents in training. You can find out by asking your doctor directly, but much of this is public information as well. For example, the *American Medical Directory* and national *Di-*

rectory of Medical Specialists lists physicians alphabetically by state and county. Also included is detailed information on their education and training, professorships they hold, and their memberships in medical societies and specialty groups. You can find these directories in the reference sections of most hospital and medical school libraries and many public libraries as well. (Not all hospital or medical school libraries are open to the public, so check first to see if special arrangements are required for visitors.)

But don't forget, you can always call the state medical licensing board, the county or state medical association, the nearest medical school, or the medical staff secretary of any hospital and ask: "Is Dr. So-and-so a member of your staff? In what department? Does he have full privileges?"

You can also find out from the state licensing board if any disciplinary actions have been taken against this physician and whether his or her license has any limits to it.

Many doctors display their diplomas, certificates, licenses, and faculty appointments in their offices. For example, the American Medical Association (AMA) "Physician's Recognition Award" acknowledges the doctor's ongoing efforts at continuing medical education. When you go to a doctor's office, don't be shy about inspecting these credentials at close range.

Most important of all, however, is your own intuitive sense after talking to the physician—is this the right physician for you?

Be suspicious if your doctor makes grandiose claims that "I always make people well" or "you can be assured of a cure if..." Be leery if he guarantees that a "special" treatment will work if you follow his "unique" program, see him twice a week, and do this, that, and the other thing—because in medicine, there are *no* guarantees.

Clues you're not getting the care you should

There are twelve warning signs that should raise a red flag in alerting you to the fact that you may not be getting proper health care or may be seeing a doctor who's not right for you.

Your doctor:

1. Doesn't seem to be listening to what you're saying.
2. Doesn't answer your questions or take time to ask if you have any. When there is an answer, it's in words you don't understand.
3. Fails to take an adequate medical history or give you a complete physical examination when it's called for. (Over a period of time, of course, your doctor gets to know your health history, and for certain types of illness, say a cold or "flu bug," may forgo a total-body-system physical and examine only those areas where you have symptoms.)
4. Doesn't help you learn more about your condition and what you can do about it, or explain why the recommended tests, treatment, or medications are necessary.
5. Neglects to inform you of potential risks, benefits, and side effects of prescribed drugs or suggested procedures and tests. (Beware if you've said you're "allergic" to a certain medication and your doctor prescribes it anyway.)
6. Doesn't respect your modesty and makes suggestive remarks while doing a pelvic examination or examining your breasts.
7. Doesn't make a follow-up appointment for you or urge you to call the office to report how you're doing.
8. Seems forgetful, peculiar, or belligerent at times, and may even have alcohol on the breath.
9. Is hard to reach, doesn't return phone calls, and, when away, fails to arrange for a replacement.
10. Is not on the staff of any community hospital or medical center.

11. Is rigid, a know-it-all, and insists on an "only" way to treat your condition.
12. Reacts defensively when you suggest a second opinion.

Getting a second opinion

Second opinions aren't new. Good doctors have always consulted with colleagues and been willing to refer patients when it was in the patient's best interests. However, eighteen years ago, patients like my retired father-in-law, for example, were much less likely to question a doctor's diagnosis, prognosis, or treatment or lack of it.

When my father-in-law's doctor told him he'd have to learn to live with his degenerating hip disease, which was causing great pain, he resigned himself to hobbling on crutches, pain medication—and another stiff drink. It didn't make sense to me, since hip replacements, which were being done successfully in England, had just been approved in selected American hospitals. And one of these medical centers was less than half an hour's drive from his home. Yet his doctor had not mentioned this to him or suggested hip replacement surgery as an option.

I urged him to get a second opinion from one of the surgeons doing this new technique. On the appointed day, I picked him up, carried him to the car, and drove him to a New York City medical center, where, happily, he was deemed a good candidate for surgery. After the operation, he lived another seven years free of pain, able to walk alone, travel, go to the theater and to restaurants—all things he thought he'd never again enjoy.

Today, it's not only doctors like me who want second (and sometimes third) opinions for patients and relatives. More and more patients and their insurance companies or other third-party payers are also insisting on second opinions before making serious treatment decisions.

But don't be surprised if your doctor doesn't welcome a second opinion.

"A lot of doctors get very threatened by the thought of getting a second opinion," says Dr. Jeffrey Millman, former director of the University of Nevada's Family Medicine Center. "They see this as questioning their ability and expertise and may say to you, 'You mean you don't trust me?' or 'You doubt my medical opinion and judgment?'"

Don't hesitate to seek a second opinion because you're afraid you'll insult, offend, or anger your physician. Remember, you have a *right* to another opinion, and *good* physicians acknowledge and respect this right. They don't think less of you for exercising it.

However, be honest and up-front with your doctor; don't go behind his back. Let him know you want another opinion, and seek his help in getting the best referral.

But don't stop there. Check out his advice with others. Some doctors will merely send you around the corner to a colleague who thinks the same way about patient treatment. Unfortunately, not all doctors keep up with medical literature, and thus they're not aware of the most recent advances in diagnosis and treatment—as in my father-in-law's case.

The more serious the diagnosis and more radical the treatment recommended, the more important it is for you to get the best medical consultation you can. In fact, for your second opinion, you may want to go to one of the nation's outstanding medical centers or clinics—where doctors see, treat, and follow the progress of many patients with serious medical conditions like yours.

If your doctor won't refer you, ask a nurse or another doctor you trust. Ask your county medical society to recommend a specialist qualified to treat problems like yours. Call a medical center or specialty clinic and ask to speak to a physician in the department which seems most likely to handle conditions similar to yours (surgery, obstetrics, medicine, oncology, etc.). Explain your situation and ask for a consultation with one of the experts in the department or ask for a referral to another doctor in your area.

Who pays for second opinions?

According to a 1984 survey by the Health Insurance Association of America, nearly 75 percent of commercial health insurers cover costs of second opinions on nonemergency surgery and pre-admission testing.

You can obtain the name of a doctor authorized to give second opinions for Blue Cross, for example, by calling its Second Opinion Referral Center in New York City, (212) 481-2658. And the Health Care Finance Administration of the Department of Health and Human Services will refer you to an agency near you which can suggest a consultant if you call its toll-free Second Opinion Surgical Hotline, (800) 638-6833; in Maryland it's (800) 492-6603.

In his book *Second Opinion*, New York internist Isadore Rosenfeld says, "No matter how devoted you are to your doctor or how much you dislike antagonizing him, you owe it to yourself to consult with another expert when you are ill and not responding to treatment, or when you are presented with a diagnosis or prognosis that may drastically alter the course of your life, or when a major operation is recommended."[7]

In addition, says Rosenfeld, "if your request for another opinion is turned down just because your physician objects on *principle* to having someone else in, it is time to change doctors. *In the final analysis, what medicine is all about is patient care, not doctor ego.*"

(If your doctor refuses to refer you to another physician, won't forward your medical records, or intimidates, threatens, or badgers you, his behavior is unethical, and in most states illegal. Report the doctor to the county medical society's ethics committee and state licensing board, as outlined in Chapter 10. Then find a new doctor.)

Interviewing a doctor—are you right for each other?

As a consumer, you've got purchasing power. Doctors need to be paid to survive. And in most large communities, there are enough doctors to go around. They're advertising in newspapers, marketing their services, and making themselves more available than ever before. One advantage of shopping around for the doctor who's right for you—and talking to him or her before you make a final choice—is that it gives each of you a chance to assess the other.

Today more and more patients are making initial appointments with doctors, not only to get a firsthand look at how the office staff treats patients but also to talk over in advance everything from the doctor's basic medical philosophy to practical concerns about services, fees, payment plans, referrals, hospital privileges, medical records, and who covers the practice when he's not around.

"If I'm going to put my life in someone's hands and share decision-making about what happens to my body," says one patient I talked to, "it makes sense to discuss beforehand my values and what's important to me—like not prolonging my life if I'm hopelessly ill, donating my organs someday, or even seeing my medical record if I want to. But when I told my doctor I'd like to see my records, he said, 'Thanks for telling me; I guess you don't trust me.' As I see it, though, the chart may be his, but the information in it is about *me* and it's mine." (For more on access to patient records, see Chapter 10.)

Your doctor doesn't necessarily have to hold the same values you do. But he should respect your values if he's going to act in your best interests.

A number of experts in medical ethics believe physicians are obliged to share *their* values with patients as well, so that the patient will know what to expect from the relationship beforehand. If your doctor doesn't bring up the subject, you should. For example, what are his views on Living Wills, removing life supports, relieving pain, or the use of placebos? (Chapter 3 deals with the use of placebos in research studies.)

If you are pregnant or are considering pregnancy, you should know your doctor's position on abortion and amniocentesis, a technique of evaluating the development of the fetus *in utero* and detecting potential problems early. Some doctors refuse to do abortions. Others feel there is no point in doing amniocentesis if a woman is not willing to consider abortion as an alternative. Others won't do amniocentesis if the purpose is to determine the sex of the child.

Though the doctor may not call it sharing values, he may say something like "My philosophy about this is..." or "Here's how I feel about..." or "Here are some things I want you to know about me if you're going to be my patient."

A charming smile and ability to put you at ease may make one doctor more appealing than another. But what you're looking for in choosing a doctor (and in the physician who covers the practice when he's away) are those qualities that will enhance trust and mutual respect. These include competence, expertise, and a commitment to act in your best interests based on your values. There must also be the ability and willingness to communicate openly *and* in a caring way.

Truth-telling—a two-way street with stop signs

Many doctors agree with Dr. Isadore Rosenfeld that "communication is now as vital a part of medicine as the diagnosis and therapy."[8] They know that the informed patient is their best ally.

With emphasis on partnership and shared decision-making between doctor and patient, it follows that sharing of information is basic to that process. But good communication is more than just a simple exchange of words. And truth-telling is, too. As Thoreau said, "It takes two to speak the truth—one to speak and another to hear."

Good doctor-patient communication is not only honest, but considerate in respect to a person's feelings, safety, privacy, and a full range of human rights and privileges. If, however, you believe that what you don't know *can* hurt you, then it's important to be aware of what your doctor may be doing under the guise of caring and sparing you further pain.

Recognize these truth-telling dodges?

According to a 1982 Louis Harris and Associates poll, 94 percent of Americans surveyed said they "want to know everything"—including dismal facts about their health. And even if they had a type of cancer which usually leads to death in less than a year, 85 percent reported they'd want a realistic estimate of how long they had to live.

Polled at the same time, however, doctors showed much less willingness to be candid in such circumstances—although the trend generally is toward greater openness with patients.

In a *Barrister Magazine* article titled "When Should the Patient Know?" Robert Veatch says that, with one possible exception, the adult patient should always know the truth—if he is capable of knowing. That exception? If the consequences of disclosing the truth would be "devastatingly and overwhelmingly negative."[9] For example, not disclosing the terminal diagnosis to an already suicidal or severely depressed patient might be justified, but only on a temporary basis.

Veatch goes on to discuss five truth-telling dodges—and I've added two others—which you should be able to recognize if you want information about your health and want to avoid care that is inadequate or confusing:

49

"You can't tell them everything."

The line of reasoning goes like this. Since it's impossible to describe the disease in detail or list *all* the complications or all *possible* side effects of drugs, the doctor says to himself, "I'll tell this patient very little." Many physicians accept this general approach as being adequate for informed consent. But I disagree. I side with ethicists who argue that the standard should be what the "reasonable person would want to know," including the possibility of death or major harm.

In her warm, sad, and very human book *Heartsounds*, Martha Weinman Lear tells what happened when her husband, Hal, tried to talk to his cardiologist about his condition following a massive heart attack (myocardial infarct). Hal was a New York physician. He knew the language of medicine; he knew the survival rates. What he wanted to know was the odds in *his* case. What he heard was the classic truth-telling dodge:

Hal: I have a wife, two kids. I want to be able to make realistic plans. Can you give me some idea of my prognosis?

M.D.: You're doing fine. Don't worry about it.

Hal then tried a different tack, quoting some findings from the Framingham Group Study (a noted long-term study of heart disease in a Massachusetts community). Again, he tried to learn the truth of his condition. This time, the cardiologist got red in the face, rose from his chair, abruptly shut Hal's medical record, and ended the office visit, adding, "It is nonsense to talk about this kind of thing. You're all right."[10]

In fact, Hal was an extremely sick man.

Truthful jargon

When a doctor told my neighbor who used to work in a shipyard that he had "mesothelioma with metastatic implants in the pleura," he came home, knocked on my door, and said, "What the hell do I have?" After calming him down, I suggested his wife call the doctor and tell him what happened. When she called, the doctor said, "I explained it all to your husband, but he must not have heard me."

Indeed the doctor may have told my neighbor the truth, but he didn't understand its meaning (cancer of the lung associated with exposure to asbestos, spreading through the chest cavity). Frank Lloyd Wright put it well: "The truth is more than the facts." And it's more than just the doctor's explaining a diagnosis to the patient—who may have unconsciously *stopped listening* the moment he heard "I'm sorry to have to tell you that you have cancer."

(This stunned and very common reaction to distressing news is sometimes called "shutdown," "selective denial," "selective hearing," or, in psychiatric terms, "dissociation." It's a way of screening out information we don't want or can't handle at the moment, and this mindset can occur with any serious medical problem. We simply don't hear anything the physician says once he informs us of the specific diagnosis— regardless of how kind, sensitive, and good at communicating jargon-free information the doctor usually is. You may panic and feel you've got to get away before you start to cry. Or you may be thinking, "Will I live to see my first grandchild born?" All the while your doctor is explaining treatment options. In truth, you may not have heard a word, but not feel free to say so. So you ask no questions and your doctor assumes you understood what was said.)

Generalizing to avoid the truth

"Am I going to die?" asks the patient with a fatal illness. "Sure, we're all going to die eventually," responds the physician, who is providing information in such a way that the real question is avoided and the patient is given a false sense of security.

Another instance of this dodge was recounted by a New

York editor whose father had a stroke from which he eventually died. "When my mother and I asked the doctor about Dad's prognosis, the reply was 'He's in God's hands.' I then said, 'That's true of all of us,' but the doctor would say no more."

Misreading the signals

Nonverbal communication can be very effective—when correctly interpreted. Occasionally, the signals are misread. For example, when a 50-year-old chief executive officer of a large East Coast corporation told his personal physician, a friend from way back, that he was thinking of retiring early, taking a leisurely cruise around the Pacific Islands with his new young lover, then settling out West, the doctor hesitated to tell him the diagnosis: cancer of the pancreas.

He interpreted what the CEO was saying as "Don't give me any bad news; I don't want anything to get in the way of my new life—no matter how short." Believing he was reading the nonverbals correctly, the doctor said nothing more during the visit. The truth of the matter is that the CEO, had he known, would still have gone on the trip and moved out West. But one thing would have been different. Before he left, he would have tried to make peace with his grown children, who still were angry with him for divorcing their mother. As it was, he died a few months later with what Elisabeth Kübler-Ross, the expert on death and dying, calls "unfinished business."

"We never know for sure."

The rationale for withholding information here is that at best, medical prognosis is an uncertain science based on probabilities, experience with similar cases, and often just plain luck. Since concepts like "60 percent five-year survival rate" apply to groups of patients with the same disease, and since a patient is both a member of that group *and* a unique person, the prognosis becomes unique to each patient.

Predicting the future under these circumstances is risky business. Since doctors often claim that they never know for sure what the prognosis in a specific case will be, it seems prudent to be vague. "The deception," says Veatch, "arises when he uses this as a rationalization for failure to disclose what he *does* know."

Self-fulfilling prophecy

Here's how an Ohio cardiologist explains this common dodge. "Many seriously ill patients are not able to grasp what is being said; they're in a state of shock. If you stopped to inform each one about potential side effects of his or her medications, it could start these patients thinking about every little thing that could go wrong and might even plant the seed for those symptoms to occur."

Medical ethicist Arthur Caplan disagrees. "While it's true that many factors can interfere with hearing what's being said, there are no studies I know of that prove that revealing symptoms produces them." And if these symptoms do occur, then you deal with them as with any others.

"A little knowledge is a dangerous thing."

But if a little knowledge is dangerous, asked Thomas Huxley in 1877, "where is the man who has so much [knowledge] as to be out of danger?" Doctors who use this argument for not disclosing information hold that the patient may be so scared by even "a little knowledge" that he will not be willing to go along with treatment or, even worse, will refuse to comply with it at all.

"People are much more afraid of what they *don't* know," says Southern California oncologist Georgia Edwards, citing as examples side effects of medications or complications of the disease. "I believe in the well-educated patient—they do what you want them to do and they get good results."[11]

Further support for this approach comes from the Cleveland Clinic, where radiologists studied 236 patients referred for angiograms (x-ray studies of blood vessels) to see if giving detailed written information about risks of these procedures would lead patients to refuse them. Only four patients refused.

"We believe," says Dr. Ralph J. Alfidi, who conducted the study, "that we have proven that the majority of patients not only have a right to know but want to know what possible complications may be expected from any given procedure. The concern that informing a patient of possible complications will result in his refusal of the procedure is now outmoded."[12]

Most experts agree, and much case law supports the view, that if you are competent, you are in the best position to make decisions for yourself. This *right to self-determination* in the medical arena was well defined in a 1914 decision by New York Supreme Court Justice Benjamin Cardozo, who wrote in the *Schloendorff* v. *Society of New York Hospital* case that "every human being of adult years and sound mind has a right to determine what shall be done with his own body."[13]

"Don't tell me—I don't want to know"

Some patients don't want to know. "Do what you have to, doc, but spare me the details," they say, in essence waiving their right to such information. But they're also saying in effect that they don't want to be actively involved in making decisions about their own health care.

"I respect that," says ethicist Arthur Caplan. "I think it's a poor decision, but I don't think you can force people to be—in ethical language—autonomous. We should make it possible, but if somebody makes an informed refusal, if they say, 'I don't care—you do it, you decide,' you can press that a little, but that's their right."

(If you don't want to know, it is your privilege to say so. But I urge you to think twice about this approach and, better yet, hedge your bets. You might say, "Right now I don't want to think about it or know the details—maybe when I feel better or have more time, I will.")

As patients, most of us want information—but down deep we hope it's not all that bad. Doctors know this. And if you want the truth, but only in small doses, it's all right to say, "Stop. I need some time to think about this. Can I call you tomorrow when I've had a little time to digest this and discuss it with my family?"

Sensitive doctors tell us the facts of our illness or condition, the likely outcome, and the risks and benefits of proposed treatment in a way that's caring and helpful. And a 1982 Louis Harris poll suggests that patients who are informed and involved in decision-making receive an improved quality of care.[14]

In *The Healing Heart*, Norman Cousins tells the story of his heart attack in December 1980. He credits his amazing recovery not so much to his doctors, but rather to his own active role in the healing process and positive thinking, stress reduction, exercise, and dietary changes.[15] He refused some treatments and procedures, such as bypass surgery, which had been suggested by his doctors, among them Dr. K. I. Shine, department of medicine chairman at the University of California at Los Angeles School of Medicine.

Commenting on Cousins's unorthodox approach in *American Health* magazine, Dr. Shine lets us in on just how uneasy he felt about the decision:

> In treating Norman Cousins, I have agreed to live with a degree of medical uncertainty that makes me uncomfortable. I will feel responsible if anything should happen to Norman arising out of a cardiovascular cause. But I cannot espouse the cause of patients' involvement in their own care and then be

unwilling to accept partial responsibility when the patient makes a decision in which I do not concur.[16]

I don't know Dr. Shine and I'm not sure I would have made the same decision Norman Cousins did when surgery was recommended. But that's not important. What does matter is that Dr. Shine is willing to share decision-making and stand by his patient, not abandoning or bawling him out, when his decision is contrary to what the doctor thinks would be the right choice under the circumstances.

That's what a sharing relationship between a patient and doctor is all about.

If you want that kind of doctor-patient relationship, too, don't settle for less—especially if you feel the same way as the seriously ill 20-year-old patient who told me: "I might never want to make that kind of decision for myself—but for my peace of mind, I want to know I can."

Resources

National Women's Health Network (NWHN)
224 Seventh Street, S.E.
Washington, DC 20003
(202) 543-9222
Victoria Leonard, executive director

Women's health advocacy organization which monitors federal health policy as it affects women, testifies before Congress and federal agencies, conducts conferences and sponsors a national resource file on all aspects of women's health care. Write for list of publications, which includes a pregnancy information packet; the booklet *How Safe Is Safe?* on how the FDA determines safety of drugs and medical devices ($1.50); and *Plaintext Doctor-Patient Checklist*, a list of questions to ask your doctor during an appointment ($1).

People's Medical Society (PMS)
14 E. Minor Street
Emmaus, PA 18049
(215) 967-2136
Charles B. Inlander, executive director

Encourages citizen involvement in national and local health care systems and institutions, and promotes self-care, alternative health care procedures, and more preventive health care, practice, and research. Provides members with information on maintaining personal health and how to prepare for doctor appointments. Publications include newsletter, pamphlets, books, and Health Action Kits.

American Association of Retired Persons (AARP)
1909 K Street, N.W.
Washington, DC 20049
(202) 728-4450
Barb Quaintance, manager of Health Advocacy Services

The nation's largest organization of working and retired Americans age 50 and over; among health-related services are a group health insurance program and mail-order pharmacy service with locations in eight states plus the District of Columbia. Write to AARP Fulfillment (P.O. Box 2400, Long Beach, CA 90801) for a list of publications and free single copies of *Strategies for Good Health, Knowing Your Rights,* and *Healthy Questions,* a publication designed to help consumers deal effectively with health care professionals.

Center for Medical Consumers
237 Thompson Street
New York, NY 10012
(212) 674-7105
Arthur A. Levin, M.P.H., director

Provides an alternate source of medical and health information to facilitate medical decision-making by consumers; maintains library of more than 1,500 books and periodicals for laypeople, and publishes *HealthFacts,* a monthly consumer newsletter.

Suggested reading

Cousins, Norman. "How Patients Appraise Physicians." *New England Journal of Medicine*, vol. 313, no. 22 (November 28, 1985), pp. 1422–24.

Hines, William. "Doc, Don't Call Me Maggie." *American Health*, February 1984, pp. 64–5. (Many patients feel put down when doctors use their first name. Do you?)

Lear, Martha Weinman. "Down with High-Handed Health Care!" *Woman's Day*, February 7, 1984. (Arrogance is bad medicine—there's no reason you have to take it.)

"Many Americans Visited Health Practitioner Other Than M.D., D.D.S.." *American Medical News*, March 22, 1986, p. 85.

Mechanic, David. "Physicians and Patients in Transition." *Hastings Center Report*, December 1985, pp. 9–12.

President's Commission for the Study of Ethical Problems in Medicine and Biomedical and Behavioral Research. *Making Health Care Decisions.* Washington, D.C.: U.S. Government Printing Office, 1982. (See Volume 1, Chapter 4, "The Communication Process"; deals with attitudes toward less than full disclosure.)

Robin, Eugene D., M.D. *Matters of Life and Death: Risks vs. Benefits of Medical Care.* New York: Freeman, 1984. (See especially Chapter 3, "What the Patient Wants or Should Want from the Doctor"; Chapter 4, "The Doctor as God"; and Chapter 12, "Making Patients Out of Normal Human Beings.")

Rosenfeld, Isadore, M.D. *Second Opinion.* New York: Simon and Schuster, 1981. (Must reading even if you love your doctor and think he or she is the best. See especially Preface; Chapter 1, "A Second Opinion—Why, When and How"; and Chapter 2, "Patient Care Versus Doctor Ego.")

Thomasma, David C., and Edmund D. Pellegrino. *For the Patient's Good: The Restoration of Beneficence in Medical Ethics.* New York: Oxford University Press, in press. (See section titled "The Good Patient.")

Veatch, Robert M. "Models for Ethical Medicine in a Revolutionary Age." *Hastings Center Report*, vol. 2, no. 3 (June 1973).

3 Knowing and Exercising Your Rights as a Patient

LUCY MILLER—not her real name—could not resist the temptation to peek inside the bulging folder on her lap. Opening the seal carefully, the 75-year-old woman quickly skimmed her medical records, which she was hand-carrying to a well-known Southern California specialist for evaluation.

There were the cardiologist's notes on a potentially serious heart problem dating back to the 1970s; also side effects from various medicines he had prescribed; serious bowel problems in 1982 had required a colostomy (but, Lucy recalled, the surgeon had never said a word about cancer to her). And the latest entry—the reason for this hastily booked plane trip to Los Angeles and consultation—was a report on an abnormal mammogram (a type of breast x-ray), which had Lucy worried because both her mother and her sister had undergone breast cancer surgery years before.

What shocked this vibrant and attractive woman most, however, was the pathology report at the time of her bowel surgery. Not only had cancer been detected then, it had already spread to two out of four lymph nodes.

No one had told her.

Angrily, she read the last sentence of a letter from the surgeon to her cardiologist and found out why: "Because of her age and her husband's age, I have not mentioned anything about any further treatment and, in fact, do not think she should have any."

Her *age?* She was only 72 then. Was that too old to be told a serious diagnosis? Would treatment then have prevented possible breast cancer now? And what did her *husband's* age have to do with *her* health?

For nearly one hundred years, the courts have recognized that every adult person who is competent—that is, of sound mind—has the right to determine *voluntarily* what will be done to his or her body. Lucy Miller, though totally competent, was deprived of her right to know her medical condition and freely make health care choices for herself. Lucy felt betrayed. "If you can't trust your doctors to tell you the truth and respect your rights," she later told a friend, "who's going to do it?"

We all know we have the right to be informed of our condition—the right denied to Lucy—but what other rights do we have that our doctor might intentionally or inadvertently deny to us?

Know your rights

You have a right to privacy and to control over what is done to your body. You have a right to be treated with respect and not to be harmed. You have a right to information about your condition so you can make informed choices. You have a right to life and, many experts argue, a right to die as well.

You have a right to reject all treatment—or to say "no" to those aspects of the treatment plan you don't want. If you have agreed to take part in a research program, you have a right to quit at any time.

You have a right to accept treatment and to expect that once a treatment plan has been agreed upon, you will get the care, medicines, tests, and procedures that your doctor has ordered for you—provided you or some third party, such as private insurance, Medicare, or Medicaid, will cover the costs.

In *emergency* situations, you have a *legal* right to medical care even if you can't afford it.

What you may not realize, however, is that regardless of who's paying, you or your advocate may have to monitor your own care to be sure you get what the doctor has ordered —when, where, how and without undue risk to your health.

Take to heart what Eugene D. Robin, M.D., says in his book *Matters of Life and Death:* "Remember that you, the patient, have the highest stake in the decision—the most to gain and the most to lose. You, the patient, if you are capable of making the decision, are the one to decide what constitutes a happy and productive life. Don't let your doctor, however well-intentioned, usurp this right."[1]

"Go wash your hands"

Consider what New York attorney Morris B. Abram had to say at a recent medical ethics conference about his experience in a large metropolitan medical center. In 1973, he was diagnosed as having acute leukemia and given very little time to live. Chemotherapy was recommended.

With his immune system depressed, it was crucial that Abram's care-givers observe sterile procedures each time they entered his room. On the walls of his room were signs reminding people to wash their hands. Yet all too often the message was ignored. And according to Abram, "It was I who, more frequently than not, had to tell the young intern, 'Go wash your hands—don't touch me.'"

When an intravenous infusion tube supplying his medication was removed two days earlier than prescribed, Abram again felt compelled to fight for his due. "I was supposed to receive seven days and seven nights of the drug by continuous infusion," he says. "I don't know if three days would have been sufficient, but I do know this: if I didn't know the orders, there would have been a problem with respect to the continuous infusion" of the drug prescribed. In this high-powered center, comments Abram angrily, there was "slippage" from shift to shift and from one intern to the next.

In a 1983 *New York Times Magazine* article, Morris Abram, whose leukemia was then in remission, summed up his approach to the disease and protecting his best interests: "I decided to fight with all my resources, take on the pain, the odds, the experimental therapies and the risks. I signed release upon release. I read medical journals and learned all I could about the latest research. I continually questioned my treatment. It amounted to a crash course in biomedical issues, though at the beginning I saw it only as a fight for my life."[2]

Fighting for one's life is a big enough task without having to remain constantly on the alert to see that care prescribed is being delivered according to doctor's orders. Yet Morris Abram's experience is not unique. Bright, informed, conscious throughout his hospital stay, and vocal in demanding his right to good care, Morris Abram could look out for himself.

But who's looking out for people like Lucy Miller? Who's looking out for the patient who is unconscious or groggy from anesthesia or drugs, or unable—for whatever reason—to monitor his own care and speak up when his best interests are in jeopardy?

The message is clear: if you are being hospitalized, be sure a family member or friend knows you are there and is able *and* willing to be your spokesperson or advocate—not in a formal sense, perhaps, but in the unofficial role of checker-upper. (For tips on how to be an effective advocate, see Chapter 4.)

"Squeaky wheels get the grease"

For many reasons, says medical ethics expert Arthur Caplan, "you need to have someone who can act as an 'amplifier'—someone who can make your voice louder when you may be talking more softly. And [hospital] staff has to know that person has the role of trusted person or friend and will be speaking for you."

Being in an institutional setting, Caplan explains, limits your autonomy, your freedom, your ability to speak for yourself. So to get more service and better quality of care, it works to your advantage to have family and friends visit and ask about you.

For one thing, Caplan says, "squeaky wheels get the grease —and I have constantly been impressed by the fact that those patients who have family members visiting them and inquiring how they're doing get better attention. The staff responds to that—and that's even true in getting access to a [donor organ] transplant. When the family comes in and says to the doctor, 'How's he doing?' or 'Aren't we getting anywhere?' that generates pressure to do something."

And without that independent voice to speak for you when you're at your most vulnerable, you can find yourself being subtly (or not so subtly) pushed into accepting a treatment or procedure that you don't want—or being made to feel guilty if you go *against* your doctor's recommendation.

That's what happened to a young woman I'll call Terry Martin, a 30-year-old aerobics instructor who was expecting her first baby. Told by her obstetrician that she was in excellent physical shape and that the birth would be normal, Terry and her husband attended natural childbirth classes and eagerly awaited her first sign of labor.

Subtle coercion or free choice?

The day Terry's contractions began, her husband was away on a business trip. A neighbor drove her to the hospital, where Terry's doctor examined her and then said unexpectedly, "The baby's head is much larger than we expected. You know, we can do a cesarean section, which will make it much easier on your baby. But, of course, if you're still set on natural childbirth, that's up to you."

The young mother-to-be consented to surgery and was thrilled when presented with a perfectly normal seven-and-a-half-pound daughter whose head circumference was thirteen inches (the average head measurement for a normal infant girl). In explaining her decision later, Terry told a friend, "I knew I'd never be able to live with myself if something went wrong just because I opted for a natural birth. If the C-section was easier on my baby, that seemed the way to go."

Quite frankly, I suspect many doctors would not find fault with the obstetrician's approach in Terry's case. And without knowing the medical facts surrounding her labor and delivery, I can't say for sure whether Terry's doctor made the right or wrong decision.

But look at it this way.

She was in excellent physical condition and not a high-risk patient. There was no reason to think that a natural labor would not progress normally and no evidence that the infant was in fetal distress. (Terry told her friend the obstetrician had not done any tests on her or the baby.) A more conservative approach would have been to allow her to go into labor, monitor her progress carefully, and do a cesarean section only if problems arose.

Many physicians say the possibility of malpractice suits affects how a doctor handles a case with even the *slightest* possibility of turning into a problem delivery. In my town, for instance, there's a 29 percent cesarean rate. This is higher than the national average of 21 percent, which itself may be too high, according to the American College of Obstetrics and Gynecology. When you consider that doing a cesarean is faster than attending a long and possibly difficult natural birth, the way in which Terry's obstetrician broached the possibility of this procedure takes on overtones of subtle coercion.

Add to that the fact that a cesarean section is major surgery and, as with any surgery, there's a chance of death greater than the risk of death from natural childbirth, and you have to question how informed Terry was when she consented simply because "it would be easier" on her baby. Was she informed about the *risks* to her infant and herself? Not only that, but when you're hooked up to IVs, hungry for something to eat, and stripped of your uniqueness, the doctor who tells you the cesarean is going to make it easier for your baby is not only putting a lot of pressure on you, he's setting you up for guilt later if you go with a vaginal delivery and your baby isn't born perfect.

What makes your consent "informed"?

Ethically, informed consent is rooted in your right to privacy, self-determination, and the promotion of your personal well-being. The legal doctrine of informed consent is your most important safeguard.

No doctor, nurse, or institution is going to force treatment on you without your consent or, if you are not competent to make health-related choices for yourself, without the consent of your proxy. To do so makes a doctor, nurse, or institution liable for criminal *and* civil action. (You'll find a detailed explanation of the legal basis for this doctrine in the American Civil Liberties Union handbook *The Rights of the Criti-*

cally Ill. Copies are available for $3.95 plus $1 for postage and handling from Literature Department, ACLU, 132 West 43rd Street, New York, NY 10036.)

But remember, signing a release form is not the same as giving informed consent.[3]

As the President's Commission on medical ethics said: "Patients who have the capacity to make decisions about their care must be permitted to do so voluntarily and must have all relevant information regarding their condition and alternative treatments, including possible benefits, risks, costs, other consequences, and significant uncertainties surrounding any of this information."[4]

Probably 95 percent of the time, the person who can best answer your questions is your physician.

Today health care takes place in many different settings— ranging from a doctor's or dentist's private office to public health departments, nonprofit community clinics, hospitals, and hospices—and health care is increasingly practiced by health care teams. You may find yourself dealing with issues of informed consent if the person treating you is a nurse practitioner, chiropractor, dentist, or physical or occupational therapist—to name but a few.

Without the following four elements, no truly informed consent can be given:

- A patient *competent* to make health-related decisions
- Disclosure of *relevant information* by the physician, including risks, benefits, and alternatives
- *Understanding* of the disclosed information by the patient
- A *choice—freely made* by the patient

(If the patient is incompetent, these criteria apply to his or her *legal guardian*. For information on criteria for competence of children, see Chapter 8. For information regarding the person who is mentally retarded or senile, see Chapter 9.)

66

The Patient's Bill of Rights

In short, you or your proxy are entitled, as a legal right, to know what treatment you are getting, what the major risks are, and who is responsible for your care. As spelled out in sections 2 and 3 of the American Hospital Association's *A Patient's Bill of Rights*,[5] this means:

> The patient has the right to obtain from his physician complete current information concerning his diagnosis, treatment and prognosis in terms the patient can reasonably be expected to understand. When it is not medically advisable to give such information to the patient, the information should be made available to an appropriate person in his behalf. He has the right to know by name the physician responsible for coordinating his care.

and:

> The patient has the right to receive from his physician information necessary to give informed consent prior to the start of any procedure and/or treatment. Except in emergencies, such information for informed consent should include, but not necessarily be limited to, the specific procedure and/or treatment, the medically significant risks involved, and the probable duration of incapacitation. Where medically significant alternatives for care or treatment exist, or when the patient requests information concerning medical alternatives, the patient has the right to such information. The patient also has the right to know the name of the person responsible for the procedures and/or treatment.

But I want to caution you: don't agree to anything you don't want. Read the fine print on any informed consent release you're asked to sign, and don't give *general* or *blanket* consent.

For example, surgeons frequently say something like this:

"Until I open up your abdomen and see what's going on there, I can't tell you what I'm going to have to do."

Your response should be: "Then tell me the five or six things you're most likely to find."

Any experienced surgeon can say, "When I get in there, I may find (a), (b), or (c) and have to do (e), (f), or (g), but there's always a slight chance I might have to do (h) or (i)." With that spectrum of possibilities made clear, you know what you're getting into and, assuming you can live with *any one of those options*, you're wise to trust your surgeon and give consent.

Of course, the law recognizes certain exceptions to informed consent. Among these are patient waiver ("Don't tell me, doc, I don't want to know"), patient incompetency, and life-threatening emergencies. If you're in the emergency room with a bullet in your skull or a knife through your chest, you're in no position to discuss risks, benefits, alternative treatments, and quality of life. But that's rare.

In most circumstances, you'll have time to consent to proposed treatment, medications, tests, x-rays, etc. And as Boston University law school professor George J. Annas reminds us in the American Civil Liberties Union Handbook *The Rights of Hospital Patients:*

> The more elective a procedure is, the more important full disclosure becomes....In order to win a lawsuit for lack of informed consent, one must convince the jury that if one knew about the risks, one would not have undergone the procedure or operation. The more elective the procedure, the more likely the jury is to find such a decision reasonable.[6]

Any risk of death, however slight, must be disclosed

You have a right to know the common and serious complications, side effects, and other risks of treatment or procedures which may pose a threat of significant bodily harm or death.

(And although the risk of a treatment or procedure may seem extremely small at times, doctors can't afford *not* to tell patients when the risk of legal liability is so high.)

In the landmark case *Canterbury* v. *Spence*, a 19-year-old man underwent a spinal operation to correct serious back problems. Although there was a low risk of paralysis in the procedure, the surgeon failed to tell his patient of this possibility. Following surgery, the young man found himself paralyzed and sued for damages. The court ruled that even a *1 percent chance* of paralysis must be disclosed—since this represents a serious, albeit remote, risk.[7]

In another case, *Cooper* v. *Roberts*, a Pennsylvania court ruled that *any* risk of significant harm to the patient must be disclosed. In that case, the physician was held liable for failure to tell his patient of a one in 2,500 risk of perforation of the stomach during a gastroscopic examination (a diagnostic procedure in which a semirigid lighted tube is passed through the throat into the stomach).[8]

Most experts in medical ethics agree a doctor does not have to inform you of lesser side effects or risks, such as a body rash or itch. Yet, if these side effects of a drug or treatment commonly occur, I would think it important that my patient by alerted to this possibility.

"I see a fair number of patients who leave their doctors because these patients aren't willing to tolerate their impotence or depression, for example, and they aren't comfortable talking to their doctor about these side effects of medication they're taking," says Loma Linda School of Medicine internist Stewart Shankel. And when they do try to discuss these problems, Shankel adds, "their doctors say, 'Well, your blood pressure's down and right where it should be.' Their focus is on the disease, not the person—and they aren't willing to change things around or try other drugs." So their patients up and quit.

You should feel free to talk to your doctor about symptoms or side effects you are experiencing from drugs and treatments—especially those problems that affect your personal relationship with your spouse or "significant other," such as impotence, lack of sexual drive, depression, aggressive or suicidal tendencies, etc. Such stresses and emotional problems are factors in your medical condition.

Your doctor's job is to help you get back your physical and emotional health, not to make value judgments about your life-style, sex life, or ability to cope.

So express your concerns. Ask questions. Insist on answers in words you can understand. Keep at it until you have enough information to weigh the pros and cons, risks and benefits of the proposed treatment—or no treatment at all.

If you find you can't communicate with your doctor, or that he ignores your concerns and questions, find another doctor who's willing to help you get your medical problems under control, and still *enjoy your life* to the fullest extent possible.

Questions to ask for informed consent

1. What's wrong with me? What's the diagnosis?
2. How serious is this condition/illness?
3. What test(s) do you plan to do?
4. Why are you doing this test? How will the information affect the way you plan to treat me?
5. What are the risks of this procedure or test? How accurate is the test, and what are the percentages of false negative or false positive results?*
6. What kind of treatment do you recommend—surgery, radiation, drugs?
7. What's the purpose of this treatment? Will it cure my condition? Is it going to relieve pain or help to rehabilitate me?
8. What are the risks of such treatment?

---

*A false negative result means the test has indicated the absence of a given disease or condition which, in fact, the patient *has;* a false positive result means the test has indicated the patient has a certain disease or abnormality which, actually, he does *not* have.

9. What are the chances that the proposed treatment will be successful in my case?
10. Will this be a long-term or short-term benefit?
11. What will happen to me if I refuse all treatment?
12. What alternative treatments are available?
13. How do they compare to the one you're recommending in terms of risks and benefits?
14. Of these other treatment methods, which do you think would be best for me?
15. If you were in my situation, which treatment would you choose for yourself or a family member? Why?
16. Do you have any information on this test or procedure which I could take home with me to read? Is there a patient information center here (or at the hospital, office, clinic, etc.) where I can get more information, see a film, or review other materials?

If you have doubts about what your doctor is recommending, ask him to explain it further. If you're still not satisfied, get a second opinion. Become an informed consumer.

Read up on your condition, its diagnosis and treatment, and anything else you feel you need to know. Remember, although much has been said in the media about excessive testing and x-rays, when medical circumstances require it, in most cases the benefit of information gained far outweighs the risks.

What you want to know is, are the tests being done to satisfy your doctor's curiosity—or to help him or her do a better job caring for you?

Ways to become better-informed

Since a well-informed health care consumer is likely to get better care, it's smart to keep up with the latest medical news. It's not hard when television documentaries, radio broadcasts, and newspaper and magazine articles focus day after day on health-related topics. But don't rely solely on mass media for your information.

Good sources of information include health newsletters, such as the *Harvard Medical School Health Newsletter* and *University of California, Berkeley, Wellness Letter*; brochures, fact sheets, and booklets published by so-called disease organizations, such as the American Cancer Society or American Heart Association; and a variety of patient-education books, articles, film strips, audiovisual cassettes, and programmed self-learning materials available through your physician, hospital, or clinic.

In addition, there are several good general medical references you may wish to consult, among them the *American Medical Association Family Medical Guide*, rev. ed. (New York: Random House, 1987); *The People's Book of Medical Tests* by David Sobel, M.D., and Tom Ferguson, M.D. (New York: Simon and Schuster, 1986); *Complete Guide to Prescription and Non-Prescription Drugs*, rev. ed., by H. Winter Griffith, M.D. (New York: H. P. Publishing Co., Inc., 1986); and *Modern Prevention: The New Medicine* by Isadore Rosenfeld, M.D. (New York: Linden Press/Simon and Schuster, 1986). One gynecologist I know gives a copy of his own book *All About Hysterectomy* to each of his patients to whom he recommends such surgery. The book was coauthored with a professional writer, a patient of his who felt she needed more information about risks, benefits, and alternatives, as well as what to expect before, during, and after surgery. Now, before a patient signs a release form for hysterectomy, she has a chance to read the book. "The majority read it," he explains, "and that gives them an opportunity to ask specific questions. It's entered into their record that they read the book, so it becomes part of the informed consent, too."

Medical journals—reading for lay people, too

Another source of information that many lay people overlook is the hundreds of professional journals that doctors and ethicists turn to for the latest in opinion, review articles, and clinical and research data.

However, unless you know just what you're looking for or have an exact reference (such as journal articles suggested as further reading in this book), ask a medical librarian for some guidance in selecting a journal or finding a specific topic. "I frequently suggest a lay person read an article in a nursing journal first," says medical librarian Laurie Potter, who's also a registered nurse. Often these publications contain overviews of a topic or review articles which are a little easier to read than a highly technical research or clinical report in the *New England Journal of Medicine* or the *Journal of the American Medical Association.*

Before you go to a medical library, call ahead to be sure you'll be permitted to use its resources. Often, special clearance or a visitor's pass is required. (Don't forget that if public tax dollars are helping to support the library, it's hard for librarians to say users *aren't* welcome.)

After you find the information you want, don't indiscriminately apply it to your own case. You aren't taking a crash course in medicine to become your own doctor or to treat yourself. You want information so you can discuss with your doctor what the best approach might be in treating your condition.

So discuss your concerns. Ask your doctor to clarify and interpret information you get from other sources. It's as easy as saying, "Doctor, I read about such and such in the [title of journal]; how does this apply to my case?"

When too much information is confusing

The whole point of having enough information is to help you make informed choices about whether or not you want to be treated. But all too often, when every risk, benefit, side effect, and alternative treatment is explained, people feel as though they're faced with a smorgasbord of choices that leaves them floundering.

Recently at a dinner party, for example, a vivacious 59-year-old widow turned to me and said, "I think I liked it better the old way when doctors *told* you what to do. Right now, I'm seeing this nice young doctor who gives me every risk, benefit, alternative, and piece of paper for patients to read that he can put his hands on—but I feel confused. I don't know what to do. Would you know what to do if you weren't a doctor?"

"I think I'd be confused as hell," I told her, "so I'd ask the doctor a question like 'What would *you* do in this case if you were me?' Or 'What would you advise someone in your family to do under these circumstances?'"

Ideally, I think a physician should present all the options, and then recommend the one he thinks is best for you. If you don't agree with his recommendation, or if you choose a procedure which he doesn't "do," he may try to change your mind, but in no case should he coerce you—or abandon you. He should help you find another doctor, although you may prefer to do this on your own.

That's what happened a few years ago, when my wife discovered a small, rocklike lump in one breast.

The surgeon who initially examined her recommended she have the lesion removed and biopsied *immediately* to determine if it was malignant. If so, he explained, she had a number of options—ranging from mastectomy to lumpectomy (a less disfiguring procedure in which the lump plus

74

additional tissue in the area of the tumor is removed, followed by radiation therapy and possibly by chemotherapy).

However, he made it clear he was not convinced lumpectomy had proved "as good" as mastectomy—and if she chose that option, she would have to get another surgeon to operate. He didn't do lumpectomies.

Second opinions can help you avoid unnecessary surgery

After talking it over, my wife and I decided the first step was to get a second opinion. An oncologist associated with the University of Nevada School of Medicine examined her and ordered a mammogram x-ray of her breasts.

After seeing the report, he assured her that with such a small tumor (and there was even the possibility the "lump" might be an encapsulated cyst rather than a tumor), there would be no increased risk to her in waiting a few days, thinking it over, and having a lumpectomy rather than partial mastectomy. In fact, he recommended that approach and gave her the names of two or three surgeons he knew who performed lumpectomies and were supportive of women who chose that method.

She also had the choice of having the biopsy done at a hospital or separate minisurgery center. She doesn't like hospitals, so she chose the latter.

Because of a urinary infection, she was put on antibiotics for the week preceding surgery. By the fourth day of medication, the "lump" had disappeared. The biopsy was no longer needed. The new surgeon's best guess was that the antibiotics had cleared up what must have been a localized infected breast cyst.

Close calls like that make you appreciate the value of accurate diagnosis, of knowing the treatment options, of second opinions from specialists who are totally *independent* of one another, of a little time, and, yes, of good luck.

If you have doubts about the surgery your doctor recommends, don't hesitate to get a second opinion. A glance at the following chart shows why. In a 1983 study, doctors disagreed with each other an average of 17 percent of the time over whether a patient should have surgery as follows:[9]

Operation	Number of times surgery proposed	Surgery opposed by 2nd physician	% of disagreement
Varicose vein	6	3	50
Breast	23	9	39
Back	29	11	38
Bunion	22	8	36
Knee	58	16	28
Prostate	17	3	18
Hysterectomy	53	9	17
Gall bladder	25	3	12
Tonsils and adenoids	43	5	12
Dilatation and curettage	43	3	7
Cataract	52	3	6
Hernia	39	2	5
Nose	25	1	4
TOTAL	435	76	17

Results of mandatory second opinions for insured employees of Owens-Illinois Inc. in 1983.

(For more on second opinions in medical and surgical matters, see Chapter 2. But don't forget, if the consulting physician examining you goes over your report and then says, "I'll get back to your doctor with my opinion," you're right back at square one—with only one opinion. You don't want the consultant's opinion relayed through your surgeon, you want it given directly to you.)

Weighing risks versus benefits

When you try to make a judgment about what to do medically, you are weighing risks against benefits. An accurate diagnosis and prognosis are essential starting points. What you are attempting to do in risk-benefit analysis, explains Victor R. Fuchs in a *New England Journal of Medicine* article, is to "consider systematically all the consequences of a possible course of action—arrayed as costs and benefits."[10]

But keep in mind this isn't merely a *scientific* balancing of costs and benefits, but also a weighing of *values*.

Although we tend to think of most risks in terms of bodily injury, the courts have long accepted the rights of certain religious groups to refuse specific treatment because they believe that in accepting it, they would risk their salvation.

Spiritual values can affect your treatment choices

You have a right to worship as you see fit. And sometimes, religious values weigh heavily in a patient's decision to refuse or consent to certain medical treatment or medications.

Members of Jehovah's Witnesses, for example, have deep religious convictions against accepting whole blood or its components needed for treatment of shock, dialysis, or some surgical procedures. The courts have upheld this right to refuse treatment by competent adults but have ruled that parents cannot make a similar decision for their children. (See Chapter 8.)

Reluctance to take medication for a heart condition that was affecting his sports performance in 1983 nearly ended the pro basketball career of San Diego Clippers player Terry Cummings. An ordained Pentecostal minister, Cummings

77

had missed eight games the preceding season because of an irregular heartbeat which caused dizziness and fainting spells during periods of exertion.

Following tests, his doctors recommended he take a powerful experimental drug to combat the heart condition—*if* he wanted to continue playing ball. But he'd been brought up to believe people didn't take medicine to cure something wrong with them, Cummings explained in a *San Diego Tribune* interview, adding, "I didn't do it for a long time and I wasn't ready to start."[11] What changed his mind, he said, was a visit from a minister friend who told him he had to understand that doctors and medicine are just another helping hand of God—and that he was free to use it.

And because the late Terence Cardinal Cooke of New York City believed his suffering could be meaningful, he chose to limit the amount of medication he was receiving when gravely ill so that he could remain conscious as much as possible and offer the pain of his leukemia "as a beautiful gift for others." Roman Catholics believe that suffering can be dedicated to a purpose, including the salvation of the souls of others, and Cardinal Cooke wanted his suffering to be "purposeful."

The case of Elizabeth Bouvia

At about the same time that Cardinal Cooke was dying nearly three thousand miles away, a 28-year-old quadriplegic woman suffering from severe cerebral palsy saw no purpose in living any longer in great pain from her arthritis. During several hospitalizations, she asked to have her pain controlled and to be allowed to starve herself to death. Doctors and hospital officials refused and finally, against her will, resorted to force-feeding her through a nasogastric tube.

The case of Elizabeth Bouvia went to court several times during the next two years—making media headlines from coast to coast as she became a symbol of the right-to-die movement. But the *real* issue at stake during many months of legal battles, including one that yielded a landmark decision, was her *right to refuse medical care.*

In February 1986, Superior Court Judge Warren Deering refused to halt the force-feeding of Elizabeth Bouvia, saying that it was fairly clear from the evidence that she had formed an intent to die. Her claim that she didn't want to commit suicide, he wrote in his eleven-page opinion, "is but a semantic distinction."

Two months later, the California court of appeal overturned Deering's decision. Elizabeth Bouvia had won the right to refuse force-feeding or any other unwanted medical treatment "even if its exercise creates a 'life-threatening condition.'" Furthermore, the higher court ruled that the trial court had seriously erred in basing its decision on the motive behind Elizabeth Bouvia's decision to exercise her right, and they concluded, "If a right exists, it matters not what 'motivates' its exercise."[12]

Whatever you think of her crusade to force her care-givers to respect her wishes, don't be confused about what the basic issues are. One issue concerns public policy. Court decisions create such policy, and the ruling that Elizabeth Bouvia has the right to refuse all treatment—including feeding—may set the dangerous precedent of establishing a corresponding duty on the hospital's medical and nursing staff to medicate and support her during the starving and dying process. Many experts believe that such a policy could seriously undermine public confidence in the healing and treatment roles of health professionals.

The other issue focuses on the rights of the competent patient to make treatment choices. Simply put, until proved otherwise, the law presumes that *each of us is competent* to make his or her own choices—and we cannot be disqualified from making decisions for ourselves until we are proved incompetent.

But there's the rub.

Medicine has many gray areas. Although some experts

claim a doctor *never* has a right to overrule a patient's wishes until a court has judged the person incompetent, there are other physicians and experts in medical ethics who believe that in a very narrow range of cases—and for a *limited* time only—overriding a competent patient's wishes is justified.

Here is an example that caused quite a furor at a recent seminar on medical ethics held on a university campus and open to the public.

What would you do?

A 40-year-old man who was diagnosed as having cancer of the colon told his doctor, "Cancer means pain, suffering, death—I want nothing done."

Firmly convinced the man's cancer was curable, the doctor didn't let him off the hook.

He called in another physician to try to persuade the man he should seek treatment. No luck. He asked a world-renowned surgeon working at Stanford University's Palo Alto Clinic to talk to the patient. No results. Finally, he called in a patient who had been operated on successfully for a similar type of cancer ten years earlier and was doing well. The patient talked to the man, who later agreed to surgery. That was twenty years ago—and he just retired from his job at a California university with plans to travel and enjoy his grandchildren. He says now he's glad he had the surgery.

Was the doctor badgering the patient to change his mind about treatment? Was the patient severely depressed when he said, "Cancer means pain, suffering, death"? If he was depressed, was the depression affecting his competence to make a life-and-death decision for himself?

Some people in the audience said that in this case, the doctor's pushing the patient to consent to surgery had worked to his benefit. But in another situation, audience members said, such pressure to consent could be a form of harassment which would only add to the patient's already considerable stress.

In this case, I believe the doctor, who had known and treated the patient for many years, was right in trying to get the patient to change his mind. Asking three people to talk to him hardly seems like harassment. I agree with those experts who argue that "weak" paternalism is justified in certain *limited* circumstances, when, for example, severe depression or the side effects of drugs cloud the patient's judgment to the point that he or she takes unreasonable and dangerous risks.

Although there is always the possibility of overestimating the negative effects of depression and drugs on a patient's competence, these are valid reasons for *temporarily* overriding the usually competent patient's right to self-determination. The rationale is that treating the patient against his wishes will restore him to a point of competence at which he can again exercise his autonomy and make decisions for himself—even if those choices are life-threatening or seem foolish to others.

At that point, patient, family, doctors, hospital officials, and attorneys often reach such an impasse that the only recourse is to go to court. And often it's differing opinions on *quality of life* that cause the hottest debate.

"Inflicting a living hell"

In the case of 70-year-old William Bartling, whose doctors were invoking "limited paternalism" in keeping him on a respirator against his wishes, there was never any hope of restoring his health or freeing him from the tubes that ran up his nose, down his throat, and into his arms and shoulder as well as through a hole cut in his neck. He had not only inoperable lung cancer, but four other diseases as well.

At stake, Bartling's attorneys argued, was the competent

patient's right to make health care decisions for himself. Mrs. Bartling testified that beginning a month after her husband entered the hospital, he began asking for the ventilator's removal. She could read his lips: "I can't take it anymore."[13] Hospital attorneys, however, claimed the real issue was the rights of physicians to follow *their* interpretation of medical ethics to preserve life.

When the case went to a California court, Bartling's right to die was upheld in a major ruling which came twenty-three hours *after* the retired dental-supply salesman had died. But by then, his lawsuit against the Glendale Adventist Medical Center in Los Angeles had already been a subject for *Donahue* and the television show *60 Minutes*—where millions of viewers had seen segments of his videotaped deposition from the intensive care unit shortly before death.

Quality of life

What constitutes a quality of life worth living is highly subjective; like so many things, it varies from person to person.[14]

Quality of life for the person who has never been sick may be nothing short of feeling great, being on the go from morning until night, and going in exciting directions in life, work, play, and relationships with others. For these people, quality of life is that top-of-the-world feeling that can make it hard to accept the fact that someone else may have lost all will to live.

For the person who is seriously ill, quality of life may be measured in days without nausea; afternoons feeling well enough to visit with friends and family; mornings with energy enough to go to school or to work, bake fresh bread, plant daffodils in the garden, or make love one more time.

When there's so little, or even nothing, left to live for but pain, suffering, and isolation, competent patients like Elizabeth Bouvia and William Bartling feel free to say they no longer want to endure the quality of life their illnesses and treatments are subjecting them to.

In other cases, however, patients who find that illness is severely affecting the quality of their life can opt for experimental procedures or medications which offer a chance for a better quality of life or even a slim hope of recovery.

Some of these courageous patients—like Dr. Barney Clark, the world's first artificial heart recipient; William Schroeder, who lived longer than any other artificial heart recipient; and the late Mary Gohlke, who was the world's longest-surviving heart-lung recipient—take enormous risks in entering highly experimental research programs.

Because of the uniqueness of their risks, they also make media headlines around the world. So, too, do their families.

Much more common, however, are patients who don't make news—those who volunteer to take part in experimental research testing new drugs, new vaccines, and new surgical procedures. Still other patients participate in sociological and psychological surveys and experiments, or epidemiological studies, i.e., studies which trace the natural course of disease in a given population.

After talking to your doctor, you, too, may decide an experimental research program offers you a chance of recovery. You may also feel it's a chance to help doctors learn more about your condition and new and better ways to treat it.

"Most patients," says University of Nevada School of Medicine neurologist John Peacock, "are usually willing to participate in a new drug study, particularly cancer patients who have previously failed to respond to a certain therapy. All medical care and medications are free to the patient during the course of the study."

No one, of course, wants to be a guinea pig. And today this is extremely unlikely because of strict federal guidelines for extensive laboratory testing before human subjects can be used in drug trials. But even so, under *no* circumstances should you ever be coerced or deceived into signing a release form for experimental research.

The best way to protect yourself is to know your rights, choose a research program with great care, and read the consent form—fine print and all—before signing and dating it. (Be sure to get a copy for yourself, as you have a right to one. See the guidelines in Appendix B.)

Take a tip from the wife of artificial heart recipient William Schroeder. Writing in the December 16, 1985, issue of *People*, Margaret Schroeder said that she would "give anything" to know whether her husband wanted to continue living after a third stroke left him unable to speak or sit up unaided. With her husband unable to express his feelings about the quality of his life, Mrs. Schroeder worried about her role as guardian of his best interests.

"If I had to do it over again," she wrote in a first-person account, "I would read the consent form very carefully and talk to someone who has been through it. I would want to put into the consent form some things that would help the family. They don't have anything that says, 'How far down the road do you want to go with this before you call it quits?' I wish Bill had written down on the consent form at what point he would want to say, 'Stop this, I've had enough.'"[15]

When entering a research program, know your rights

The opening words of the Nuremberg Code of 1946 are: "The voluntary consent of the human subject is absolutely essential." Although written in reference to Nazi wartime medical experimentation, those words hold generally true. Since then, many national and international bodies have expanded these guidelines. Newer codes include the U.S. Guidelines on Human Experimentation of 1971 and the World Medical Association's Helsinki Declaration of 1975, both of which spell out in more detail the definition of informed consent and rules for protection of human subjects in experimental research.

In America today, *all* institutions which carry out legitimate human-subjects research follow these guidelines.

More to the point, all institutions in which research is carried on must have an Institutional Review Board (IRB) or similar committee responsible for reviewing and approving all human subject research proposals, consent forms, and protocols. (A protocol is a document which specifies in detail how patients will be selected for research projects and how the procedure or testing will be carried out.)

Here's what this means to you. As stated in the revised U.S. Guidelines on Human Experimentation (1974), you should receive the following:

- A fair explanation of the procedures to be followed, and their purposes, including identification of any procedures which are experimental
- A description of any attendant discomforts and risks reasonably to be expected
- A description of any benefits reasonably to be expected
- A disclosure of any appropriate alternative procedures that might be advantageous for you
- An offer to answer any inquiries concerning the procedures
- An instruction that you are free to withdraw your consent and to discontinue participation in the project or activity at any time without prejudice to you

In other words, you can leave the program whenever you want and can't be "punished" or penalized in some way for dropping out. (But don't forget the Schroeders' experience. Consider signing a Durable Power of Attorney for Health Care Decisions, explained in Chapter 4, so that your spouse or other proxy can remove you from a research program if you become incapacitated and are unable to express your own wishes.)

In addition, you should be neither required nor requested to give up any of your legal rights or to release the institution or its agents from liability for negligence. "If you have any

85

questions or problems with your experimental treatment or program," advises Dr. John Peacock, "report them to your program's IRB or review committee—anonymously, if you prefer."

Ask about placebos

Know what you're getting into from the start. For example, in some research studies, some of the subjects receive a standard treatment or drug while others are assigned to a control group which receives a placebo.

(A placebo is a pharmacologically neutral or inert substance given under the guise of medicine. In research studies, placebos are used as a control to evaluate the effectiveness of an experimental drug or treatment. Ideally, neither the researcher nor the subject knows who is getting the placebo or the experimental drug at any time during the study.)

Ethically, placebo studies should not be carried out when there is a well-recognized and effective treatment for a condition, because to do so places the subject at high risk unnecessarily. Many protocols call for an independent group to monitor the progress of the study and its subjects. In cases where there is significant difference between the response of one group of human subjects and the other, the independent reviewers have the power to break the code and see that all subjects receive the more effective treatment or drug.

But you should not be put into a placebo control group without knowing from the outset that it's possible you might be assigned randomly to such a group rather than to the treatment group. Don't wonder about it, ask. "Is there a placebo group in this research program I'm entering and is there a chance I'll be randomly assigned to it?"

You have a right to know.

Once you're accepted

Once you're accepted in a research program, your right to privacy and strict confidentiality should be guaranteed—*unless* you agree to take part in hospital public relations efforts or give your doctors or hospital officials permission to disclose information about you and your condition to others.

"It is imperative that you know as much as possible about your personal role in a research project before agreeing to participate," advises Eugene D. Robin, author and professor of medicine and physiology at Stanford University School of Medicine. "Evoke the Golden Rule. Ask the doctor soliciting your participation if he himself would participate in the study under similar circumstances...or if he would permit members of his own family to participate."[16]

But check it out with others as well. For example, here's what one university professor told me influenced his decision *not* to encourage his wife to go into an experimental program for multiple sclerosis: "I consulted with outside physicians and, most important, with the research director of the MS society."

Remember, research programs are designed and carried out to obtain *new* knowledge about specific diseases, treatments, or classes of patients. You may not meet the criteria for entry into a particular program. In short, you don't have a "right" as such to be a human subject in a research study—no matter how desperate you may be *or* how altruistic.

Genetic engineering—who profits if your cells are valuable?

It's rare, but suppose you're one of a small group of research patients whose cells prove useful in making genetically engineered products or medicines. Do you own the unwelcome

87

"disease information" stored in your tissues? Do you have a right to share in any profits the research institution may reap from your cells and tissues?

According to leading research officials who testified before Congress in May 1985, patients have little or no right to any resulting profits. Furthermore, an official of the National Institutes of Health told the committee that federal regulations require only disclosures of potential risks to the patient—*not potential profit.*

Under consideration was the case of a 40-year-old Seattle seafood sales manager who sued the University of California–Los Angeles Medical Center for compensation for emotional and mental distress and a share in potential royalties for a cell line cloned and patented from spleen cells taken from his body during treatment for cancer in 1976.

According to newspaper accounts, John Moore's doctors claim he signed over all ownership rights to material produced from his spleen cells which have been cloned and patented and today are being used for research into cancer, acquired immune deficiency syndrome and other diseases. Moore apparently did sign such an informed consent release in April 1983. But five months later he changed his mind. Signing another form, he stated he did not want to sign over rights to products developed from his cells.[17]

What it boils down to is that you should know what potential benefits you're retaining or giving away when you sign a consent release. If you're not sure, *seek advice*—including that of your attorney.

When your medical problem puts you in the news

Cases like Moore's and those of Elizabeth Bouvia and William Bartling are the ones that go to court, set legal precedents, and help shape public policy. Ethical dilemmas arising from space-age technology also make headline-grabbing news.

Life-and-death outcomes, last-minute searches for donor organs, and tearful family members making desperate pleas for help are irresistible real-life drama. Both hospitals and media garner a large and sympathetic audience. And who of us isn't cheering on the patient in his or her battle against disease—especially when that person is a child.

Odds are that your story will not be headline news.

Reporters will not be camping on your doorstep or hounding you, your family, or your doctors for exclusive interviews. Nevertheless, you may find yourself dealing with the media for other reasons. For example:

- You may have exhausted your personal funds and need community support to cover doctor and hospital bills.
- You may need help in raising funds to pay for your travel to a highly specialized research center, or, like one potential heart-lung recipient, you may need help finding housing while you wait for a donor organ to become available.
- You may be grateful for the medical or hospital care you've received and want to tell your story to give hope to others or, possibly, to help the hospital in its public relations efforts.
- You may be convinced current rules, regulations, or laws affecting your medical situation should be changed and feel that the media are the best forum for your ideas and suggestions.

One grieving couple, prevented by law from donating the organs of their dying infant born with anencephaly (a fatal condition in which only the primitive brain stem is present), were willing to tell their story to the *San Francisco Chronicle*.[18] They know other babies' lives will be saved by organ transplants from infants like theirs—*if* one section of California's brain death law is amended to allow organ donation from babies born with anencephaly.

If your case is a test case in medicine and law, you may be

bombarded by phone calls from strangers who disagree with your position; letters from ultraconservative or extremely liberal groups; or notes from school children or fanatics or self-appointed guardians of the public interest. Don't underestimate the stress all of this puts you under. Consult Appendix I for pointers on working with the media. Take heart from the feedback you get from those who *support* your position.

And if you're taking your case to the media because you need help in raising funds, don't be surprised when the bonus is, as one mother put it, "an incredible outpouring of love and support and prayers from total strangers. Sometimes you forget so many people are out there rooting for you and your child."

Resources

Thinking of Having Surgery?
Surgery, Dept. HHS
Washington, DC 20201

Published by the Department of Health and Human Services, this excellent and free brochure concerning second opinions can also be obtained by calling the government's Second Surgical Opinion toll-free Hotline, (800) 638-6833; in Maryland, it's (800) 492-6603.

Suggested reading

Abram, Morris B. "Ethics and the New Medicine." *New York Times Magazine*, June 5, 1983.
Crawshaw, Ralph, M.D., *et al.* "Oregon Health Decisions: An Experiment with Informed Community Consent." *Journal of the*

American Medical Association, vol. 254, no. 22 (December 13, 1985).

Drane, James F. "The Many Faces of Competency." *Hastings Center Report*, April 1986, pp. 17–21.

Gruson, Lindsey. "Value of the Placebo Being Argued on Ethical Grounds." *New York Times*, February 13, 1983, p. 24.

Hull, Richard T. "Informed Consent: Patient's Right or Patient's Duty?" *Journal of Medicine and Philosophy*, vol. 10 (1985), pp. 183–97.

Katz, Jay, M.D. *The Silent World of Doctor and Patient*. New York: Free Press, 1984. (Each chapter deals with a different facet of informed consent: historical, legal, professional, psychological, scientific, and philosophical—unifying them into a compelling argument for genuine dialogue between doctor and patient.)

Preston, Thomas, M.D. "Warning: Doctors Can Be Hazardous to Your Health." *Cosmopolitan*, October 1982, pp. 236–39.

Robertson, John A. *The Rights of the Critically Ill*. New York: American Civil Liberties Union, 1983. (Includes chapters on human experimentation; the right to treatment, to control of medication, and to refusal of treatment; and the right to commit suicide.)

Robin, Eugene D., M.D. *Matters of Life and Death: Risk vs. Benefits of Medical Care*. New York: Freeman, 1984. (Discusses flaws in the health care system and encourages readers to evaluate the medical expert's opinion more critically to avoid serious errors in their own care.)

Schroeder, Margaret. "An Affair of the Heart." *People*, December 16, 1985, pp. 58–63.

Starr, Paul. *The Social Transformation of American Medicine*. New York: Basic Books, Inc., 1982. (See "The Generalization of Rights" in Chapter 4, pp. 388–93.)

4 The Living Will, The Durable Power of Attorney, and Naming a Proxy— the Pluses of Thinking Ahead

RECENTLY, after returning from St. Louis where her brother had been in an intensive care unit for six days before he died, my wife said, "We've got to sit down, talk, and make some decisions—sign a Living Will or whatever it takes to ensure we won't be hooked to a respirator if we don't want to be. And the kids need to know how we feel about it."

Like many other couples, we had a will that wasn't up to date. Our five children, for example, now were all over twenty-one and therefore no longer needed the guardians we had appointed for them years ago. Since we drew up that will, we'd even become grandparents—and hadn't given any thought to where our children's "issue" (legal terminology for that bright little grandchild smiling back at us from picture frames around the house) would fit into the parceling out of whatever we left behind.

Furthermore, we hadn't spelled out our wishes regarding health care if we were ever unable to make decisions for ourselves. From time to time, we had talked about signing Living Wills and making out a Durable Power of Attorney for health care, but we had never gotten around to doing it.

"You realize," one woman told me after her husband died suddenly and without a will, "that being 'too busy' is the dumbest excuse in the world for not doing what down deep you know you should do—it's going to catch up with you sooner or later. Here I am now looking all over the place for business papers, insurance policies, bank books, safety deposit box keys, and other things that I should have been able to put my finger on all along. It just always seemed there'd be plenty of time to organize those papers and talk about a will later on—now it's too late."

The pluses of thinking ahead

Most of us shove thoughts of illness, accidents, and death to the back of our minds. We refuse to think about them when life is going along smoothly.

But a crisis is not the time to be running around hunting for important papers, telephone numbers, and safety deposit box keys. Nor is it the time for making decisions based on hunches rather than information that could have been gathered more easily beforehand—with plenty of time, thought, and good legal, medical, and fiscal advice.

"Whatever the limits of free will, we are not free to choose not to die," says Rex Julian Beaber, assistant professor of family medicine at the University of California–Los Angeles Medical School. "If we can face this limit and overcome the denial of death, we can exercise our only real freedom. We can choose how we will die."[1]

But that requires facing up to our own mortality.

Certainly two young skiers I'll call Judy and Scott never gave it a thought as they headed for Lake Placid ski resorts a few years ago. Having just announced their engagement at Christmas, they had decided to fly across the country to celebrate the New Year with East Coast friends. On the drive back to the airport, their rental car hit black ice, spun out of control, and rolled down a snowy gully. Scott walked away from the accident unhurt; Judy didn't.

On impact, her head had hit the windshield. "It didn't seem that bad," Scott says now, "but she must have hit at just the wrong spot, because she never came to." Medical tests in the hospital showed very little brain activity. Yet for weeks, Judy remained on life-support systems. Seeing her like that, Scott says, was horrible. "I began to ask, why? Why is all this life-support stuff being done when there isn't any hope of recovery? But the machines were on," he says, "and I learned that once they're hooked up, it's hell to get them unhooked."

The problem was that Judy had no family or next of kin who could tell doctors what she would want for herself under these circumstances. She had never signed a Living Will or a more sophisticated document known as a Durable Power of Attorney for health care. And Scott was not yet her husband. If he had been, he would have been the person with whom doctors would have consulted in making decisions involving life supports for Judy. As her fiancé, however, he had no say in the matter and could only stand by frustrated and heartbroken—and watch.

A month later, Scott arranged for Judy to be taken back to a hospital in Minnesota, where they lived. Eventually, a hospital ethics committee recommended that her doctors withdraw all treatment and allow her to die.

"Once you've seen someone like that," says Scott, "you say to yourself, 'No way. I don't ever want all those tubes and wires for myself.' I've taken care of all the paperwork—Living Will, directives to my doctor, you name it—and I hope to God I never go through anything like that again."

If it's important to you to die with dignity and in peace, and to maintain some control over future legal and medical decisions made on your behalf, then look at the positive side of doing some advance planning now.

Basically, this falls into two categories: estate planning and health care decision-making.

The purpose of this chapter is to help you make those health care decisions, spell out the details of your wishes, and consider appointing another person to act for you if an illness should ever render you incompetent to make certain choices for yourself.

Because legal matters are extremely important in this type of personal planning, I urge you to discuss specifics that apply to you and your family with your own attorney, physician, family members, and anyone else whose opinion you respect and want. Be sure your loved ones and your doctor and attorney know how you feel about life-saving treatment when there is no hope for recovery and what kinds of procedures you would be willing to accept if you were ever unable to speak for yourself.

Remember, you are free to say, "I want it all—every last thing medicine can do for me till the very end." You're also free to say "no" to any treatment and to change your mind whenever you wish.

Here are some guidelines to start you thinking and help you understand what's involved in health care decisions now which will go into effect later.

Choose your doctor carefully.

Discuss with your physician your values, concerns, and wishes regarding your medical care should you become unable to make decisions for yourself.

In their book *For the Patient's Good: The Restoration of*

Beneficence in Medical Ethics, David Thomasma and Edmund D. Pellegrino point out that patients who do *not* discuss their values with their physicians and express their wishes regarding life-support systems when there is no hope for recovery leave their doctors with no alternative but to make decisions for them. Such decisions are based *solely* on what the doctor thinks is in their best interests—basically, *medical* criteria.[2]

Be selective in the health care setting you choose—whether it is home care, hospital, hospice, or nursing home.

The ancient Greeks believed hospitals should be pleasant places because a pleasing environment would augment the healing process for people who were ill. In today's cost-conscious hospital, pleasing environments are getting harder and harder to find. But if you know in advance that you must enter a hospital, check its track record for success in treating conditions like yours.

Statistics, of course, can be misleading. A recent report from the Department of Health and Human Services, for example, stated that in 1984, 142 of the nation's hospitals had abnormal death rates among Medicare patients (usually over 65 years of age), while overall mortality rates were lower than expected in 127 facilities.[3] But lower-than-average death rates do not necessarily mean better patient care; it could mean that very ill patients are transferred to other hospitals or routinely discharged before they die. And the study was widely criticized because it also included death rates in hospices, which care *only* for dying patients.

The report, however, does provide consumer groups with another means of assessing hospital care. And as competition for your business escalates and third-party payers attempt to cut costs, you'll see more of this type of comparative analysis—though doctors and hospitals are sure to resist such public disclosure.

As a result, you'll be in a better position to shop around for the best success rate, quality medicine, and value for your health care dollar. Remember, though, if you belong to a pre-paid group insurance plan, your choice of physicians and hospitals may be limited—unless you're willing to pay out of pocket for other options.

Given extra time, you can also look into an institution's policies and guidelines—and plan accordingly.

You may decide one hospital offers more in an emergency situation, another in handling elective procedures. I know of one expert in medical ethics who has instructed his wife to take him to an emergency room close to home if he has a relatively simple problem, like a laceration that needs stitches, but to a second hospital a few miles away for a serious emergency, like a heart attack, which would require hospitalization.

Once you go to an emergency room for treatment or enter a hospital for a procedure, however, you're basically saying "I want to find out what I've got" or "I want to get better."

That's when a conflict can arise, explains one emergency room physician, who says, "Hospitals are geared to healing, curing, doing things *to* people and sending them back home. If your condition is terminal and you're dying, the *last place* you may want to go to is the hospital."

Tell your doctor, family, and friends how you feel about the use of life-support systems after hope for your recovery has passed, and also if you wish to donate your organs.

America's best-selling baby-care author Benjamin Spock, for example, said in a *Parade* magazine article that he wants jazz, ragtime, and lively hymns played at his funeral, in a church full of cheerful people—and after that, a convivial cocktail party someplace close by.

Spock, who was 81 at the time, said that he wasn't ready to

die but wanted relatives to be aware of his wishes. "I don't fear dying as long as it's not very painful or lacking in dignity," he wrote.⁴ But he added that if he was in unbearable pain, he'd want to be put out of his misery.

Make your wishes known through advance directives, such as a Living Will (Directive to Physicians) or a Durable Power of Attorney for Health Care.

Eight months before he died in March 1986, Senator Jacob Javits went before a Capitol Hill Forum to endorse so-called Living Will legislation.

"The contemplation of death should be a timely thing of beauty and not a thing of disgrace," said the New York Republican, who suffered from amyotrophic lateral sclerosis, the degenerative nerve disease better known as Lou Gehrig's disease. Laws allowing people to have some control over their death, he said, are "the highest form of humanitarianism and love."⁵

Confined to a wheelchair and dependent on a breathing tube hidden under a red-flecked cravat, Javits said he was practicing what he preached—and formalizing his wish to die when his brain stopped functioning. He not only had signed a Living Will but had given his wife, Marion, the authority to decide when medical treatment should stop. Jacob Javits recognized that the time would come when he would need an advocate (or proxy) who legally could speak for him and make medical decisions on his behalf.

Don't leave your future to chance

You may be tempted to say, "I'm in good hands—my doctor knows me and I know he doesn't believe in prolonging the dying process." But don't forget, your personal physician (and even some of your family members) may not be around when you are seriously ill and admitted to a hospital.

A case in point. My mother-in-law's doctor has reassured her that he doesn't believe in putting elderly people on a life-support system if it offers no hope for recovery. "But what will happen," I asked her, "if your doctor is sick or out of town someday when you have to go to the hospital? Will the physician covering your doctor's practice *know* you don't want any heroic measures?"

After thinking it over, she decided to formalize her wishes through a Living Will and Durable Power of Attorney for Health Care Decisions, naming her daughter as her agent or proxy. But she also knows she can make additions, changes, or deletions by dating and clearly initialing them on the documents—or revoke these directives at any time if she changes her mind.

By not making clear what you would want for yourself in such situations, you leave it to chance that someone else will make the decision to resuscitate you again and again, force-feed you even though you don't want it, and, in the process, add cost upon cost to your health care through additional tests, medications, surgical procedures, or prolonged hospitalization.

Here's how one nurse sums up the problem: "The greatest dilemma facing [doctors and nurses in] critical care today is deciding when to use our amazing modern medical technology and when *not* to use it. We shouldn't try to keep everyone alive 'forever' just because we're able to."[6]

A number of nationwide polls have shown that the right-to-die philosophy is favored by some 68 to 81 percent of Americans.[7] However, what others feel about the terminally ill person's right to refuse medical treatment is not the issue. What's important is how *you* feel about accepting or forgoing such procedures for yourself.

Laws affecting your right to die

Let's look at the pros and cons of advance medical directives and *why* such directives are needed when the courts have repeatedly ruled that "every human being of adult years and sound mind has a right to determine what shall be done with his own body."

You have a constitutional right to be left alone—to refuse any form of medical treatment you don't want.

This right is virtually absolute, unless you are being treated in a hospital emergency room. In that case, even if you have a copy of your Living Will or Durable Power of Attorney on your person, doctors and nurses are not obliged to comply with your wishes. (See Chapter 3 for more on informed consent in emergency settings.) Despite this exception in an emergency, you should protect your best interests through these documents.

Living Will laws

Since 1976, when California passed the nation's first natural death statute, thirty-eight other states plus the District of Columbia have followed suit passing some form of "Living Will," "right to die," or "death with dignity" statute.

The Living Will authorized by such laws and generally referred to as a Directive to Physicians is a legal document which must be signed by you and duly witnessed. It permits you to specify your wishes regarding treatment and procedures you may or may not want if you become terminally ill or if your condition is hopeless and there is no chance of regaining a meaningful life.

If you are thinking about signing a Living Will, check to see if your state has passed a natural death statute (see chart) and obtain a copy of the Living Will form valid in your state.

WHEN STATES PASSED...

Living Will laws	Durable Power of Attorney for Health Care**
1976 California	
1977 Arkansas, Idaho, Nevada, New Mexico, North Carolina, Oregon, Texas*	
1979 Kansas, Washington	
1981 Alabama	
1982 Delaware,* Vermont, District of Columbia	Pennsylvania (specifies only consent, not refusal)
1983 Illinois, Virginia*	Colorado (no specificity regarding terminating treatment)
	California (authorizes refusal of life-sustaining treatment for incompetent principal based on prestated wishes of principal; grants immunity to the attorney-in-fact and physician for compliance with principal's wishes)
1984 Florida,* Georgia, Louisiana,* Mississippi, West Virginia, Wisconsin, Wyoming*	

1985   Arizona, Colorado,
        Connecticut,
        Indiana,* Iowa,*
        Maine,
        Maryland,
        Missouri,
        Montana, New
        Hampshire,
        Oklahoma,
        Tennessee,
        Utah*

1986   South Carolina

1987   Alaska, Hawaii

*Optional designation of a proxy.
**Although all states have Durable Power of Attorney laws, many hospitals and physicians will not usually honor them unless they are amended to include health care decisions. For this reason, a number of states have passed or are considering separate legislation to create a Durable Power document specifically covering health care decisions.

You can do this through an attorney, your county medical society, your local hospital, and possibly your own doctor. You can also obtain an up-to-date Living Will valid in your state (and instructions for filling it out) by writing to the Society for the Right to Die, Concern for Dying, or the Hemlock Society. (For addresses, see the Resources section at the end of this chapter.)

Even if your state has *not* yet passed a Living Will law, consider signing a standardized form anyway. It will serve as an important indication of your wishes if a conflict should arise about whether or not to stop, start, or alter life-saving treatment for you. (For a fuller discussion, see Chapter 9.)

Currently, there is no uniform right-to-die law, although one was approved and recommended in 1985 by the National Conference of Commissioners on Uniform State Laws. All existing laws require that you must be at least 18 years old and "of sound mind" to complete a Living Will, which usually states that you, the signer, "willfully and voluntarily make known my desire that my dying shall not be artificially prolonged under the circumstances set forth."

Here, for example, is how a standardized Living Will declaration[8] would deal with your directives regarding use of life-sustaining procedures:

> I direct that life-sustaining procedures should be withheld or withdrawn if I have an illness, disease or injury, or experience extreme mental deterioration, such that there is no reasonable expectation of recovering or regaining a meaningful quality of life.
>
> These life-sustaining procedures that may be withheld or withdrawn include, but are not limited to:
> surgery/antibiotics/cardiac resuscitation/respiratory support/artificially administered feeding and fluids
> I further direct that treatment be limited to comfort measures only, even if they shorten my life.
>
> (You may delete any provision above by drawing a line through it and adding your initials.)
>
> Other personal instructions:
>
> [This portion of the document provides space to add any other directions you want. However, if you live in California, Georgia, Idaho, or Oregon, you must follow the format exactly as outlined in the appropriate state law.]
>
> These directions express my legal right to refuse treatment. Therefore, I expect my family, doctors, and all those concerned with my care to regard themselves as legally and morally bound to act in accord with my wishes, and in so doing to be free from any liability for having followed my directions.

The standard form also contains a Proxy Designation Clause which allows the signer to appoint someone to make treatment decisions for him if he's unable to do so. But it's not necessary to designate a proxy for the Living Will to be in effect.

Finally, you must sign your Living Will and have it duly witnessed according to the law in your state. This usually means either a notary or two other people have watched you sign the document.

Signing a Living Will, however, is no guarantee that your wishes will be followed.

Some physicians refuse to honor Living Wills if, in their judgment, continued treatment may be of some benefit to the patient. Not only that, many state laws provide criminal and civil immunity to the physician if he acts in good faith—either in abiding by your wishes *or* overruling them for medically valid reasons.

(Thirty-six states and the District of Columbia have Living Will laws. In six states, the law is *permissive* rather than binding—the physician does not have to abide by the incompetent patient's previously expressed wishes. In the other thirty-one jurisdictions the physician who does not want to comply with the patient's prior directives must transfer that patient to another doctor.)

Additional limitations imposed on Living Wills, which vary from state to state, further reduce their effectiveness. In some states, for example, the Living Will must be renewed annually. In Nevada and twenty-three other states, the Living Will contains a clause invalidating it during pregnancy. But in five of these states, this exception applies only if life-sustaining procedures will help the fetus develop to the point of a live birth.

What it boils down to is this: know what your state's statutes call for and ask an attorney who is knowledgeable about living wills for advice. Then insist your Living Will be filed in your medical records—both in your doctor's office and at the hospital. If your doctor tells you he doesn't like to put *legal* documents in his office records (as one patient was told when she asked to have a copy of her Living Will inserted in her chart), you may want to consider changing doctors.

Although completing your Living Will may give you the feeling of being in control of future decisions about your medical care, most experts are concerned that this may not be enough. They recommend that you also execute a Durable Power of Attorney for Health Care.

Durable Power of Attorney for Health Care

The Durable Power of Attorney for Health Care allows you to name someone as proxy with authority to make medical decisions for you according to your previously expressed wishes if you become incompetent or unable to make those decisions for yourself.

An ordinary power of attorney is a way of authorizing another person to make decisions and take actions on your behalf—for example, selling your car for you while you're away on vacation. If you become incompetent, however, this power of attorney lapses. A "Durable" Power of Attorney signifies the ongoing authority given your proxy (that is, the person you designate) which remains in effect (or in most states, only becomes effective) *after* you become incompetent.

(All fifty states now have statutes recognizing and defining Durable Power of Attorney. But only four states—California, Colorado, Nevada, and Pennsylvania—have passed statutes authorizing a Durable Power of Attorney for Health Care. In addition, nine states allow for designation of a proxy on the Living Will form itself.)

As your "attorney-in-fact," this person is legally authorized to speak for you as though you yourself were able to give, withhold, or withdraw consent to any recommended treatment. The Society for the Right to Die suggests the following reasons for having a Durable Power of Attorney:

1. To give or withhold consent to specific medical or surgical measures with reference to the principal's condition, prognosis, and known wishes regarding terminal care; to authorize appropriate end-of-life care, including pain-relieving procedures
2. To grant releases to medical personnel

3. To employ and discharge medical personnel
4. To have access to and to disclose medical records and other personal information
5. To resort to court, if necessary, to obtain court authorization regarding medical treatment decisions
6. To expend (or withhold) funds necessary to carry out medical treatment

You'll find a copy of California's Durable Power of Attorney for Health Care form in Appendix F. A look at this document should help you understand what is required to execute one legally. However, state statutes vary considerably and are frequently amended. Because of this and the great power conferred on your attorney-in-fact through such a document, it's crucial to get the advice and assistance of a well-informed lawyer in drawing up a Durable Power of Attorney for Health Care Decisions.

Many people are uncomfortable relinquishing power over their bodies to someone else. But there are definite advantages to giving this authority to someone you know, respect, and trust—and who knows you, what you value, and how you feel about medical treatment and life-sustaining procedures. And in no way does signing either a Living Will or a Durable Power of Attorney for Health Care affect your right to insurance or health care services. In other words, the execution of such documents cannot be construed as suicide under the law or used to invalidate insurance policies you already have or purchase in the future.

While no one can force you to sign advance directives for health care, your other option is to simply leave it all to chance—and hope you luck out. Coming from a gambling town, however, I have to say the odds aren't in your favor.

The great myth is that everyone has a loving family and longtime personal doctor who will be around to make decisions when needed. But the fact is that in a crisis, you are much more likely to be under the care of *one or more doctors you've never met before*, and each of these specialists has one or more partners or other doctors taking calls for him or her.

Not only that, you may have no family or be estranged from living relatives by divorce, hard feelings, or life-styles that other family members disapprove of. Even if you have friends who are closer to you than your family, remember, they will not be able to make health care decisions for you unless you have given them *legal* power to do so.

At this point, with a valid signed and witnessed Living Will and Durable Power of Attorney, you may feel you've taken care of everything. But consider what happened to Morrice Henderson, 68, who entered a hospital for major vascular surgery for which he was given a good prognosis for recovery.

"Don't you people pay attention to Living Wills?"

A few months earlier, Morrice and his wife, Marilyn, a well-known novelist, had enjoyed a cruise along the eastern coast of South America, then spent some time in New York City. Both caught colds, but it was the pain in Morrice's leg which worried them most.

When it persisted after their return to Nevada, Morrice consulted a doctor, who diagnosed a complete blockage of the major artery in the left leg plus large aneurysms (blood-filled dilations) in his abdominal aorta. He advised Morrice to see a surgeon as soon as possible. A few weeks later, Morrice entered a hospital for bypass surgery for the aneurysms.

A month after the successful surgery, the bypass ruptured, necessitating emergency surgery, with less than a 10 percent chance of survival. What happened from that point on, Marilyn explains, was a "nightmare" of complications, hepatitis caused by a blood transfusion, fever of unknown origin, and "poor nursing care because of understaffing and indifference."

Morrice was gravely ill.

Outside his room one day, Marilyn saw a cart with "what looked like an old World War I gas mask" on it. When she asked the nurse what it was, she learned "it was in case Morrice had to be coded"—a hospital term for the emergency call which summons a special team to resuscitate a patient in cardiopulmonary failure. "But he's not supposed to be coded," Marilyn angrily told the nurse, who, according to Marilyn, said, "Oh, okay," and took it away.

As soon as she saw one of Morrice's doctors, Marilyn reminded him that copies of her husband's Living Will and Durable Power of Attorney were sitting right in his medical chart. "I had insisted they be attached to his record because we knew his chances were very poor as he went into the second surgery," explains Marilyn, adding that she then asked the doctor, "Doesn't anyone pay any attention to these things?"

To her astonishment, the doctor explained that the Living Will and Durable Power of Attorney did not mean that a patient is automatically designated "no code" (see What You Should Know about Cardiopulmonary Resuscitation, page 119).

What had happened was as follows: In his Durable Power of Attorney for Health Care, Morrice had checked and initialed the following statement as being a true reflection of his desires:

> I do not desire treatment to be provided and/or continued if the burdens of the treatment outweigh the expected benefits. My attorney-in-fact is to consider the relief of suffering, the preservation or restoration of functioning, and the quality as well as the extent of the possible extension of my life.

He and Marilyn believed that this would be enough to cover all possible situations. In fact, it wasn't. To *ensure* that Morrice's wishes would be carried out, one more step had to be taken: the doctor had to write a "Do not resuscitate" order on the Doctor's Order Sheet. Marilyn had assumed this would *automatically* be done following her discussion with Morrice's doctor at the time of the emergency surgery. But this assumption, though common, is false.

Remember, wishes expressed in a Living Will or Durable Power of Attorney for Health Care lead to action in the hospital *only* when they are translated into a doctor's specific order.

Once Marilyn raised the issue with Morrice's doctor, he took bright orange tape, wrote NO CODE on it, and plastered it boldly on the cover of the chart where no one could miss it.

A patient's medical chart can quickly become several inches thick when multiple surgeries and hospitalizations are required.

"Nobody reads what's in the back of the chart," says Marilyn. "Morrice was given narcotic drugs which made a wild man out of him—although his doctor had written early in the record 'nonnarcotic drugs only.' And there were so many other doctor's orders which were ignored," says Marilyn, "that I had to fight to see he got the treatment he was supposed to. At one point, the nurses had a meeting to decide what to do with 'that terrible Mrs. Henderson.'"

Finally, Marilyn decided enough was enough. Three of Morrice's doctors agreed he was not improving, but still wanted to run more tests. She said no and took her husband home, where he died twelve days later. However, shortly before Morrice left the hospital, Marilyn was told by a friend that a male nurse who had cared for her husband said, "I hope if I'm ever sick in a hospital, I have someone like Mrs. Henderson to fight for me."

Enlisting the right support

Virginia Turk also came up against the system when she tried to take her father, 76, home from a hospital. He had suffered a stroke a number of years before and now was hospitalized because of chronic lung disease. He kept telling his family, "I want to go home," and Virginia promised him he would. But his doctor refused to sign discharge papers.

Since private insurance carriers and Medicare will not cover costs if a patient is removed from the hospital against medical advice (AMA) and because next of kin are still liable for those bills, the Turk family tried to explain why they preferred to have their father die at home. They also offered to sign any type of permission or legal papers the doctor might need to release him from liability for Mr. Turk's welfare. The doctor still would not release him. "It's not a matter of philosophy of life," he told Virginia, "it's one of medical ethics—I can't allow a patient to go home to die."

Within twenty-four hours, the doctor had changed his mind.

Virginia Turk is a specialist in case management for the elderly and patient advocacy. She knew what to do and took her dilemma straight to the hospital administrator and chairman of the hospital's board of trustees. She had also discussed her father's situation with the hospital's Utilization Review Board, which oversees length of stay for Medicare patients.

"I told them," Virginia says, " 'If I have a doctor's permission to take my dad home, you get paid. If the family doesn't have the release, you don't get paid because we'll have to declare bankruptcy.' And they said, 'We'll get right on it and get another doctor to evaluate your father's situation.' "

By noon the next day, her father had been discharged. Mr. Turk died two weeks later at home, where he wanted to be, with family, with friends, where he could eat his favorite foods and where home care nurses provided help the Turks needed.

Virginia Turk and Marilyn Henderson were not afraid to speak up, fight for their loved one's rights as a patient—and keep at it until they got the action they wanted.

The doctor who said that "medical ethics" would not permit him to allow a patient go home to die was *uninformed.*

The attitude of Mr. Turk's physician is not uncommon.

The idea of allowing a person to die when there is no hope for recovery still troubles many people, including health professionals who see their role as doing all they can to save life. In part, the problem arises from confusion over terms, such as active and passive euthanasia.

Allowing people to die—is that euthanasia?

Euthanasia, writes Robert G. Twycross in the *Dictionary of Medical Ethics*, "literally means death without suffering. The word is now generally restricted to mean 'mercy killing,' the administration of a drug deliberately and specifically to accelerate death in order to terminate suffering."[9] This is commonly referred to as *active euthanasia*.

Active euthanasia is illegal in all countries except the Netherlands, which permits doctors to practice "aid in dying" under strict criteria and subject to thorough investigation by the government. Many Americans who watched a January 1986 *60 Minutes* television program on Dutch physicians and euthanasia availability have wondered if it's possible to travel to Holland to request such aid in dying.

"While I understand the great desire by some Americans with terminal illnesses for positive help," Professor Pieter Admiraal, Holland's most outspoken practitioner of voluntary euthanasia, explains in a Hemlock Society newsletter, "it is pointless...approaching me. I cannot help them. I will only give euthanasia to a patient I have come to know well and whose request I respect. Also, I have to work within the criteria laid down by the courts."[10]

Currently, the Los Angeles–based Hemlock Society, which takes the stance that terminally ill patients have the right to end their own lives in a planned manner, is supporting euthanasia legislation which will be introduced in the California, Arizona, and Florida legislatures.

If passed, this law, known as the Humane and Dignified

Death Act, would permit a physician to end the life of a terminally ill patient upon the competent request of that patient. (The society defines the "terminally ill" person as one who is likely to die within six months, and "physician aid-in-dying" as active voluntary euthanasia. Remember, suicide is not a criminal act anywhere in the United States; but in every state, *assisting* another person in a suicide is a criminal act—a felony murder.)

Passive euthanasia refers to the withholding of medical treatments when such treatments are futile and only burden the patient and prolong the dying process with no hope of altering the outcome. Experts in medical ethics no longer use the phrase "passive euthanasia." Instead, they speak of *forgoing life-sustaining treatment* when it is futile. As Dr. Twycross reminds us, "a doctor has a duty to sustain life where life is sustainable; he has no duty—legal, moral or ethical—to prolong the distress of a dying patient."[11]

Nor is it practicing euthanasia to relieve a terminally ill patient's suffering with very high and frequent doses of pain-killing medication even if these drugs pose a significant risk of hastening his or her death. To relieve suffering is what good medicine is all about.

The 1980 *Declaration on Euthanasia* by the Sacred Congregation for the Doctrine of the Faith, approved by Pope John Paul II, further states that "one cannot impose on anyone the obligation to have recourse to a technique which is already in use but which carries a risk or is burdensome. Such a refusal is not the equivalent of suicide; on the contrary, it should be considered as an acceptance of the human condition, or a wish to void the application of a medical procedure disproportionate to the results that can be expected, or a desire not to impose excessive expense on the family or the community.

"When inevitable death is imminent...it is permitted in conscience to take the decision to refuse forms of treatment that would only secure a precarious and burdensome prolongation of life, so long as the normal care due to the sick person in similar cases is not interrupted."[12]

Slippery-slope argument—won't permitting one thing lead to something worse?

The argument here is that taking a first step that is itself ethically justified—allowing a gravely ill patient to die peacefully while controlling his or her pain—may lead to the acceptance of other actions which are *not* justified, such as the intentional overdosing of such patients. Carried to its extreme, claim supporters of this line of reasoning, the slippery slope with no stop signs will allow society to intentionally do away with *any* undesirable group of people—as occurred in Nazi Germany. Therefore, the *first* step should not be taken.

Addressing this issue, the President's Commission for medical ethics states:

> For such an argument to be persuasive, however, much more is needed than merely pointing out that allowing one kind of action (itself justified) could conceivably increase the tendency to allow another action (unjustified). Rather, it must be shown that pressures to allow the unjustified action will become so strong once the initial step is taken that the further steps are likely to occur. Since such evidence is commonly quite limited, slippery slope arguments are themselves subject to abuse in social and legal policy debate....Obviously, slippery slope arguments must be very carefully employed lest they serve merely as an unthinking defense of the status quo.[13]

Who will speak for you?

You may not agree with the President's Commission. You may believe that any form of euthanasia is a violation of the commandment "Thou shalt not kill." You may believe that doctors who allow patients to die by forgoing life-sustaining treatment are unjustifiably playing God.

This is all the more reason for you to be explicit in making your wishes known.

Nearly everyone agrees that people in sickness tend to get cut off from their strengths and resources because their illness and the health care system put them in such a *passive* role. Certainly, anyone entering a hospital, hospice, or extended care facility of any kind should have someone—whether family member, friend, nurse, legally appointed proxy, or paid case management specialist—who can take on the role of advocate, watchdog, checker-upper, errand-person, and "squeaky wheel that gets the grease."

Such an advocate, suggests Boston University law professor and ethicist George Annas, should be able to assist the patient meaningfully in maintaining both dignity and autonomy. The advocate must be able to do such things (all at the patient's direction) as get the patient's chart for the patient to review, get a physician qualified to give a second opinion, delay procedures when informed consent is in doubt, delay undesired discharge, and forbid any experimental or teaching use of the patient without the patient's permission or knowledge.[14]

Is there someone who could do all this for you if you were ever incapacitated or unable to speak for yourself? Have you ever thought about asking someone to be your advocate if you needed hospitalization?

Most Americans confronted with that question would have to answer no, either out of unwillingness to face the fact that they might be in a position to need an advocate or out of mixed feelings about who would be the right person for the job.

Factors to weigh in choosing your advocate or proxy

Basically, what you're looking for in an advocate for yourself, explains University of Nevada–Reno bioethics professor Barbara Thornton, "is someone who knows you well, who isn't afraid to speak up and be assertive for your sake, someone who isn't intimidated by doctors or made queasy in a health care setting."

Although legally a family member will be called first in case of emergency, a family member may not always be the best choice as your advocate.[15] For example, I've known family members who couldn't bring themselves to step foot in an intensive care unit where a relative lay dying. It was too painful to see a loved one like that. Nor could they talk about the situation—their shock was so great.

Certainly, people have the right to grieve in their own way and decide whether or not they want to be with relatives who are dying. So keep this in mind when choosing your proxy or advocate. Select someone who will be able *and* willing to be there and speak for you.

Here are some additional pointers on choosing an advocate:

Look for someone who's assertive, knows your values, and understands you.

Choose someone who will respect what's important to you. This person most likely will share similar values and beliefs. But more important is whether or not your proxy would be comfortable *abiding by your wishes*—say to forgo life-

115

sustaining treatment if there were no hope of your recovery —when perhaps, he or she would make a different choice if his or her own life were at stake.

Don't assume anything; talk it over first. Just because you've asked your best friend or twin sister to be your proxy doesn't necessarily mean he or she thinks the same way you do. And you don't want your proxy *imposing* his or her views on you. You want your proxy to carry out *your* wishes.

Take into account how available this person can be on short notice—and whether he or she has time to be your advocate.

No one plans to have a heart attack, stroke, or accident; medical emergencies usually occur when least expected. Although you can't expect your advocate to be on call twenty-four hours a day, year in and year out, you do want someone who can be at your side fairly quickly when needed. (As backup, you may want to consult your lawyer about naming one or more alternate attorneys-in-fact.)

For this reason, and because traveling across the country is expensive, consider naming as your proxy or advocate someone who lives within a reasonable distance of your home— and has some time to give to your affairs. You can pick an assertive lawyer, for example, but if he or she is too busy with other clients, the attorney is going to have difficulty finding time to check on you in the hospital or nursing home as often as you'd like.

Consider your potential advocate's health and emotional stamina.

You'll need someone who may have to put in long hours at the hospital or social agencies on your behalf, and be able to think clearly when under emotional and physical stress. You want an advocate who isn't shy about asking questions, a person who won't be intimidated when doctors, nurses, hospital officials, social workers, or attorneys get annoyed because he or she is aggressive in trying to get the best possible care for you.[16]

At this point, you may be asking: "Don't doctors and other care-givers get annoyed with pushy people?"

"Yes, but don't worry about it," advises medical ethics expert Arthur Caplan, who's heard of extreme cases in which pushy family members alienated everyone, but doesn't consider this to be a common problem. "Almost always," he says, "the annoyance leads to better things for the patient."

Choose as your advocate someone who's informed (or willing to learn more) about patient rights and how to safeguard them.

Look for a person who doesn't give up easily, who will help you get information when no one in the system is willing to "talk" or act. Choose someone who isn't afraid of "bothering a busy doctor" if it means helping you to feel better, steer clear of doctor-nurse power plays, and keep from falling through the cracks of hospital or social agency bureaucracy.

Make it easy for your advocate to help you.

While it's possible that you'll never be sick a day in your life or need to call upon your advocate for help, you can't count on it. Take the necessary steps now which will simplify his or her job later—and you'll make it easier for your advocate to be the truest friend in need *and* deed that you've ever had.

First, be sure your own paperwork on all documents dealing with your estate and health care is up to date. Give your advocate a list of your Blue Cross/Blue Shield and other health insurance policy or health care plan numbers. Include names, addresses, and telephone numbers of your doctors, employer, attorney, landlord, relatives, friends, neighbors, and anyone else who might need to be notified if you become ill or incapacitated. Make a photocopy for yourself. Then if the original gets lost, you won't have to hunt up names and numbers a second time.

Give your doctor, attorney, and advocate a copy of your Living Will (and Durable Power of Attorney for Health Care, if you have one). If your advocate is not familiar with these documents, take time to explain their purpose and importance. This is a good time to let him know how strongly you feel about accepting or rejecting life-support systems if there is no hope for your recovery.

Be sure your advocate knows that a copy of these documents should be entered into your medical record. Don't forget, the fact that a Living Will and/or Durable Power of Attorney for Health Care are attached to your hospital chart is *no guarantee* that your wishes will *automatically* be carried out.

If you have opted against use of life-support equipment when you become terminally ill or there is no hope of your recovery, remind your advocate that he may have to initiate discussion with your doctor about not "coding" you. Furthermore, he may have to insist that the doctor write a "Do not resuscitate" order on the Doctor's Order Sheet in your record *or* get another doctor to handle your case.

Finally, be informed and exercise your rights.

Informed patients, says one expert in medical ethics, "are their own best advocates. They know their own bodies, what they need and what's important to them. More than that, they're not afraid to ask questions or change doctors if the doctor-patient relationship breaks down."

In short, when it comes to your future, *you* should be in

charge. If you're not, someone else will be. And that person may be the very one you would *not* want making life-and-death decisions for you at some future date. If that thought sends chills up your spine, don't procrastinate. Act today.

WHAT YOU SHOULD KNOW ABOUT CARDIOPULMONARY RESUSCITATION

Terms

CODE   Emergency efforts to maintain a patient's heart and lung function. Also known as cardiopulmonary resuscitation (CPR). It involves providing the patient with oxygen (usually by endotracheal tube and a respirator), massaging or electroshocking the heart, and using drugs to maintain heartbeat. Code does not refer to other treatments the patient may be receiving at the time of the emergency, such as IV fluids or antibiotics.

NO CODE   A doctor's order written in the patient's chart to avoid all emergency efforts as described above. Frequently it is termed DNR (do not resuscitate).

SLOW CODE OR PARTIAL CODE   A doctor's order to delay or use only partial emergency efforts to restart the patient's heart. One type is the chemical code, in which no electric shock or respirator is used, only drugs. Another type may involve electric shock but no other efforts. (Most experts believe that if it's appropriate to resuscitate a patient, these efforts should be complete, unrestricted, and wholehearted—*not* partial or slow.)

CALLING A CODE   Signaling a team of trained hospital personnel with equipment to restore a patient's breathing and heartbeat. Unless a patient's chart contains a specific no code/DNR order, a code will automatically be called in most hospitals when a patient has a cardiopulmonary arrest.

Deciding for yourself—questions to ask

Your condition may be such that you are at high risk to have a cardiopulmonary arrest, following a heart attack or major surgery, for example. Your doctor may raise the issue of whether or not to "code" you if this should occur. But don't bet on it. You or your advocate may have to bring up the subject. Regardless of who does, these are important questions to ask, because life-support systems are not always "the beginning of the end." A respirator is often used as a temporary measure to tide a patient through a crisis or to maintain the patient until the underlying medical problem can be dealt with. Indeed, many patients survive resuscitation and go on to enjoy meaningful and productive lives.

1. Am I likely to survive the resuscitation?
2. If I survive resuscitation, will I be the same, better, or worse than I am now?
3. Am I likely to be left in coma?
4. Am I likely to ever be well enough to go home?
5. Will I feel pain during the resuscitation?
6. Am I likely to wake up connected to a respirator, and if so, for how long?

The answers will depend on your medical condition and your doctor's judgment about the relative risks and benefits of resuscitating you. Don't forget, *you* can always refuse treatment you don't want. But if you're unable to speak for yourself, your advocate will need a Durable Power of Attorney for Health Care to say yes or no for you.

___

Resources

Society for the Right to Die
250 West 57th Street
New York, NY 10107
(212) 246-6973
Alice V. Mehling, executive director

A nonprofit organization working for recognition of the individual's right to die with dignity; supports judicial and legislative action; educational and informational program directed to general public, clergy, health-related professionals, etc.; publishes and distributes literature. Membership dues: $10. Write for list of publications and free copy of Living Will Declaration for your state and two free brochures: *You and Your Living Will* and *What You Should Know About Durable Power of Attorney.*

Concern for Dying
250 West 57th Street
New York, NY 10107
(212) 246-6962

A nonprofit educational group involved with patients' rights.

The National Hospice Organization
1901 North Fort Myer Drive (Suite 902)
Arlington, VA 22209
(703) 243-5900

Clearinghouse for information on hospices; publishes a nationwide directory and will provide information to consumers who call or write.

The Institute for Consumer Policy Research
256 Washington Street
Mount Vernon, NY 10553
(914) 667-9400

A branch of Consumers Union, the institute provides for $4 a 45-page summary of its report *Life Support: Families Speak About Hospital, Hospice and Home Care for the Fatally Ill.*

Hemlock Society
P.O. Box 66218
Los Angeles, CA 90066
(213) 391-1871
Derek Humphry, executive director

A nonprofit organization supporting the option of active, voluntary euthanasia for the terminally ill; informational program aimed at raising public awareness through news media, public meetings, clarifying existing laws on suicide and assisted suicide; seeks to pass legislation to permit a dying person to lawfully request a physician to help him to die; publishes and distributes literature. Membership: $20; senior citizens, $15. Publications include *Assisted Suicide: The Compassionate Crime; Jean's Way: A Love Story; Let Me Die Before I Wake*, the only guide to self-deliverance for the dying in the United States.

Suggested reading

Altman, Lawrence K., M.D. "Hospital Patients Can Suffer Twice When Staff Adds Insult to Injuries." *New York Times*, February 22, 1983, p. C-1.

Clifford, Denis. *The Power of Attorney Book*. Berkeley, Calif.: Nolo Press, 1985.

"Debate Grows over Living Wills." *Hospital Ethics*, November/December 1985, p. 12.

"Hospices: Not to Cure but to Help." *Consumer Reports*, January 1986, p. 24. (Answers commonly asked questions families ask about hospice care for patients and help and counseling for survivors.)

Lamerton, Richard, M.R.C.S., L.R.C.P. "What Helps Dying Patients: Some Common Fallacies." *Nursing Life*, September/October 1985, pp. 43–44.

Lewis, Flora. "Dignity in Death." *New York Times*, September 25, 1984.

Malcolm, Andrew H., "Extending Life or Prolonging Death? The Dialysis Dilemma." *New York Times*, March 23, 1986, p. E-24.

———. "Many See Mercy in Ending Empty Lives." *New York Times*, September 23, 1984, p. 1.

Manber, Malcolm. "Our Guide to the Best Health Care." *Family Circle*, April 27, 1982, p. 34. (Panel of experts lists twenty of nation's top hospitals, four leading general clinics, and several noted medical centers specializing in treatment programs for specific conditions and diseases.)

Mazzawy, Mary, R.N., M.S. "What Do Dying Patients Need Most?" *Nursing Life*, September/October 1985, pp. 43–44.

Otten, Alan L. "New 'Wills' Allow People to Reject Prolonging of Life in Fatal Illness." *Wall Street Journal*, July 2, 1985, section 2, p. 1.

President's Commission for the Study of Ethical Problems in Medicine and Biomedical and Behavioral Research. *Deciding to Forego Life-Sustaining Treatment.* Washington, D.C.: U.S. Government Printing Office, 1983.

Rollin, Betty. *Last Wish.* New York: Simon and Schuster, 1985. (The former television reporter tells how she secretly conducted research to help her gravely ill but intelligent and competent mother commit suicide.)

Sacred Congregation for the Doctrine of the Faith. *Declaration on Euthanasia.* June 26, 1980.

5 Transplanting Human Organs and Tissues—a New Lease on Life

SINCE Adam donated a rib to Eve, giving and receiving body tissues and organs have become both simpler on one hand and more complex on the other. While potential donors need only indicate they want to donate their organs in a Living Will or card attached to their driver's license, many legal, ethical, medical, economic, and religious considerations figure in the debate over organ donations.

Among the questions: Who should donate organs? Who should receive them? Who should pay? And should financial incentives or mandatory laws play a part in increasing the pool of sorely needed organs and tissues for transplantation?

Recent improvements in the technology of both human organ transplants and artificial organ implants—especially the use of antirejection drugs such as cyclosporin—make these once unique gifts of life increasingly common as organ donation moves from macabre and experimental to acceptable and praiseworthy in the public eye. Today, donating human organs is seen as an act of dignity, grace, and love.

In June 1987, when my kidneys failed, one of my sisters

donated a kidney to me. After the transplant surgery, she told me that she considered herself and her gift as representing the love of my whole family—since several of my brothers, other sisters, children, and even my wife, had offered to give me a kidney. After testing all potential family donors for blood and tissue compatibility with me, surgeons at the University of California–San Francisco transplant center selected my sister Evangeline as the closest match. Both of us went through the surgery without complications and I am grateful to have been given a new lease on life.

Not everyone, however, is fortunate enough to have someone who is willing and able to donate an organ, and must depend on the availability of cadaveric organs. Although currently the demand for such organs exceeds the supply, Americans are becoming more aware of the need to donate.

In a 1984 *Glamour* survey, for example, an overwhelming 88 percent of respondents said they'd be willing to have their organs donated after death. More than half already had donor cards. A typical comment: "When I consider how lucky I am to have a healthy heart, liver, two perfect kidneys and 20–20 vision, I have no trouble renewing my donor card and sharing my good fortune." Another reader who didn't have a donor card said the questionnaire made her realize she should go out and get one because "it would be gratifying to know that another person will live as a result of my death."[1]

The most personal gift

Though seemingly in good health, San Francisco teenager Felipe Garza, Jr., 15, mysteriously predicted his impending death and told his parents he wanted his heart to go to Donna Ashlock. Donna, his 14-year-old schoolmate, had a fatal heart condition and only a few months to live without a heart transplant.

Three weeks later, a blood vessel ruptured in Felipe's brain and he lapsed into coma, from which he never awoke. A respirator kept his heart functioning, even though medically he was brain-dead. When the Garza family was told of his condition, they decided to comply with Felipe's wishes. Speaking later to reporters, Felipe's father said, "We granted his wish to give his heart to Donna. It won't be the same without him, but since she has his heart, we at least have something of him."[2]

Worldwide attention focused on the dramatic tale. Within twenty-four hours, media requests for exclusive rights to Donna's story came pouring in to her family. Although the timing and crassness of some of these offers offended the Ashlocks, they hoped the publicity would encourage other potential organ donors.

Shortly after Felipe's burial Donna's father told reporters his own life had been dramatically affected too. "You betcha my life has changed, I'll be a donor to anybody," he was quoted as saying. "Once I die, they can take what they want from me. I used to say, 'No way,' but I've changed my mind."[3]

Why people donate organs for transplant

An opportunity to turn personal and family tragedy into a gift of life for someone else is one of the most common reasons family members choose to donate a relative's organs. Many families find it helps in their grieving to know some good will come from that person's death.

"Janie Fernandez," a 23-year-old part-time college student, didn't tell her family about her decision to donate her organs for transplant. She simply signed a donor card when she obtained her driver's license.

That chance to donate her organs came suddenly and unexpectedly in October 1983, when an automobile accident caused irreversible brain damage and Janie's death. Although the first her parents knew of her wishes was when doctors showed them their daughter's license with the donor card, they gave permission. Something good could still come from their loss.

As a final compassionate act, organ donation can relieve another person's suffering and give special meaning to the life of the deceased. It may involve keeping a promise or honoring a Living Will—even if family members don't approve of organ donation themselves.

Finally, when suicide is involved or when family relationships have been abusive, violent, or bitter, giving the gift of life to someone else may be seen as a way to begin the healing process among the surviving family members.

Not enough donor organs to go around

Newspapers and television tend to devote major coverage to heart, liver, and pancreas transplants because these are the dramatic life-giving ones. But these are far less common than, for instance, kidney transplants. In 1985, 7,695 kidneys were transplanted, but only 719 hearts.[4]

A look at the following table shows how rapidly the number of transplants performed in the United States is growing and what the average cost is for each procedure. Also listed are the one-year survival rates and approximate number of people waiting for specific organs.

Furthermore, as better means of preventing organ rejection are developed and surgical techniques improve, it will be feasible to do more transplants of all kinds in many more patients. For example, a recent report from the University of Chicago Medical Center indicates that for the first time in the United States, doctors were able to transplant successfully a portion of an adult liver into a 3-year-old boy in coma from liver failure.[5]

Initially, surgeons considered this a temporary measure to save little John Genna's life until a child-size liver could be

TRANSPLANTS PERFORMED IN THE UNITED STATES

	1981	1982	1983	1984	1985	Avg.[1] cost	1-year survival rate	People waiting (approx.)
Heart	62	103	172	346	719	$ 57,000-110,000	80%	100[5]
Kidney	4,885	5,358	6,112	6,968	7,695	$ 25,000-30,000	91%[3] 96%[4]	8,000[6]
Liver	26	62	164	308	602	$135,000-238,000	65%	300
Pancreas	—	35	61	87	Not available	$ 30,000-40,000	35-40%	30
Corneas	—	18,500	21,250	24,000	Not available	$ 4,000-[2] 7,000	(90% success rate)	4,000

[1]Many variables account for range of cost in transplantation procedures, i.e., lack of uniformity in reporting component costs, complications, medication regimen, method of reporting or non-reporting payment of surgeons (salary, fee, no charge), graft rejection, readmissions, infections, geography.

[2]Outpatient procedure average cost is $4,000–$5,500. Inpatient procedure average cost is $5,000–7,000; 2-3 day inpatient stay maximum.

[3]Transplant with kidney from a deceased donor.

[4]Transplant with kidney from a living related donor.

[5]According to the National Heart Transplantation Study conducted by the Battelle Human Affairs Research Centers, 14,000 people could benefit from heart transplants.

[6]May include some duplicate counting due to some patients being on more than one kidney transplant waiting list or including some patients who were not removed from waiting list after transplant.

Sources: American Council on Transplantation
Battelle Human Affairs Research Centers
Health Care Financing Administration

obtained and a second transplant operation performed. However, the human liver has the remarkable ability to regenerate, and doctors now believe the "temporary" liver may never need to be replaced. The success of the boy's operation, says a hospital spokeswoman, "could open up a whole pool of available livers for children."

Yet even now, the supply of available donor organs for transplant is not keeping pace with growing lists of potential transplant recipients. In part, this is because of the medical-legal-ethical fear of pressuring families into consenting to something they do not feel right about; in part, because many people are unaware of the need for donated organs, and hospitals are reluctant to discuss the need with them.

(Ironically, the success of new seat belt laws in reducing highway deaths has also contributed to the dramatic decline in the number of human donor organs available for transplant.)[6]

According to the Northern California Transplant Bank, there are fifteen human organs and tissues which can now be transplanted, some more successfully than others. These include the heart, lung, kidney, liver, pancreas, cornea, sclera (white part of the eye), bone, dura mater (fibrous covering over the brain), fascia lata (fibrous covering over the muscle), middle ear, cartilage, skin, bone marrow, and pituitary gland.

In addition, it's possible to donate one's entire body for anatomical study or research. Each organ and each tissue has a strict protocol which carefully defines donor requirements and circumstances.

From a single donor, doctors are able to recover as many as six life-saving organs and nine tissues with potential to improve the quality of life. But each year, the number of organ donations falls far short of the need for them.

Recent figures from the Office of Organ Transplantation are discouraging. Of the twenty thousand Americans declared brain-dead in 1984, only 15 percent donated organs for transplant.[7] The other 85 percent went to the grave with approximately 85,000 usable life-saving organs, to say nothing of 34,000 corneas and multiple other tissues.

But there's a paradox: although the Gallup poll indicates 50 percent of Americans surveyed would be willing to donate their organs after death, and 53 percent would consider donating those of a relative, too few actually do—either because they are never asked or because they don't voluntarily sign organ donor cards. Some patients who have been waiting for donor organs for more than a year are trying to change that situation.

Laura Beryl Gray, for instance, is one of twenty people currently waiting for a heart-lung transplant at Stanford University Medical Center in Palo Alto, California. She's been writing legislators urging them to support laws which would increase the supply of donor organs. She's concerned that the families of so few deceased hospital patients who could donate organs do.

"Little of this gap," she points out, "is due to public ignorance or prejudice. The major reason is that people are *never asked.* In practice, whether there is an 'Organ Donor Card' or not, no doctor in the United States will take organs without the *expressed* consent of the next of kin. Frequently that consent is never sought. Lives are painfully lost for the lack of asking."

Demand for organs outstrips supply

Although we're bombarded by media appeals for organ donations, letters to Dear Abby, nightly television filled with dramatic stories of heart and liver transplants, and smiling pictures of teenage actor Gary Coleman urging us to sign donor cards, most of us don't. We pass it off. But Coleman can't. His body has already rejected two transplanted kidneys and he's on dialysis while waiting for a third.[8]

"We read about Felipe Garza wanting Donna Ashlock to have his heart when he dies and something in us wants to believe love will find a way," says 33-year-old heart-lung candidate Laura Gray. "But life's not like that—and for too many patients waiting for donor organs, time's running out."

So far, relying on people's willingness to think about donating beforehand and following through on paperwork (usually in the form of donor cards) hasn't been effective in meeting the need for donor organs.

Many European countries have dealt with the shortage of available transplant organs and resolved the medical-legal dilemma by limiting who's eligible for an organ transplant and by "presumptive laws." Under these laws, physicians are permitted to recover all usable organs at the time of a patient's death *unless* specifically prohibited by the patient or by his next of kin.

But in America, the impetus has been to strengthen the voluntary aspects of organ donation through public education, increased professional awareness of need, and so-called "required request" laws—since typically, doctors have been slow to identify would-be donors and alert transplant surgery networks.

National network for organ transplantation

The National Organ Transplant Act, passed in 1984, authorized the establishment of a national network to increase the pool of available organs for transplant and help solve problems and abuses in the nation's network system—among them, long waiting lists and reports of wealthy patients buying their way to the top of the list. The law also made it a felony to sell human organs.

A National Center for Organ Transplantation was established within the Health Resources and Services Administration of the Public Health Service, and, as authorized by law, members have been appointed to the National Task Force on Organ Transplantation.

The center is supporting the development of a computerized network to link and expand the more than one hundred procurement programs that now match available donor organs to patients waiting for transplants and handle the logistics involved.[9] Most of these programs also maintain twenty-four-hour hotlines to answer questions from both health professionals and family members about organ donations.

The new, consolidated computerized matching system unifies the two major nationally recognized networks: the United Network for Organ Sharing (UNOS) in Richmond, Virginia, which concentrates mainly on matching kidney transplants, and the North American Transplant Coordinators Organization (NATCO), located in Pittsburgh, Pennsylvania, which matches other organs such as livers, hearts, heart-lungs, lungs, and pancreases.

UNOS will maintain a round-the-clock, toll-free telephone service. It will also establish a computerized list of individuals nationwide who are waiting for organ transplants and coordinate a national system to match available organs with patients on the waiting list.

New laws require next of kin be asked

Don't be surprised if you are approached about donating organs of a family member who is declared brain-dead. Laws in more than 30 states and a new federal law that covers about 97 percent of the nation's hospitals now require that families be asked.

Under these so-called "required request" laws, hospitals must develop procedures in which medical personnel will ask families of patients declared brain-dead about organ donations. Details vary from state to state, but the California law, for example, calls for "reasonable discretion and sensitivity" as well as regard for religious beliefs in seeking consent from next of kin. If the family prefer not to discuss the topic, the subject is closed.

However, many people don't like the term "required request," either because they have legitimate religious or moral qualms about organ donation, or because the word "required" gives the impression the government will seize human organs with or without permission. Laura Gray, for instance, thinks "Assured Organ Donation Option" might be a term less threatening to the public and more in tune with the intent of the laws—namely, to ensure a family is aware of the option and to overcome the reluctance to suggest donation that doctors and nurses often feel.

As one doctor told us, "If the law says I *have* to talk about donation, I can say that—it gets me off the hook and I don't appear ghoulish and uncaring to the family when someone they love is dying."

Why next of kin say no

Reasons why people refuse to donate organs vary with ethnic, racial, and religious groups. Some feel that "this person's suffered enough already" and think organ donation will disfigure the donor's body or cause delay in funeral arrangements. But there is no disfigurement. Removal of organs and tissues is a sterile, surgical procedure; the body remains otherwise intact. Other people fear that the organs will be taken from someone who is still alive. They are confused about the meaning of brain death.

Is the brain-dead person really dead?

When my brother-in-law was on a respirator in an intensive care unit in a hospital in St. Louis, doctors declared him brain-dead and requested the family's permission to remove his usable organs. His wife and children consented. However, my mother-in-law, who is in her 80s, confided to us that she wished doctors could turn the respirator off *first*—and then remove her son's organs.

But to be of use to anyone else, a human organ must be functioning when it's transplanted into the recipient. This means that the organ must receive a steady supply of blood-carrying oxygen and other nutrients until the moment it is removed from the donor's body and either transplanted at once into the recipient's body or carefully preserved for shipment elsewhere.

However, no organs or tissues can be removed for transplant until the person is declared legally dead.

In most but not all states, the legal definition of death includes "brain death," i.e., the person has suffered catastrophic brain injury resulting in irreversible cessation of all functions of the entire brain—including the brain stem, which controls heartbeat and breathing. But even though all brain activity has permanently ceased, the heart and lungs can continue to function on artificial life-support systems.

The concept of brain death is difficult to accept—not only for family members but for health professionals, too, who see the patient's chest moving in and out as though "breathing," albeit on a ventilator. Despite this artificially maintained heart and lung function, which may even keep skin temperature warm and cheeks pink, the person is dead. He or she experiences *no suffering or pain.*

Chapter 9 contains a complete explanation of the meaning of brain death and the criteria for making such a determination. It's important to note here, however, that to eliminate any potential conflict of interest, the determination of brain death must be made by two physicians who have absolutely nothing to do with the request for organ donation or removal of those organs.

(In certain so-called "coroner's cases," such as homicide, suicide, suspected criminal acts, death in a hospital within twenty-four hours of admission, or death from unknown cause, the coroner's permission must also be obtained before any organs can be removed.)

Who pays for organ donation?

Occasionally, you'll hear that the donor or his estate is charged—either for removing the organs or for the cost of the transplant to another person. This is incorrect. All expenses for the procurement, transportation, and transplantation of donated organs are paid either by the recipient or by third-party payers such as insurance companies.

According to the Office of Organ Transplantation, under Medicaid, states are permitted to determine coverage policy for particular organ transplants, and if they provide coverage, the federal government will match expenditures. Transplant procedure coverage varies from state to state. But a recent survey showed that most states offer Medicaid coverage for transplant costs, either as a part of a formal policy or on a case-by-case (exception) basis.

Currently, Medicare covers kidney, heart, and corneal transplants in approved transplant centers. Medicare also covers liver transplants for eligible children with congenital liver disease (biliary atresia) and bone marrow transplants for eligible persons with aplastic anemia or leukemia. For adults, liver, heart, pancreas, and heart-lung procedures are regarded as experimental at this time and therefore are not covered by Medicare. Some medical centers carrying out specific research protocols will cover costs of experimental transplantation.

Initially, costs of organ donation are picked up by the transplant facility that recovers the donated organs and tissues.

Usually, a highly specialized team of surgeons, nurses, and technicians travel to the donor hospital (where the donor has died or has been declared brain-dead) for this procedure. But it depends on the organ to be used. A local surgeon trained in kidney removal, for instance, may perform the surgery and ship the organ to the transplant center. When the donation is a combined heart-lung transplant, the donor is moved to the transplant hospital, where those organs are removed and immediately transplanted into the recipient.

"The donor is charged for all of the costs up to the time of donation when we're called in," explains North American Transplant Coordinators Board member Brian Broznick. "After that, we pay all costs, such as anesthesia, drugs, surgical fees, and transportation—we send a team. Costs are then charged back to the third-party payer—Medicare, Medicaid, Blue Cross, Blue Shield, or private health insurers, depending upon the age of the recipient and organ to be transplanted."

If any charges for organ donation appear on the donor's hospital statement, he or she should refuse to pay them. Under no circumstances should the donor's relatives ever be charged for this humane act, which offers life and hope to someone else.

Screening for AIDS

All human blood, tissue, and organ donations for transplant are now screened for exposure to AIDS (acquired immune deficiency syndrome). Such testing provides security against the small risk of contracting the AIDS virus through organ transplantation. To date, only two patients have contracted the AIDS virus from transplanted organs taken from a donor who had AIDS, but in whom the initial testing for the virus was falsely negative because of multiple blood transfusions.

The American Hospital Association also urges people at high risk of getting the deadly acquired immune deficiency syndrome not to donate tissues, fluids, or organs.

Key facts to remember

If you are considering donating your organs (or those of a family member who has been declared brain-dead), there are six important considerations you should keep in mind.

Consent for organ donation must be voluntary.

You cannot be forced to donate organs. The gift of life must be given freely, and all fifty states have passed the uniform anatomical gift act, which permits those 18 years of age and older to make provisions for donating all or parts of their bodies for transplantation or medical research. Persons under 18 years old must have a parent's or guardian's consent.

You can make your wishes known orally or in writing,[10]

through a duly witnessed donor card, Living Will, or Durable Power of Attorney. Chapter 4 explains why the Durable Power of Attorney is the most effective way to ensure your wishes will be carried out, and you'll find sample forms in Appendix F.

Your family are also permitted to donate your organs after your death. As stated by law, next of kin are, in order of priority, the surviving spouse, adult children, parents, siblings, the executor of your estate, or any other person authorized to dispose of your body. Note that although some states, such as California, do not recognize "common-law" marriage, others do. Be sure to talk over your wish to donate your organs with your doctor, your attorney, *and* your close relatives whose consent will be sought as well.

You can change your mind at any time.

Suppose you decide you *don't* want to donate your organs, but you've already signed a donor card or other document saying you do. To revoke your gift, simply inform your doctor directly or state your wishes orally in the presence of two people. You can tear up your donor card, cross out that portion of your driver's license, destroy whatever other document you may have signed, or simply amend it.

You can also set limitations on your willingness to donate, e.g., to family members only. The other side of the coin, of course, is that if you need an organ, body tissue, or bone marrow transplant, you can't strong-arm someone into being a good Samaritan—through either the courts or the media.

Confidentiality is the donor's right.

You have a right to privacy—unless you choose otherwise. A case in point is leukemia patient William Head's unsuccessful 1983 lawsuit in which he sued the University of Iowa for the name of a woman who, he claimed, offered him the possibility of a life-saving bone marrow transplant.[11] University attorneys fought the case on grounds that it represented a threat to the confidentiality of hospital records and could "irreparably damage" future programs.

Head learned of the California woman's existence when he contacted the university's experimental bone marrow transplant registry. Later, he was inadvertently told by a technician that there was one candidate who, with further testing, might be a "perfect match." The California woman had been tissue-typed as a potential donor for her child, who later died of leukemia.

But she refused to have her name revealed or to donate bone marrow to anyone but family. The case was struck down on grounds that the identity of the potential donor was secret and confidential, and her name could not be revealed.

A similar case in Pittsburgh was turned down because the court ruled that potential recipients had no legal right to expect altruism.

Sometimes the circumstances surrounding a death are such that family members will refuse to consent to organ donation because they fear the media will reveal their names and what happened. Pioneering human heart transplant surgeon Christiaan Barnard recounted this story at a national conference in Washington, D.C.: "I remember we once asked the father of a girl who had committed suicide if we could use the heart for a patient. And he said, 'I don't mind giving the heart of my daughter. But if I do, the fact that she committed suicide will be in the newspapers, so for that reason I have to refuse.' "[12]

Sadly, the gift of life in a usable heart was lost.

Not all donated organs are acceptable for transplant.

Even if you want to donate an organ, certain medical and technical criteria may rule out the use of one or more donated body parts. For example, the Northern California

Transplant Bank sets the following age guidelines for donor organs:

Heart:	newborn to 40 years
Heart and lung:	12 to 40 years
Kidney:	1 to 60 years
Liver:	3 mos to 50 years
Pancreas:	14 to 45 years
Eye:	newborn to 65 years

For research purposes, however, there are virtually no age limits. And as transplant technology continues to improve, even current requirements for acceptable organs will undoubtedly change. (Consult your regional transplant program for criteria which may affect your plans to donate an organ.)

Among medical reasons which currently determine usability of donated organs are conditions such as insulin-dependent diabetes, hypertension, a history of serum or infectious hepatitis, malignant neoplasms (cancer), a severe infectious disease at the time of death, preexisting kidney disease, and death on arrival at the hospital. In addition, infections and incompatibility—wrong size, different blood or tissue type—can eliminate a donor organ. (Although cancer rules out most donations for transplant, it generally does not affect the use of eyes for transplant or organs for research.)

Most areas of the country, of course, are within a few hours' flying time of the nearest transplant center. But bad weather and other factors, such as the ability of the donor hospital to maintain the donor's body, can also limit the use of donated organs.

Gifts of life can create bonds—wanted and unwanted.

In organ transplantation, writes Renee C. Fox in the *Encyclopedia of Bioethics*, "what is interchanged is so extraordinary—a literal as well as symbolic gift of life—that donor, recipient and kin become linked in ways that are at once mutually enhancing and self-transcending. But the exceptional nature of what they share may also create a symbiotic relationship between them that fetters rather than frees them. The recipient can never totally repay the donor for his priceless gift."[13]

The very nature of gifts involves giving, receiving, and reciprocating. We are encouraged to give freely and generously to others, not only on religious grounds but civic and cultural ones as well. Giving freely of oneself has always been the ultimate good in the Judeo-Christian tradition.

Yet being our "brother's keeper" as well as "stranger's keeper" takes on new overtones in the light of advances in transplant techniques and their success rates.

Since a person can donate one kidney or bone marrow without undue risk to his or her own health, living donors are most often twins, a brother and sister, or a parent and child. Recently, for example, Utah Senator Jake Garn, 53, was able to give one of his kidneys to his 23-year-old daughter, who suffers from progressive kidney failure caused by diabetes, and doctors say her body has a good chance of accepting the new kidney.

Statistically, however, only one in four donated kidneys now comes from a living relative—the others are cadaver organs obtained from brain-dead individuals. Although success rates are best between well-matched, living related donors and recipients, cadaver transplant success rates are improving steadily because of new drugs, such as cyclosporin, which inhibit the rejection of donated organs. Moreover, dramatic improvements in transplanting cadaver organs between unrelated people and an acute shortage of kidneys for transplants have led many doctors to suggest that friends and spouses of patients in kidney failure be permitted to give an organ to a loved one.[14]

Transplant professionals recognize the emotional bonds that can evolve from giving and receiving gifts of life. As a result, most transplant teams have counselors available to help recipients and families deal with their feelings about the organ donation. For example, a patient may feel guilty for having accepted an organ or have the impression of a changed body image. He may be concerned that he's taken on, along with the transplant, a number of the donor's traits—good or bad.

In turn, a donor may fantasize that the recipient is in some way a "rebirth" of himself. If the transplant fails, *both* can feel rejected.

For these and other reasons, transplant teams have established the policy that, with the exception of the living relative donor, the identity of the dead donor and the live recipient remain unknown to each other and their families. However, the transplant team will send a letter to the donor's family thanking them for the donation and letting them know, without revealing names, who received the organs or how they were otherwise used.

For example, after my brother-in-law's organs were donated, the family received a letter of condolence and thanks which included the following information:

> We hope it is of some comfort to you and your family to learn that a 34-year-old man from Missouri received a kidney and pancreas transplant. He is the father of a 3-year-old and has been suffering from renal failure and diabetes for several years. At last word, his transplants are functioning and he is doing well. The recipient of the other kidney is a 37-year-old man from Illinois who is also doing well. The heart and liver were unable to be taken for transplantation; however, the heart was able to be sent to a cryopreservation lab, where the valves can be frozen for use when needed in local patients who require valve replacements. In addition, the Red Cross has informed us that bone was obtained for future use in young cancer patients who might otherwise have required amputations and the corneas were successfully transplanted in the St. Louis area.

It's illegal to sell human organs.

The National Organ Transplant Act prohibits the sale of human organs. Violators of this provision of the law will be fined a maximum of $50,000 and/or imprisoned for a maximum of five years. Furthermore, no organ transplant team which receives federal funds will knowingly jeopardize its status by being a party to the buying and selling of human organs.

Having said all that, I need to point out that there are well-known exceptions—mainly, the categories of tissues that we usually think of as being "replenishable." For example, in the United States it's legal to buy and sell blood plasma and sperm. And even now, there is emerging a market in *rare* blood and tissue types used in biogenetic manufacturing. If you know you have the sought-after blood or tissue type, you're free to sell it.

"There's also a black market for organs," says ethicist Arthur Caplan. "However, it usually involves donors from *outside* the United States." (It's legal to sell organs, for example, in India and Brazil, but the difficulty in recovering usable donor hearts and lungs generally rules out these organs for sale. For the most part, it's the kidneys, corneas, skin, and bones which are sold.)

"People willing to sell their organs," says Caplan, "come to the United States and either use 'brokers' or lie about their relationship to a 'newly found relative' who's actually buying the organ from them. And there are entrepreneurs," Caplan adds, "with lots of little gimmicks to try to take an end run around direct sales—one of which is donating dollars to a charity in the donor's name if he'll give the recipient the right to take an organ when he dies."

The federal government is now considering various proposals to clamp down on such activities. "In theory, there ought to be no laws that would stop competent adults from selling whatever they want," says author and bioethicist

Daniel Callahan, "but the potential for abuse is just too great."[15]

It's not hard, for example, to envision murder for donor organs or a parent's taking his or her own life to bail out a family financially.

A few years ago, for instance, when the attempted suicide of a West Coast father of four resulted in his being declared brain-dead, friends urged family members to find out if his organs could be sold to help pay off the enormous debts facing his family—debts which, in fact, had contributed to the suicide in the first place.

National Kidney Foundation officials and a number of experts in medical ethics agree with Callahan that selling body parts demeans the relationship between donor and recipient. Other experts see selling in a different light.

Some claim it would increase the supply of organs; others argue that individuals should be free to use their bodies as they wish. Those who support selling body organs claim a relationship cannot be demeaned where none exists and ask what is immoral about selling part of oneself.

In America today, such arguments are moot. It's a crime to buy or sell human organs. "The notion of a free market, a business enterprise in merchandising organs is an unseemly and inhuman one," writes nationally syndicated columnist Ellen Goodman. "But in the end, the problem isn't whether we can buy life, but how we can be persuaded to give it."[16]

If you or someone you care about has a condition which might be improved or remedied with an organ transplant, you will need answers to the questions listed below.

Questions to ask your doctor

1. What is my condition?
2. How much time do I have left *without* a transplant?
3. What are the risks of a transplant for me?
4. What are the benefits of a transplant for me?
5. Will I get back to normal? Be able to return to work?

6. What will be the quality of my life?

7. Will I be free of "machines," such as dialysis equipment or respirator?

8. Will I have to take medications afterward? For how long?

9. What are the side effects of these drugs?

10. Is the procedure experimental, or accepted clinical practice?

11. How much will it cost? Will Medicare, my insurance, or some other program cover costs of surgery, hospitalization, and follow-up, or will I have to pay out of pocket?

12. After the transplant, can I (have a baby) (father a child) while on immunosuppressant drugs?

13. Am I eligible for a transplant? (If not, what other treatment options do I have?)

If answers to these questions lead you and your doctor to agree that an organ transplant is worth a try, he or she will refer you to a regional transplant center for further evaluation and a mutual decision to go ahead. The transplant team will evaluate your medical condition *and* the likelihood of a transplant being of value to you.

From your point of view, however, there are questions you need to have answered so that your consent is both informed and freely given. (And if you are considering an organ transplant, you might ask the transplant team the same questions you've already asked your own doctor. In a decision as important as this, a second opinion never hurts.)

Questions to ask the transplant team

1. Now that you've evaluated me, would an organ transplant help me? What are the benefits?

2. What are the risks—with or without transplant surgery?

3. How successful is your program? What are your one-, two-, and five-year survival rates?

4. What will the procedure entail? Will there be any special pretransplant preparations, such as blood transfusions, medications, etc.? (If a kidney will be donated by a living

relative, will he or she have to undergo special pretransplant procedures too?)

5. Where will the surgery be done—in my hometown, or do I have to travel to another hospital?

6. Assuming a good result, how soon before I'm up and around? How soon before I go home?

7. What will my life be like with the best results? And with the worst results?

8. What will this procedure cost?

9. Will I have to take medications for a long time? What will they cost?

10. If the quality of my life is worse than I can tolerate, will I be free to refuse further treatment or stop medications?

11. If the first transplant isn't successful, would I be eligible for a second organ?

12. If so, would I have priority on the waiting list or start over again at the bottom?

13. How do I get an organ? (If you need a kidney transplant, ask whether you should consider a "cadaver" organ or one donated by a living relative.)

14. How do I get on a waiting list?

15. Who decides when my turn comes?

16. While waiting, do you recommend an artificial organ as a "bridge" until a human donor organ is available?

17. Should I arrange to have available "donor designated blood" prior to the transplantation? (Blood donated by a friend or relative for a specific patient.) If so, what do I need to do next?

18. Do you have a patient educator or counselor in your program who could explain some of the details of your program to me and my family, and talk to me about some of the feelings I might experience after surgery or once I am back home?

It's frustrating to be a good candidate for organ transplant and not be on the top of the list for the next available human donor organ. Although each patient's case is different, there are some problems and frustrations common to nearly everyone who's waiting *and* his or her family.

How do you get your name on a transplant list? What are these registries that hold the power of life and death?

Getting on the list

Waiting lists of potential organ recipients are maintained at regional and local transplant centers, by organ procurement programs, and by the two networks NATCO and UNOS, now joined in a single national network. Included in these registries are data on the transplant candidate's blood and tissue type, size, and weight. In special categories, such as bone marrow transplants, the names of potential donors are kept on file as well.

At present, there are no national criteria for who can do transplants or which institutions can establish transplant programs, and no standard rules or regulations for accepting patients in a program or ranking them on a waiting list. But the Health and Human Services Task Force on Organ Transplantation is working to develop such policies and procedures, based on the experience of many transplant surgeons from coast to coast.

Currently, each regional transplant center uses its own discretion, based primarily on sound medical criteria and an evaluation by the transplant team of the urgency of the patient's need, the chances of success, and his or her ability to recover from a transplant procedure. Age, tissue compatibility, and how long a patient has been waiting are also taken into account.

Following the 1985 *Pittsburgh Press* exposé that well-paying foreigners were sometimes given priority over Americans at one of the nation's leading transplant centers, many institutions established an "Americans first" policy.[17] Some medical experts have suggested setting a quota system for foreigners or placing them at the bottom of the list. Americans have even less chance of obtaining a donor organ overseas, since fewer transplant centers exist and eligibility is even more restricted.

Will advertising or public appeal help?

When time is running out, it makes sense to consider going public.

At one time, newspapers as diverse as the *Los Angeles Times* and *Burlington County* (New Jersey) *Times* occasionally carried ads, mostly for kidneys. (In one case, a hundred people responded to an ad placed by a man in Detroit willing to pay $3,000 for a kidney.) You can still *place* such ads. However, since selling organs is now illegal, chances of a response based on pure altruism are almost nil.

In the past, media appeals have helped increase organ donation overall. But they don't always result in a donor organ suitable for the person for whom the appeal is made. That's because clinical factors enter into the decision as well. For certain donations, such as kidney or bone marrow, however, you can appeal to tissue-compatible relatives and friends.

If you're of the nothing ventured, nothing gained school, you have nothing to lose by letting others know your need is desperate. Talk it over with neighbors, friends, coworkers. You might also consider taking your case to the public at large and special-interest groups.

That's what Jamie Fiske's father did in 1982 when he became the first lay person to address the American Academy of Pediatrics. Fiske appealed to thousands of doctors nationwide to help find a potential liver donor for his gravely ill 11-month-old child. Three major networks and newspapers from coast to coast ran the story.

Among those watching television that evening were Laird and LeAnn Bellon of Alpine, Utah. Six days later, when their son was the victim of a car accident and declared brain-dead, the Bellons decided to give his liver to Jamie. The girl, who

had been diagnosed as having biliary atresia (a fatal liver condition that strikes six hundred newborns each year), became
one of the nation's youngest and best-known liver transplant
recipients.[18]

But this route depends on luck, and that, in part, depends
on how "newsworthy" your story is. Furthermore, some
media watchers believe media appeals may be losing their
effectiveness with the public.[19] And many people feel that
circumventing the "system" is inherently unfair to all the
other patients waiting in line.

The media can help in fund-raising

Of course, a different situation exists when it comes to a
media appeal for help in *raising funds* for surgery, doctor's
bills, transportation to a medical center, housing while
awaiting a donor organ, and the like. Organ transplantation is
so prohibitively expensive that most families need more than
the amount private insurers or third-party payers can cover.
(A heart transplant costs approximately $95,000, for example,
and a liver transplant about $130,000.)

"If you don't have the resources, or a place to stay while
you wait for a donor organ to become available," comments
one patient waiting for a donor organ, "you can't do much.
That's when an ad in a newspaper or alumni journal and taking your story to the media can really help." (See Appendix I
for guidelines on working with the media.)

Would you? Could you? Should you?

Thousands of patients awaiting transplants and their families
are hoping a donor organ will become available before time
runs out. Each of us has the power to bring that possibility a
step or two closer. Consider what you can do today:

Become a potential donor. If you haven't already signed your own organ donation form, do it now. Free donor forms are available from many organizations, including the National Kidney Foundation, American Red Cross, and other groups listed at the end of this chapter. Closer to home (except in Pennsylvania, Delaware, and the District of Columbia), you can obtain donor cards from your state department of motor vehicles, your local hospital, and many county or state medical societies.

One drawback to donor cards or Living Wills is that they may not be on your person when a crisis comes. Not only that, family members often don't know where to begin to look for your personal papers.

Be sure you discuss your wish to donate your organs with your doctor and relatives. This will make it easier later on when your physician approaches your family to ask for their consent. Don't forget, without their permission, no organs will be taken on the basis of a donor card alone.

Encourage others to sign donor forms. "What signing these cards often does is to generate a discussion of organ donation among family members and that's a valuable contribution," explains Jeffrey Prottas, Ph.D., a professor at Brandeis University's Health Policy Center in Waltham, Massachusetts.[20] Furthermore, knowing how family members feel about organ donation may be crucial if someday you, as the next of kin, are asked to donate *their* organs when they die.

Ask your doctor to urge colleagues and other patients to consider the need for organ donation. Transplant procedures are one way of making people well again. But surgeons and patients are frustrated by the serious shortage of donor organs, which prevents this surgery from ever taking place. Your doctor can do much to increase awareness of the need for organ donation and bring about change in hospital policies so that the greatest number of usable organs and tissues are re-

149

covered. A natural time to bring up the subject is when you're talking to your doctor about your wishes to donate your own organs.

Lobby your legislators. Nineteen states are now in the process of either drafting or submitting bills which would require hospitals to request organ donations from the families of brain dead patients. Support for such legislation has come from a number of groups including the American Red Cross, National Kidney Foundation, and National Task Force on Organ Donation. "Let your legislators know that you support these laws and appropriate brain-death statutes," says Arthur Caplan, an expert on the ethics of organ donation. "Public education alone won't suffice to solve the problem of a shortage of organs. Without a clear, unambiguous law clarifying the definition of death, health care professionals will still be wary of involving themselves with organ donation. And the law can no longer afford the luxury of trailing so far behind medical science—not when so many lives hang in the balance."[21]

Help educate the public. Finally, almost every community has one or more nonprofit or voluntary organizations involved in educating the public about organ donation. Many of these also include counseling and support services for families who have donated or have someone who needs an organ transplant. To offer your support and volunteer to help, consult your telephone directory for the address and number of local organ procurement agencies, eye banks, blood centers, or a local chapter of the National Kidney Foundation.

In addition, the American Council on Transplantation (ACT) is an independent, private federation of organizations, health professionals, and others interested in organ donation. ACT has begun a national education program to increase organ donation. Call ACT's toll-free number (800-ACT-GIVE) for information, donor cards, and referral to local agencies.

Resources

Questions and Answers on Organ Transplantation (free booklet)
Office of Organ Transplantation
Health Resources and Services Administration
5600 Fishers Lane, Room 17–60
Rockville, MD 20857

Suggested reading

Caplan, Arthur L. "Ethical and Policy Issues in the Procurement of Cadaver Organs for Transplantation." *New England Journal of Medicine,* vol. 311, no. 15 (October 11, 1984), p. 981.

Manninen, Diane L., Ph.D., and Roger W. Evans, Ph.D. "Public Attitudes and Behavior Regarding Organ Donation." *Journal of the American Medical Association,* vol. 253, no. 21 (June 7, 1985), pp. 3111–15.

Pekkanen, John. *Donor: How One Girl's Death Gave Life to Others.* New York: Little, Brown, 1985. (The story of a lovely, loving 17-year-old declared brain-dead twelve hours after being hit by a car and how her death brought fresh hope for four donor organ recipients—the youngest 3 years of age, the oldest 68.)

Making Babies — Conflicting Rights *in Utero* and Beyond

ACCORDING to the National Center for Health. Statistics, one in eight American couples is infertile —that is, unable to become pregnant after one year of regular intercourse without contraception. And of the four million infertile couples who want children, it's estimated that about 25 percent could benefit from a promising artificial procedure in which a baby is conceived *in vitro*—outside its mother's body in a small glass laboratory dish.[1]

Since July 1978, when tiny Louise Brown made headlines as the first so-called "test-tube" baby, more than a thousand *in vitro* babies have been born worldwide. Today, improved success rates have made the *in vitro* fertilization (IVF) procedure an accepted treatment for infertility—though it still can take several attempts and cost as much as $38,000 to give an infertile couple a one-in-three chance of becoming parents.

While it may come close to being a miracle, IVF isn't an easy one to bring about. Creating an *in vitro* baby involves careful evaluation of a woman through blood tests and ultrasonography of the ovaries, injections of the drug Pergonal for twelve to fifteen days to stimulate her ovaries, and surgical removal of from four to seven eggs at the time of ovulation. While she is still in the recovery room, her spouse or partner provides sperm, which is placed with her eggs in a petri dish for fertilization

After a short incubation period, the developing embryos (usually three or four) are implanted in the woman's uterus. With her prior agreement, the remaining embryos can be frozen (cryopreservation) and later thawed for another attempt at implantation if the first fails to produce a pregnancy.

"I could never give up an embryo for experimentation"

Mike and Shauna Poulsen, who suffered from infertility and feared they would never have children of their own, were ecstatic when they learned the IVF process had worked for them. The Poulsen twins, born by cesarean section in April 1984, made not only family history but Wyoming's as well. They were the state's first *in vitro* twins.

The Poulsens had decided to begin adoption proceedings after a tubal pregnancy requiring emergency surgery to save Shauna's life had left her with only one fallopian tube, which was blocked. Surgery to clear the tube failed. "But I wasn't going to give up hope until I exhausted every possibility," Shauna says. "When I first started, I checked out nearly all the *in vitro* fertilization clinics in the United States and England."

But it was a newspaper clipping sent by English friends that alerted the Poulsens to the Northern Nevada Fertility Clinic in Reno, which has one of the highest pregnancy success rates in the country.

During a preliminary visit to Reno, "we filled out forms and had psychological and medical interviews," recalls Shauna. "They asked about our moral character and if we had a stable marriage." Out of the three hundred couples interviewed when the clinic first opened, only seventy were accepted, and the Poulsens were thrilled to be among them. "It was a super program, and it was closer to us and cheaper, and their methods met our ethical standards."

One of the first questions Shauna had asked the Nevada doctors was "What are your ethical standards?" Their response that she could choose the number of eggs she wanted to have fertilized and that *all* the resulting embryos would be placed in her uterus at the same time was exactly what she wanted to hear. "It was fine with me that none would be frozen—there wouldn't be anything left over to play with."

The Poulsens would not have participated in some of the other test-tube-baby programs Shauna looked into because they asked that one embryo be donated for experimentation. "I couldn't do that," she says. "It would be like giving my baby away."

Hope—but no guarantees

"I can't promise you a pregnancy," clinic administrator Virginia Marriage tells hopeful couples who inquire about treatment at the Northern Nevada Fertility Clinic. "But I can promise, you'll have the best chances in the country—and you'll be treated with respect." Marriage, who interviews and counsels all couples accepted in the Nevada program, is appalled by the callous and insensitive way in which some couples are subjected to all kinds of indignities before they ever get to the final step of asking for *in vitro* fertilization.

If you are entering such a program, you and your spouse or partner will give up much of your privacy. You will be exposed in every sense of the word—physically, mentally, and emotionally. Your sex life will be an open book—at least to the health professionals in the program you select. Although many of these procedures are necessary if you are going to achieve your goal of becoming pregnant and having a baby, it is stressful to be literally and figuratively undressed over and over—and without any guarantee of success.

"I'm very honest with them," explains Marriage, "and lay my cards on the table: two couples will go away without a pregnancy; only one couple out of three will be successful."

According to a 1985 report in the *British Medical Journal,* 135 of the 244 women who became pregnant in eight Australian IVF programs ultimately gave birth, and about 20 percent of these had multiple births. Although the study found a premature rate three times higher than normal pregnancies, there was no evidence that the procedure carries a greater risk of major birth deformities.[2]

In most test-tube-baby programs, couples have the option of repeating the process up to three times. (If pregnancy has not occurred by then, statistically, it's not likely to—and the whole process is stressful, expensive, and generally not covered by medical insurance programs.) Despite these drawbacks, thousands of women in fertility programs from coast to coast are now eagerly awaiting the chance to try for a nine-month miracle of their own.

Some women already have had two *in vitro* babies; a few "repeaters" plan to try for number three.

One of these is Gerri Guiler, 34, who was told by doctors in 1979 that she would never be able to bear children. "For me, it's not an emotionally draining experience," she says, "because I was lucky to have gotten pregnant both times on the first try at implantation." Having had a healthy boy and girl by *in vitro* fertilization, she doesn't feel the process is at all unnatural—though some relatives who don't understand what the procedure involves have made some strange comments.

"God has given the doctors a gift to help women who have not been able to achieve this goal," says Gerri. "But I draw the line on certain things—I don't believe in abortion, don't even go along with the freezing of an embryo. To me, that [stage] is when life begins. All these doctors are doing," she explains, "is taking the eggs and bypassing one part of my body that won't allow me to become pregnant naturally— the fallopian tubes. It doesn't bother me that my son is called a test-tube baby. For me, it's being able to fulfill a dream, and my husband says at least our kids will know that we wanted them really, really badly."

Carol and Dennis Day, a deeply religious Mormon couple, also see the hand of God in the *in vitro* process.

The Days' triplets, born in 1984, were the first for the test-tube-baby program at the University of California–San Francisco. "Unlike a lot of people," Dennis Day was quoted as saying in the *San Francisco Chronicle*, "we don't subscribe to the idea that you should leave everything to God. We believe you should do what you can for yourself and then let God decide the outcome."[3]

Carol Day had already borne three children by a previous marriage, and her husband had five. She had been sterilized. But the Days wanted at least one child together. Surgery to reverse the sterilization and open the blocked fallopian tubes was unsuccessful, and the Days consulted doctors at the University of California program. In the *in vitro* procedure, four fertilized eggs were reimplanted in Carol Day's uterus in hopes at least one would survive. In fact, three survived. "We'd hoped for one anyway," said her husband later, "and we really wanted twins, so three was a really unexpected blessing."

Because several embryos are reimplanted in the mother's womb at one time, the possibility of multiple births is higher than average. And with the recent report of an English woman who gave birth to what is believed to be the world's first set of *in vitro* quintuplets, interest has flared anew in the process and its ethical implications.

Still troublesome are the medical, legal, and moral questions surrounding experimentation on embryos, who owns them, and what to do with unused embryos which have been frozen. If either natural parent dies, for example, or the couple divorces, or makes a decision not to have the embryo transferred for some reason, should the orphan embryo be implanted in a surrogate mother? Do orphan embryos have legal status, and if so, can they be subject to donation, disposal, or custody?

This was the quandary Australian doctors faced in a test-tube-baby program at Melbourne's Queen Victoria Medical Center.

Australia's orphan embryos

In 1981, California millionaires Mario and Elsa Rios had entered the Australian program, where her eggs were surgically removed and fertilized. The first attempt at transferring an embryo was unsuccessful. But doctors had frozen two other embryos for possible use in future attempts at pregnancy. Elsa Rios, however, felt she wasn't "emotionally ready" to try again and decided to postpone a second attempt at implantation. Before that could take place, the Rioses died in a plane crash in Chile, Mario's homeland.

Their deaths in 1983 brought world attention to the plight of the orphan embryos and raised the issue of whether they should be destroyed or raised to maturity, when they could inherit a share of the couple's estate. Further complicating the matter was the disclosure that Mario Rios was not the biological father of the embryos, as sperm from an anonymous donor had been used to fertilize Elsa Rios's eggs.

The Rioses had not left wills, and it seemed likely that a son from Mario Rios's previous marriage would inherit the estate. At the time, a lawyer handling the case told the *New York Times*, "This is a legal problem no one has ever faced before....Do the embryos have rights? Are they living beings? The doctor told me they are in a state of suspended animation. They have no organs, no heart, no lungs, and cannot be seen by the human eye. They have no functions by which we define existence."[4]

When does life begin?

All religions have moral teachings in the area of contraception, abortion, pregnancy, and when life begins. Some of these religions leave the specific application of these teachings to the individual; others hold their members to strict behaviors under pain of sin. At the root of these moral concerns is the issue of when life begins.

Many people believe life begins at the moment of conception, and consequently that the potential embryo should be accorded all the rights of a person—rights which should be respected and protected. Fertilized eggs and embryos should not be manipulated, experimented upon, dissected, frozen, or altered in any form.

Others hold that the fourteenth day after fertilization is the critical time, since this is when embryos normally implant in the mother's uterus and the development of critical organs, such as the primitive nervous system, begins. From this perspective, the embryo's potential for personhood is viewed as the beginning of human life.[5]

Thomas Aquinas, the thirteenth-century theologian, believed that the soul entered the fetus at the moment of quickening, when the fetus began to move inside the mother's womb at about four months.[6] The Sikh tradition holds that the soul of a human enters the body on the 120th day after conception.[7]

The U.S. Supreme Court in its 1973 landmark decision on abortion (Roe v. Wade) considered viability (the ability to live outside the uterus) as the crucial factor in establishing the legal rights of the fetus. (In anatomical terms, the transition from embryo to fetus is not abrupt, but generally takes place at the end of the seventh week when the original embryonic mass of cells has developed into a recognizable human form.)

All of these views address three fundamental questions for

which there are no answers acceptable to everyone: When does life begin? What is an embryo? What rights, if any, does it have?

Despite the fact that there is no consensus, *in vitro* fertilization, the freezing of embryos, and research in reproductive technology continue. In the United States, there are no uniform laws, rules, or guidelines for these procedures. Nor is there a national commission (comparable to those in England, Australia, and the Netherlands) to develop public policy, recommend laws, or establish rules for ethical behavior. At present, the only laws related to parenthood and reproduction are state laws—and these vary considerably.

Ethical standards

In 1979, the Ethics Advisory Board (EAB) of the Department of Health, Education and Welfare, now Health and Human Services (HHS), proposed guidelines for experimentation on human embryos. These guidelines were never formally approved by Congress or adopted by HHS, but they do provide a framework for possible future laws.

The EAB concluded that "the human embryo is entitled to profound respect; but this respect does not necessarily encompass the full legal and moral rights attributed to a person."[8] Thus, they said, experimentation was justified on human embryos up to fourteen days after fertilization—but not beyond. The President's Commission on bioethics endorsed this position in 1983.

The following year, the American Fertility Society developed guidelines to govern the ethical behavior of its members—the physicians, scientists, and others participating in the development of new reproductive technology and fertility programs. These guidelines were revised in September 1986.[9]

If you plan to enter an IVF program, be sure you know what will happen to extra embryos which are not implanted into your womb. Will they be frozen for future use by you or, with your written permission, for use by others? Or will the embryos be subject to experimentation? The latter was a big factor in the Poulsens' choice of a Nevada fertility clinic instead of some other programs which request the donation of an embryo for experimental purposes—something Shauna Poulsen felt morally she could not do.

Since no one knows how long-term freezing will affect an embryo, most fertility programs hold frozen embryos for no more than two years (some only one year), at which time they are either implanted into a woman or thawed and destroyed. Recent technological advances, which allow researchers to freeze a woman's *eggs* and later thaw and fertilize them for immediate use, may eliminate the whole issue of frozen embryos and what to do with them.

In the Rioses' case, the embryos remained in storage at the Australian medical center until a government-appointed committee studying the ethics of *in vitro* fertilization could make a recommendation. When the committee recommended that state officials authorize the destruction of the embryos, worldwide public outcry was such that lawmakers in the state of Victoria passed an amendment calling for an attempt to have the Rios embryos implanted in a surrogate mother and then placed for adoption. (Under Victoria law, a donor embryo does not belong to the donors of the genetic material but to the parents to whom the child is ultimately born.)[10]

Today, prior agreements are nearly always made with couples whenever embryo freezing is being considered.

"My feeling," explains Dr. Geoffrey Sher, codirector of the Northern Nevada Fertility Clinic, "is that some agreement with couples considering the procedure should be made from a legal standpoint. And where there are embryos that are not used or don't have parents they belong to, consent should be given in advance so that those embryos can be transferred to other needful parents who can't produce eggs or sperm."[11] A specialist in high-risk pregnancies, Sher says that the Nevada clinic does not discard any healthy embryos. "In our practice, all fertilized, healthy embryos are replaced in the mother."

Remember, you have the right to donate an unused egg or embryo for research purposes. You also have the right to donate an extra egg or embryo as a gift to another woman who is infertile. But neither of these options should be forced upon you as a condition for acceptance in a fertility program.

Choosing a fertility program

In your eagerness to have a baby and be accepted in a fertility program, don't overlook the risks involved as you concentrate on the benefits. You should take part in a detailed informed consent *process* in which the risks and the benefits—and your rights and those of your embryo(s)—are clearly spelled out in advance.

This process takes place over time, but it starts as soon as you contact a fertility clinic and begin to receive "Dear Patient" letters, information packets, detailed questionnaires, and so forth. In many programs, couples are also interviewed and evaluated psychologically. Signing the legal consent forms is the last step.

Here are some guidelines to help you select a fertility program which meets your medical needs and ethical standards:

First, locate a good fertility clinic. Most are university-based or university-affiliated, with qualified obstetricians who specialize in infertility. But there's no clearinghouse for information on fertility programs, and the American Fertility Society does not yet have an accrediting body to establish a level of expertise. "That means anyone can put up a clinic, and the consumer has no place to go to check it out," says Northern Nevada Fertility Clinic administrator Virginia Marriage, adding that nationwide there are 120 fertility clinics, most of which have only a 1 to 2 percent pregnancy rate.

*Second, decide what kind of medical treatment you're will-
ing to accept.* For example, you may be willing to take a fertility drug which triggers your ovaries to produce as many
eggs as possible, but you know from the start IVF is not for
you. Or perhaps, as a couple, you would gladly try to have an
in vitro baby, but draw the line at surrogate motherhood or
artificial insemination by a donor.

*Third, make sure you know what you're getting into—par-
ticularly what the risks are.* If you can't visit the clinic personally, get as much information as you can—the more the
better. "In checking on a clinic or program's success rate,"
warns Marriage, "don't be misled by general statistics that
reflect national averages. The top five American *in vitro*
clinics have success rates of 20 percent or higher.[12] But what
you want are the specifics of the group you're investigating."
Beware of the clinic that will not share its statistics with
you.

Questions to ask in evaluating a fertility program

1. How many women have gone through your program?
2. What percentage of your patients get pregnant? (Is this based on ultrasound confirmation at five weeks, or simply a "chemical" pregnancy confirmed by blood tests?)
3. What is the miscarriage rate of women in your program?
4. What percentage of women have given birth to a live in-fant? (For example, in two and a half years, seventy-one babies have been born to couples in the Northern Nevada Fertility Clinic program, which claims that 35 percent of women who undergo IVF there become pregnant. Since some miscarry, however, there is only a 25 percent chance per each IVF that a woman will have a baby.)
5. What are the criteria for admission to your program?
6. What can I expect if I enter your program?
7. What are the costs? Does your quote include any hidden costs for extras?

8. What are the ethical standards of your clinic?

9. Do you participate in any experimental programs? Would my eggs or embryos be used without my consent?

10. Do you have a psychological support system? If so, what does this entail?

11. Is staff available seven days a week, twenty-four hours a day? (You don't want to go there Monday through Friday, and be on your own over the weekend!)

12. What kind of rooms or facilities do you have for patients during the twenty-four-hour period of bed rest following the embryo transfers?

13. If I become pregnant, where do I go for prenatal care? Where do I have my baby—in my hometown or at your clinic?

14. Will I be expected to take part in any public relations or publicity efforts for your clinic?

15. Could you put me in touch with some of your patients who have had *in vitro* babies...and some who haven't been successful in your program?

Doctors don't usually release patients' names without their permission. But after their stories appeared in local newspapers, Shauna Poulsen and Gerri Guiler received many phone calls from women who had similar fertility problems and wanted to know more about the *in vitro* process. Both women were happy to share their experiences with these strangers.

"It's still a very private thing," says Gerri Guiler, "but if you can, try to talk to someone who's been successful and to someone who hasn't succeeded. You're going in there with the idea you'll be one of the lucky ones, but you have to keep in mind it might not work for you. Someone who's been successful is going to say the program is great. If you talk to someone who's disappointed but *still* gives you a favorable view of the whole procedure *and* the doctors *and* all the caring she received, then you've got a really good opinion of the clinic to go on."

NEW WAYS OF CREATING BABIES

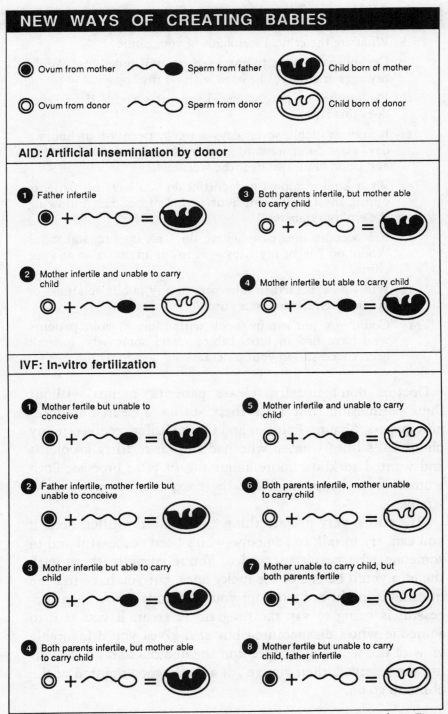

Ovum from mother ⬤
Sperm from father ~~~⬤
Child born of mother

Ovum from donor ◎
Sperm from donor ~~~○
Child born of donor

AID: Artificial inseminiation by donor

1 Father infertile
⬤ + ~○ =

3 Both parents infertile, but mother able to carry child
◎ + ~○ =

2 Mother infertile and unable to carry child
◎ + ~⬤ =

4 Mother infertile but able to carry child
◎ + ~⬤ =

IVF: In-vitro fertilization

1 Mother fertile but unable to conceive
⬤ + ~⬤ =

5 Mother infertile and unable to carry child
◎ + ~⬤ =

2 Father infertile, mother fertile but unable to conceive
⬤ + ~○ =

6 Both parents infertile, mother unable to carry child
◎ + ~○ =

3 Mother infertile but able to carry child
◎ + ~⬤ =

7 Mother unable to carry child, but both parents fertile
⬤ + ~⬤ =

4 Both parents infertile, but mother able to carry child
◎ + ~○ =

8 Mother fertile but unable to carry child, father infertile
⬤ + ~○ =

Other options

In vitro fertilization is certainly one of the most dramatic developments in helping infertile couples to conceive. But other options for childless couples range from adoption and foster parenting to artificial insemination and surrogate motherhood. A look at the accompanying chart shows twelve ways of achieving pregnancy and having a baby other than through natural intercourse.

Opinions vary as to whether these methods should or should not be used. Objections to some of these procedures are based on ethical and/or legal grounds. But social, economic, and medical reasons also come into play. (For example, sperm from a donor with AIDS or hepatitis is medically unacceptable; and on social and economic grounds, population control experts decry enhancing fertility when predictions are that world population will double by 2025.)[13]

Artificial insemination and surrogate motherhood raise special concerns. Both of these methods force us to look anew at issues of personal identity, parenthood, and family.

Artificial insemination

About one-quarter of American men now have sperm counts so low that they are considered functionally sterile.[14] Among methods which counter this medical problem, artificial insemination—either by husband or by donor—is the most widely used. And in some cases in which a fertile man must undergo medical treatment or chemotherapy which will result in sterility, banking his frozen sperm beforehand can allow the couple to still have children later.

Shauna and Mike Poulsen, for example, would like to try for another *in vitro* baby. But last December, Mike was diagnosed as having leukemia. Since then he's undergone chemotherapy, and this summer he will receive a bone marrow transplant following extensive radiation, which is likely to leave him sterile. "What we're considering," explains Shauna, "is banking some of his sperm until this is all over. That way, we'd still have the chance of having more children. Then, if he recovers and he's fine, we're considering going back" to the fertility clinic.

Few ethical problems, and no legal ones, arise when the sperm is the husband's.[15]

Artificial insemination is gaining wider acceptance: twenty-six states already have laws legalizing artificial insemination, and an estimated 250,000 children have been born in the United States so far by this method.[16] In addition, twenty-five commercial and university-based sperm banks nationwide store human semen which has been frozen for future use. Among these commercial banks, for example, is the Repository for Germinal Choice in Escondido, California, sometimes called the "Nobel sperm bank" because among its donors are three Nobel Prize winners.

While supporters hail the repository as a godsend for women who want bright and healthy children, opponents cite the California facility as one more proof that uses of modern technology have gotten totally out of hand. This raises other fears, such as possible attempts to create a master race of superior individuals by preselecting their genetic potential (the science of eugenics). Although no one yet knows for sure whether heredity or environment has more influence on human beings, at this point scientists believe inherited intelligence is important, but its potential can be undermined by poor health, nutrition, and upbringing and lack of motivation.

Your dreams for your baby may not include world leadership, an Olympic gold medal, or a Nobel Prize. But you should be concerned about proper screening and selection of sperm donors. Your health and that of your future child depend on such screening.

Be sure your physician obtains *frozen* sperm from a *reputa-*

ble sperm bank that supplies general information about the donor such as race, age, and physical characteristics, and routinely screens donors for AIDS, hepatitis, and other transmissible diseases. "Anyone using fresh semen [for artificial insemination by a donor] is taking a chance [of getting the AIDS or hepatitis virus]," says Jerome K. Sherman, M.D., president of the Reproductive Council of the American Association of Tissue Banks.[17]

Often available as well is information about the donor's genetic history and health. The donor has the right to remain anonymous, but it's not absolute. Find out what your state law says about artificial insemination, including the rights of the donor *and* the child.

For example, only half the states have passed laws making the consenting husband of the woman inseminated the lawful father of the child. In a recent case, the genetic father and donor of the sperm won the right to visit his child against the mother's wishes because the insemination procedure had not been performed by a physician as required by California law.[18]

In Nevada, for good cause, the child, the mother, and the man presumed or alleged to be the child's natural father *all* have a right to bring action in court to determine the existence of the father-child relationship.[19]

Writing in the *Journal of the American Medical Association*, medical geneticist Sherman Elias and law professor George J. Annas state that even if we assume that parenthood by artificial insemination is acceptable to society, "we ignore the relevance of legitimacy, lineage, and individual identity tied up in kinship, and thus bypass fundamental questions about the definition of fatherhood and its role in the family and the life of the child."[20]

In addition, researchers are now exploring the long-term emotional effects on donors, many of whom are young medical students who have not yet started their own families and don't realize what it means to be a father.

Speaking at a 1985 meeting of the American Fertility Society, attorney Lori Andrews pointed out that some critics claim that sperm donors may later feel remorse about having created children "who are out there somewhere in the world, might be in need and cannot be contacted. Psychologists," she says, "are now suggesting that these haunting feelings might be comparable to those of women who have undergone abortions earlier in their lives."[21]

The American Fertility Society guidelines set the limit of successful pregnancies from one donor at fifteen—with no more than five pregnancies in any one city. Not every sperm bank goes along with these limits, but the society believes these guidelines will avoid the statistical probability of half sisters and brothers marrying each other in the future. (One California doctor who reportedly donated sperm leading to thirty-three pregnancies in Washington, D.C., while he was in medical training there thirty years ago now advises his children—all in their 20s—not to marry anyone born in the District of Columbia!)

Surrogate wombs—for love or hire

Surrogate motherhood generally works as follows. A couple sign a contract with another woman, who provides the egg and agrees to bear the husband's child through artificial insemination. After delivery, the genetic mother turns the baby over to the couple for adoption by the husband's wife. In some cases, the surrogate mother's motivation is profit; in others, generosity and the wish to give someone else a truly priceless gift.

For example, with the consent of her husband, a Detroit woman agreed to be artificially inseminated with her brother-in-law's sperm because her 34-year-old sister was unable to conceive. Three attempts were unsuccessful. On the fourth try, she really delivered—triplets.

The surrogate mother, Jeanette Wilks, 32, had taken no fertility drugs. Nor was there a family history of multiple births. "This was supposed to be something between two sisters, then the triplets came into it," Associated Press reports quoted her husband, Martin Wilks, as saying. "She loves her [sister] so much she just wanted her to have children. My feeling is that it was great.... They're very giving people, very kindhearted."[22]

But most surrogate mothers aren't sisters.

Baby brokering—who's looking out for the baby's welfare?

The majority of surrogate births are brokered by physicians and attorneys for a fee (usually $10,000) paid by the couple who want an unrelated surrogate to give birth to their baby. This raises many ethical issues about the rights of women to sell their bodies as incubators and the buying and selling of infants. An even more fundamental legal issue is: Who are the parents of children born following this type of contract?

Syndicated columnist Ellen Goodman spins out a scenario in a column titled "Where Did I Come From?"

> Baby Girl Who (as in "Who" does this baby belong to?) was conceived last August. The egg and sperm of a couple from New York got together in a petri dish in Cleveland. What came from this union was an embryo, which was implanted into the womb of a woman from Detroit.
> The genes of the first woman and her husband were nourished and carried in the uterus of the second woman, who was paid $10,000 for fetus care. Then, on April 13, in Ann Arbor, Baby Who was delivered into the arms of the New York couple.[23]

Surrogate mothers and "open adoptions" are two of the most dynamic legal issues today, according to family law expert Sanford Katz, and these issues are changing almost too rapidly for judges and lawyers to keep up. Yet producing "contract" babies is hardly a new phenomenon: Genesis 16 tells us that Hagar, as surrogate for Abraham's wife, Sarah, gave birth to his son.

Speaking at a National College of Juvenile Justice conference, Katz explained that in cases where a surrogate mother, after entering into a contract with a couple, later decides she *doesn't* want to hand over the infant to them, the legal rights of each depends on state law and the presiding judge. And in that situation, he warned, "it's a battle between the best interests of the child and [what is stated in] the contract." Other factors may also enter into it—such as "to what extent did [the natural mother] know what she was doing when she agreed to the arrangement."[24]

Baby M—the landmark surrogate child-custody case

In the widely publicized case of Baby M, William Stern, 40, and his wife, Elizabeth, a 41-year-old pediatrician who suffers from multiple sclerosis, thought they had found the perfect woman to bear their child. Mary Beth Whitehead, a 29-year-old housewife with two school-age children by her husband, Richard, claimed she didn't want any more children of her own but did want to help a childless couple by becoming a surrogate.

The Sterns agreed to pay her $10,000 plus medical expenses. Mrs. Whitehead signed a contract, agreed to be artificially inseminated with Stern's sperm, and promised, among other things, that she would not "form or attempt to form a parent-child relationship" with the resulting baby. Her feelings, however, changed dramatically in the delivery room.

After the baby's birth on March 27, 1986, Mrs. Whitehead decided to keep the child, but she and her husband didn't know how to inform the Sterns. Forfeiting the fee, she took her baby daughter home from the hospital and later fled to Florida. But authorities caught up with the mother and infant, whom she had named Sara, and returned the baby to the temporary custody of the Sterns.

In the unprecedented court battle to obtain permanent custody of the child, whom they've named Melissa, the Sterns claimed that Mrs. Whitehead is emotionally unstable and unfit to be the baby's mother. Four of the five mental health professionals whom the court hired to examine the two families recommended that the infant should be raised by the Sterns. Among other things, they cited the Whiteheads' financially troubled marriage and several impulsive acts by Mrs. Whitehead, including threats that she would kill herself and the baby, and defiance of the court order to give Baby M to the Sterns.

In deciding the case, New Jersey Superior Court Judge Harvey R. Sorkow became the first judge to enforce a surrogate agreement. After lengthy hearings, he ruled that the surrogate parenting contract with its requirement that the biological mother surrender her parental rights was "valid and enforceable." He awarded permanent and "sole custody" of Baby M to William Stern citing the infant's best interests, arranged for Elizabeth Stern to immediately adopt her husband's child, and denied visitation rights to Mrs. Whitehead. However, the New Jersey Supreme Court reinstated the surrogate mother's right to visit her daughter, pending a decision on her appeal.

Sorkow's decision has left many people uneasy. Troubling issues range from what it means to be a parent and the way in which the court-appointed psychiatrists evaluated Mary Beth Whitehead and her family, to the bartering of human life and the strong belief that a mother should not sell her child —even a child conceived through artificial insemination. As one lawyer commented: "There was not one state in fifty that was ready for this scientific revolution—this is the case that will set the standard."[25]

Should fees for surrogate mothers be outlawed?

Increasingly, state legislatures and courts are addressing these questions of parenthood and contracts to deter the growth of a black market for babies. Several states are considering prohibiting surrogate births for a fee, and it is likely that all states will begin to take action on at least two questions: Is it permissible to commercialize the conception, birth, and adoption of children born through surrogate motherhood? Who should be identified as the parents of the resulting child?[26]

"The mother who gestates a child should be considered the child's legal mother for all purposes," writes George Annas in the *Hastings Center Report*, in recognition of the risks she assumed during her pregnancy and her "greater biological contribution to the child."[27] Such a definition of motherhood would allow the surrogate mother to honor her contract or to change her mind and keep her baby.

Annas argues that regardless of whether the surrogate mother enters a contract or does it as a free gift of love, as in the Wilkses' case, she is *the mother* until she formally relinquishes parental rights to the adopting parent. Furthermore, he says commercialism should be outlawed—and I think he's right on both points.

As new state laws are developed, Elias and Annas suggest in part that three objectives be met:

- Primary consideration should always be given to the welfare and "best interests" of the potential child, rather than to the donors, the infertile couple, or the physician or clinic.
- Complete and accurate records should be kept of *all* participants. These records should be kept confidential, but in a manner that makes future access by the child possible if this is determined to be in the child's best interests.

· Uniform and complete standards for donor selection and screening, including genetic screening, should be developed and made public.

Yet even if such standards had been in existence in 1983, it's unlikely they would have prevented the paternity nightmare that developed in the Malahoff-Stiver situation—a classic "contract baby" case in which everything that *could* go wrong did go wrong and lawmakers vowed to make sure "this horror" wouldn't happen again.

The baby no one wanted to claim

When Alexander Malahoff, 46, hired 26-year-old Judy Stiver to bear his baby through artificial insemination, neither had any reason to expect that nine months later "Baby Stiver" would be born with a severe strep infection and microcephaly—an unusually small head, often associated with mental retardation.

After doctors told Malahoff the baby's retardation was severe and he might live only a few days, he ordered that medical treatment for the potentially fatal infection be stopped. Judy Stiver, however, wanted treatment continued. The hospital filed suit and won a court order to treat the infant.

Meanwhile, initial blood tests indicated Malahoff was not the father. Additional tests—the results of which were made public on *The Phil Donahue Show*—totally ruled out the possibility Malahoff could have fathered the child. Malahoff, who by then had separated from his wife, refused custody of the infant and sued the Stivers, claiming loss of a child's love and breach of contract in that the couple had not abstained from sexual intercourse for the prescribed time before and after the insemination took place. He also withdrew the $10,000 fee he had promised Judy Stiver for carrying the child.

At first, she disputed the test results and refused to take

the child home. Baby Stiver was placed in foster care. Later, despite the fact she had insisted earlier that she felt no maternal bond to the infant and had borne him solely for the money, Judy Stiver and her husband, Ray, agreed to assume responsibility for the boy. The Stivers then sued the attorney who had arranged the surrogate contract and the doctor who had performed the artificial insemination, saying he had not properly instructed them.

If there was any socially redeeming aspect to this no-win drama in real life, it was the attention focused on the nation's childless couples who desperately want children, the plight of the "surprise" baby who is not perfect, and the need for states to enact laws either to prohibit surrogate parenthood or to regulate it so that the child's welfare comes first.

As of May 1987, there has been no state legislative recognition of the surrogate mother contract. But currently, a number of states are addressing the issue of whether or not to approve such contracts.

Because the legal rights of the surrogate mother and baby depend on each state's adoption and contract laws and their interpretation by a local judge, Reno attorney Don Purke advises anyone considering these options to get the best possible legal advice.

Purke not only has arranged private adoptions and contracts for surrogate mothers, he has had personal experience with both. He and his wife both had children by previous marriages but wanted a second family of their own.

They decided on surrogate motherhood, and Purke donated his sperm to artificially inseminate "Kathy," the surrogate mother who since then has borne two of his daughters. Kathy then completed the contract by relinquishing custody of each child to Purke and allowing his wife to adopt the infants. The girls, now preschoolers, know "Aunt Kathy," who visits the Purkes on special occasions and brings her own children to the birthday parties of their half sisters.

Providing the womb, but not the egg

The Purke daughters, of course, share Kathy's genes. But in another case, that of the Boffs, Shannon Boff's *genes* were *not* part of the bargain when she agreed to be a surrogate mother for $10,000.

In her case she supplied only the uterus. The egg and sperm of another couple (the genetic parents) were united in a petri dish and then implanted in Shannon's uterus. Under Michigan state law, Boff's name, and that of her husband, would normally appear on the child's birth certificate. However, the genetic parents wanted their own names on the document and took the case to court. The judge ruled in favor of the genetic parents, since both couples wanted it that way.[28]

But what if the two couples had disagreed? And what would have happened if amniocentesis had indicated the child would be born with severe genetic defects?

The latter raises concerns about who is responsible for making decisions about the fetus *in utero*—for example, whether to consent to intrauterine surgery or treatments, or whether the fetus should be aborted.

If you decide to enter into a surrogate motherhood agreement, as either a genetic parent or a surrogate mother, get expert legal advice about your state's laws on adoption, buying and selling of children, artificial insemination, and surrogacy. Each party to the contract should have an independent attorney looking out for his or her best interests. And there are experts who insist the *unborn child* needs an advocate, too. Be sure that whatever contract you agree to is detailed and covers all possible risks and options and the rights of everyone involved—including the infant.

Should surrogate parenting be outlawed?

Many people believe *all* surrogate parenting should be outlawed. Others would allow altruistic surrogacy (such as in the Wilkses' case, in which Jeanette volunteered to bear a child for her sister, who was infertile) but would abolish all brokered surrogate parenting for a fee—as England has done.

In an *AMA Medical News* opinion piece, pediatrician Burton Sokoloff argues that measures intended to legalize surrogate mothering attempt to deal with the rights and responsibilities of the parties to the contract, but in no way consider the best interests of the child so conceived. He questions the effect of the surrogate mother's pregnancy on her own children as they see her hand over her new baby to the infertile couple. How certain are these children that they won't suffer the same fate—being given away for some uncomprehended reason?

In arguing that surrogate mothering should be outlawed in the United States before it gives rise to a new "cottage industry," Sokoloff says, "Contract law is more at home in the business world than in the nursery; artificial insemination statutes were designed to legitimize, not bastardize, a child; and adoption procedures were established to facilitate giving up an unwanted child rather than to orchestrate its conception."[29]

But there are other ethical issues related to the best interests of the fetus and the pregnant woman—and these relate to *all* pregnant women regardless of how the fetus was conceived.

Fetal testing, fetal surgery

Good prenatal care often includes fetal testing and genetic counseling. Only a woman's doctor, who knows her medical and obstetrical history and physical condition, can tell her what the risks and benefits are of specific tests designed to reveal whether her baby is healthy and developing normally. These tests include ultrasound, x-rays, amniocentesis, fetoscopy, blood hormone levels and alpha-fetoprotein (AFP) screening, and a new technique known as chorionic villus sampling (CVS).

Prenatal Tests

Amniocentesis   A procedure by which amniotic fluid is withdrawn through a needle inserted through the pregnant woman's abdomen directly through her uterus into the amniotic sac surrounding her baby. This fluid and the cells contained in it can be analyzed for various chromosomal and other fetal abnormalities. It is usually done at around fifteen to sixteen weeks to detect fetal defects and late in pregnancy to evaluate fetal maturity and the likelihood of the child's being born without developing respiratory distress.

Ultrasound (sonogram)   Ultrasonography refers to the directing of high-frequency sound waves painlessly through the mother's abdomen to produce images of the fetus on a screen or photograph. Because of the different densities of various parts of the developing fetus, the deflected sound waves allow doctors to "see" the size, shape, and position of the fetus, to evaluate many of its organs, and to determine its sex. Ultrasound is most useful in detecting multiple pregnancies, major abnormalities, and treatable conditions of the fetus and, near the end of the pregnancy, the size of the infant's head relative to the mother's pelvis.

X-ray   Although all x-rays should be avoided whenever possible and especially in the first trimester of pregnancy, they are sometimes used to determine the age of the fetus and the ability of the mother to deliver vaginally. The use of x-rays during pregnancy has generally been replaced by ultrasound, which poses fewer risks to the mother and fetus.

FETOSCOPY   A procedure in which a hollow tube is inserted into the uterus to observe the fetus, its placenta, and the amniotic fluid. Blood samples and biopsy of fetal tissues, such as muscle or skin, can be taken for analysis. This procedure carries the highest risk of miscarriage, but may be critical in diagnosing certain structural abnormalities in the fetus as well as rare fetal blood disorders, such as hemophilia.

CHORIONIC VILLUS SAMPLING (CVS)   The newest of the intrauterine diagnostic tests, CVS involves the insertion of a catheter through the woman's vagina and cervix to remove a sample of the chorionic membrane, which surrounds the fetus. Cells from this membrane, which are genetically identical to the fetus, can be studied in the laboratory for certain genetic defects, such as Down syndrome.

ALPHA-FETOPROTEIN (AFP)   This relatively new blood test analyzes the alpha-fetoprotein circulating in the mother's blood as a result of neural-tube defects in the fetus. AFP levels are useful in detecting major nervous system disorders, such as spina bifida and hydrocephalus. Because of false-positive results (see Chapter 3) this *screening* procedure, if positive, must be confirmed by amniocentesis and ultrasound.

HORMONAL TESTS   Measurement of hormones produced by the placenta and found in the mother's blood often provides data which are useful in evaluating placental function and maturity.

When performed by qualified doctors, these tests and procedures yield important and helpful data about your pregnancy. And in most cases, the risks are far outweighed by the benefits. The greatest benefit is information which gives you peace of mind that nothing is wrong or alerts your doctor to potential problems and allows you to give truly informed consent for treatment.

Some of these tests *do* pose risks, such as miscarriage, fetal damage, and inaccurate test results. Ask your doctor what the risks are in your case. The ethical dilemma, then, is whether or not to consent to a given test or procedure in the first place. (Furthermore, if you are a surrogate mother, will someone else have authority to make health-related decisions for you and your fetus by virtue of the contract you have signed, or will you make all such decisions?)

For example, after you know the test results, you may wish to obtain an abortion. Or if you're opposed to aborting a defective fetus, you may wish to consent to certain tests which will lead to intrauterine treatments or special precautions and preparations for labor and delivery, such as having medical specialists on hand to start appropriate emergency treatment right after birth.

(Radical and experimental methods of operating on the fetus *in utero* now allow doctors in selected research centers to correct hydrocephalus, or excessive fluid in the brain, and hydronephrosis, or blocked and dilated kidney. Doctors foresee the day when they'll be able to do "open-uterus" surgery to repair diaphragmatic hernias and perform fetal bone transplants.)

If you have a strong family history of genetic abnormalities or diseases like Tay-Sachs disease, sickle-cell disease, or cystic fibrosis, for example, or so-called sex-linked disorders like hemophilia or muscular dystrophy, be sure to inform your physician so you can get genetic counseling and appropriate testing. (For more on genetic counseling, see Chapter 7.) If your doctor doesn't do such tests, ask for a referral.

Your doctor's answers to the following questions will help you give informed consent to whatever tests or procedures are recommended.

Questions to ask before undergoing a prenatal test

1. Why are you doing this test or procedure? Is it to get information which will help me and/or my fetus, or is it simply for research purposes?

2. Will the results reveal something that can be treated?
3. How will the results affect the way you treat or care for me and/or my fetus during the pregnancy? During labor and delivery? After I give birth?
4. What are the risks to me and/or to my fetus?
5. Will the results lead to a consideration of abortion?
6. How soon should the tests be done? When will you have the results?

If any of these prenatal tests or procedures indicates that you or your fetus has a significant problem, you will face some difficult choices—whether to consent to surgery or other treatments *in utero*; whether to confront a difficult labor, delivery, and postnatal period; or whether to end your pregnancy through abortion.

The abortion dilemma

In 1981, shortly before being named Surgeon General, Dr. C. Everett Koop, commenting on abortion, said, "Nothing like it has separated our society since the days of slavery."[30] Indeed, a recent Gallup survey shows the nation evenly divided 45–45 on legalized abortion, with 10 percent having no opinion.[31] Today, the ongoing "pro-life" and "pro-choice" debate over abortion has not only escalated, but also become violent—as evidenced by the bombing of abortion clinics nationwide.

In the 1973 landmark case *Roe* v. *Wade*, the U.S. Supreme Court, in a 7–2 vote, declared restrictive abortion laws in two states to be unconstitutional invasions of the right of privacy. As a result of that decision, states were prohibited from outlawing abortions and a whole new set of rules regarding the procedure came into being. The decision said that states cannot place restrictions on a woman's right to an abortion during the first three months of pregnancy. In other words, she may go to a doctor to end pregnancy at any time during the first trimester.

Furthermore, the court held that during the second trimester, the state still has no authority to prevent abortion, though because the operation is more difficult at this time, states can regulate certain of the medical aspects involved. However, during the third trimester, when, medical experts generally agree, the fetus is capable of living outside the womb, states can impose restrictions on a woman's right to abortion unless the operation is necessary to protect her life or health.

In a 1983 reaffirmation of its ruling, the Supreme Court (by a 6–3 majority) struck down several state laws and local regulations that made abortions more difficult to obtain. And in June 1986, the court again reaffirmed its decision legalizing abortion, warning states against intimidating women into giving birth. Court watchers see the closeness of the 5–4 vote in the 1986 case as an indication of the deepening rift among the high court's members over this highly controversial social, political, and legal issue.

Although as a physician, I could in conscience rarely ever perform an abortion, I empathize with any woman who faces the dilemma of whether or not to terminate a pregnancy that she is not sure she wants. I recognize that there is much more to the issue than the well-being of the fetus, though this is certainly of major concern. A woman's health, ability, and willingness to be a parent are also critical factors which enter into her decision.[32]

"In my experience, most women don't make up their minds to end a pregnancy right off the bat," says the president of one pro-life league. "A woman or young girl finds out she's pregnant, needs help, panics, doesn't know where to turn or what's available to her by way of resources. She's tremendously influenced by a friend or someone else who can say, 'Look, here's a place to go for a pregnancy test, a place where they'll help you and give you some information about your options.' A woman may be considering abortion, but it's not without its dangers, and to give consent in an informed way, she should know what they are."

In a few pages, it is impossible to cover all aspects of the abortion issue. However, there are several excellent books and articles which can help you better understand the ethical, medical, and legal arguments for and against abortion. (See suggested readings at the end of this chapter.)

The following are some things you should know if you are pregnant and unsure of your next step:

No one can force you to have or not have a child.

That would be a violation of your constitutional rights. Clearly, these rights would be seriously violated whether you were forced to have an unwanted child or forced to consent to an abortion.

Although you have a legal right to abortion, there are limits to this right.

For example, the Supreme Court decision restricts third-trimester abortions, allowing them only for the purpose of saving a mother's life or health.

Legally, you will not need your spouse's consent to abortion, as that requirement has been declared unconstitutional by the U.S. Supreme Court. However, in some states, if you are unmarried, under 18 years of age, and seeking an abortion in the first twelve weeks of pregnancy, you will have to obtain parental or court consent unless, as the Supreme Court put it, "the abortion is certified by a licensed physician as necessary in order to preserve the life of the mother."[33]

But state laws vary and are constantly changing. Some states permit a minor to make her own decision about abortion; others require parental permission or parental notification. With the exception of Utah, Montana, and Idaho, the other thirteen states which require parental consent or notification provide for a court-bypass option. This allows a minor to maintain her privacy by going before a judge for a hearing—if her parents' knowledge of the abortion would cause serious problems for her.[34]

To learn what your state law says, check with your doctor or one of the resource groups listed at the end of this chapter. You can also call the toll-free National Abortion Federation Consumer Hotline, (800) 772-9100.

Your doctor cannot be forced to do an abortion.

Remember, the whole effect of the Supreme Court decision is to emphasize freedom of choice—and that includes your doctor's choice *not* to do abortions if he or she has medical, moral, or religious objections. In that case, your doctor should refer you to another physician who does not have such objections. (However, if the new "month-after" abortion drug—known as RU 486 and now being tested with remarkable results in France—is approved for routine prescriptions in the United States, it may be possible for women to induce an abortion safely at home without surgical intervention by a doctor.)

You have a right to continue your pregnancy—even if it is the result of rape or incest.

Many women, however, choose not to, for obvious reasons. In fact, the "Jane Roe" of the famous *Roe* v. *Wade* case was a divorced 21-year-old Texan who claimed she had become pregnant in 1970 as a result of gang rape—a story she later said was untrue.

A high school dropout who was working at night as a waitress, she couldn't obtain an abortion locally because the Texas law permitted it only "when the mother's life appeared to be threatened by the continuation of the pregnancy." She didn't have the money for an illegal abortion and was too poor to travel to California, where abortion was legal. When she consulted an attorney about placing her future baby for adoption and getting financial help in the meantime, the lawyer suggested she challenge the Texas abortion law. By the time the Supreme Court agreed to hear *Roe* v. *Wade*, however, her child, whom she had put up for adoption, was already two years old.[35]

You have a right to know what the abortion procedure entails, what its potential benefits and risks to you and the fetus are, what you can expect during the recovery period, what total fees will be, and what signs of complications you should look for.

In getting this information, you should not be harassed or intimidated into making a decision for *or* against the procedure. Friends, family, and others you consult may try to persuade you one way or another, but your informed consent must be free and not coerced.

California investigators, for example, are following up on reports that a pregnant 14-year-old who went for help to a "free pregnancy center" in San Francisco was talked out of having an abortion by counselors who tried to get her to leave home under a reportedly false pretext, to continue the pregnancy without telling her parents, and then put the baby up for adoption through the center—although it is not licensed by state adoption agencies.[36]

You have a right to know what your prenatal, childbirth, and support options are.

Because you represent not one but *two* patients, it's doubly important that you take part in decisions involving your well-being and that of your unborn child—unless there is a medical emergency which makes this impossible. (See Appendix C, "The Pregnant Patient's Bill of Rights.")

If you feel you will be unable to care for your newborn, remember, there are hundreds of couples on waiting lists nationwide who would be happy to adopt a child like yours. There are county and state agencies which arrange for adoptions and also attorneys who handle private adoptions. One lawyer I know encourages mothers to meet potential adoptive parents and select the couple she thinks would raise her child as she would like it to be raised.

But there are also thousands of single mothers doing an excellent job of raising babies they decided to keep. I see many of these women in a pediatric clinic where I care for patients. I also care for children with disabilities—children whose parents decided, even after amniocentesis indicated the child would be abnormal, that they could not go through with an abortion.

The point I want to stress is that if you've just learned you're pregnant and are not certain you want to be, you are in a very vulnerable position. Don't rush into a major life decision.

You may not have a lot of time to think about it, but you almost certainly have a few days (or perhaps a few weeks) to get information from your doctor and groups like Planned Parenthood, Alternatives to Abortion International, pro-life leagues, and Catholics for a Free Choice, an independent group of Roman Catholics who, contrary to their church's teachings, support the Supreme Court's abortion decision. (For more information on these and other groups, see the Resources section at the end of this chapter.)

Many of these groups hold a strong position for or against abortion. This can put you in a difficult position in learning about *all* your options—unless from the start you know exactly what type of counseling or information you are seeking. You may want to contact several groups and compare their advice. If you find a center or group that is not up-front and honest about its purposes, you should report it to your local district attorney, state officials who regulate adoption agencies, *and* the Better Business Bureau.

That's what a 26-year-old San Francisco bookkeeper did after going to a center which advertises free pregnancy tests in the Yellow Pages.

Carla Abbotts only wanted a quick test to find out if she was pregnant. But even before the test was run, a woman who never identified herself asked whether she would have an abortion. When Abbotts said she probably would, she was told she would have to watch a presentation while she waited for results of the pregnancy test. That's when she was subjected to a slide show of bloody fetuses and bruised women supposedly injured during the abortion procedure.

Infuriated, Abbotts turned off the slide projector. When the counselor returned, according to Abbotts, the woman again tried to dissuade her from considering abortion.

"The more I thought about it, the madder I got," Abbotts was quoted as saying in the *San Francisco Chronicle*.[37] "If they revealed themselves as a right-to-life organization that gives slide shows on their views on abortion, I would go somewhere else," said Abbotts, who has filed a civil suit in which she asks only that such centers advertise openly that they are anti-abortion clinics. "At a vulnerable time like that, you shouldn't get such misleading information."

Viewpoints for and against abortion

In making your decision for or against abortion, you need to consider the medical, social, personal, and moral aspects of your choice. Viewpoints you'll hear most often fall into three categories.

Pro-life

Pro-life advocates will tell you the rights of the fetus come first. This position is based on the belief that life begins at conception and the embryo and fetus represent innocent life which must always be respected, protected, and preserved.

A number of recent court cases have tested this philosophy to the extent that even a brain-dead woman must be maintained by life-support technology if it would allow her fetus to develop to viability. In one case, the woman's husband and sister-in-law authorized maintaining her dead body for nine weeks after they decided she would have wanted it that way. A premature baby boy, with "excellent" chances of survival, was delivered.

In another case, the woman's boyfriend, who claimed he was the father, sued to prevent doctors from removing a respirator "because this would result in the death of the infant and would deny the unborn child and the father rights protected by the state and federal constitutions."[38]

Many state legislatures have recognized this uncommon dilemma in developing their Living Will laws. Nineteen states invalidate the Living Will during pregnancy and allow the physician to overrule the Living Will and permit the pregnancy to progress to term and a live birth. Another four states invalidate it only "as long as the fetus could develop to a point of live birth with continued application of life-sustaining procedures." (For a fuller discussion of the Living Will and Durable Power of Attorney for Health Care, see Chapter 4.)

Pro-choice

Pro-choice advocates who support a woman's right to make her own choice hold that a woman's right to privacy, to control her reproductive processes, and to make decisions about her body are all the considerations that fundamentally matter—and no other justification need be given.

As shown above, these rights may be limited if a pregnant woman is declared brain-dead or becomes incompetent to make her own health-related decisions. (Although it hasn't yet been tested in court as far as I know, a Durable Power of Attorney for Health Care which delegates decision-making about her fetus to a proxy may ensure that a pregnant woman's expressed wishes will be respected. Among these might be whether she would want to be kept on a ventilator for the sake of her fetus or if she would agree to a cesarean section.)

Case-by-case

Those who argue for balancing conflicting rights on a case-by-case basis believe that you should try to weigh and balance your needs and rights against those of your embryo or fetus. For example, if amniocentesis has revealed that your embryo is genetically defective or has been severely damaged by drugs, alcohol, medications, or a viral infection, such as German measles, the quality of life of your expected offspring might be the deciding factor. Few obstetricians, however, will perform amniocentesis in the early months of pregnancy unless a woman is willing to consider aborting a defective fetus —and no one recommends this potentially risky procedure simply to determine the sex of the child. The risks outweigh the benefit.

On the other hand, your mental or physical health and economic and social situation (suppose you're single, unemployed, and living below the poverty level of income) also are factors which may determine whether you are able to care adequately for your expected child.

In weighing the pros and cons of continuing your pregnancy or having an abortion, you may hear people say, "You're too young, too immature" or "No way can you afford to raise the baby—go get an abortion." Those opposed to this position will tell you, "It's irrelevant, because you can put your baby up for adoption."

Even though you're caught in the middle of these arguments and feel confused and maybe angry, or perhaps panicky, you still must make a choice. After you feel you've gotten the best medical, social, and spiritual advice available, all you can do is make a decision *you can live with*.

Many state laws require that hospital emergency rooms

provide appropriate anti-pregnancy treatment, such as dilatation and curettage (D&C) or estrogen therapy, to women who have been raped. However, when a hospital, based on its expressed religious values, will not provide preventive treatments, that hospital should refer you rapidly to another facility or physician prepared to provide the treatment you choose.

If you have been raped, or if you are considering an abortion for any reason, you will need to ask your doctor the following questions.

Questions to ask your doctor before you have an abortion

1. Is it too late to prevent ovulation or fertilization with drugs?
2. Is it too late to prevent implantation with drugs or a D&C (dilatation and curettage)?
3. Am I pregnant? If so, for how many weeks?
4. Are you sure? Should the tests be repeated?
5. What's the chance I will spontaneously abort—that is, have a natural miscarriage?
6. What are the possible risks to me if I have an induced abortion?
7. Will having an abortion now make it more difficult for me to become pregnant and have a child in the future if that's what I want to do?
8. What does an abortion procedure involve?
9. If I decide to have an abortion, when must it be done?
10. Will you do it? If not, where do I go?
11. What will it cost? Does this include everything—medication, tests, anesthetic, prescriptions, the follow-up exam?
12. Whom can I call for advice?

If you decide to have an abortion, it's important that you go to a reputable clinic that is staffed with licensed physicians who have admitting privileges at a local hospital and that provides twenty-four-hour coverage to handle any questions or complications that you may have after the procedure.

If you decide to continue your pregnancy, get prenatal care as soon as possible, and if you smoke, stop today.

Like the decision to have an abortion, deciding to maintain your pregnancy is a moral choice and carries with it the ethical responsibility to do what is best for your developing fetus and future child. Chances are you will have a normal baby, but you can increase the chances of giving your baby a normal birth and healthy head start on life by being careful, being informed, getting prenatal care, and maintaining your own good health.

Resources

American Fertility Society
2131 Magnolia Ave., Suite 201
Birmingham, AL 35256
(205) 251-9764
Herbert H. Thomas, M.D., medical director

Forum for presentation of scientific studies; provides information on the medical specialists in infertility nearest you.

Resolve, Inc.
P.O. Box 474
Belmont, MA 02178
(617) 484-2424
Beverly Freeman, executive director

Offers counseling, referral, and support to persons with problems of infertility.

Permanent Families for Children
67 Irving Place
New York, NY 10003

(212) 254-7410
Elizabeth Cole, director

A clearinghouse of information about adoption in North America, especially for children with "special needs."

Alternatives to Abortion International
8 Cottage Place
White Plains, NY 10601
(914) 683-0901
Ellen Walsh, director

Clearinghouse for information to assist a person with a problem pregnancy; offers practical services and positive and life-protecting personal, medical, and emotional support.

Catholics for a Free Choice
2008 17th Street, NW
Washington, DC 20009
(202) 638-1706
Frances Kissling, executive director

Public education on being Roman Catholic and pro-choice regarding abortion and contraception; write for list of publications.

National Abortion Federation
900 Pennsylvania Ave., SE
Washington, DC 20003
(202) 546-9060
Barbara Radford, executive director

National professional forum committed to making safe, legal abortions accessible to all women; operates toll-free hotline for information on how to choose an abortion facility, (800) 772-9100.

Planned Parenthood Federation of America, Inc. (PPFA)
810 Seventh Avenue
New York, NY 10019
(212) 541-7800
Faye Wattleton, president

Operates more than 735 centers nationwide that provide medically supervised family planning services and educational programs; provides leadership in making effective means of voluntary fertility regulation, including contraception, abortion, sterilization, and infertility services, available and fully accessible to all.

National Association of Surrogate Mothers
9200 Sunset Boulevard, Suite 620
Los Angeles, CA 90069
(213) 655-2015 or (213) 276-2121
Person to contact: Hilary Hanafin, Ph.D.

Newly formed group to educate the public; to lobby for legislation; to suggest guidelines to all surrogate programs, including careful screening of surrogate mother applicants and ongoing psychological support; to advise prospective parents; and to provide support to surrogate mothers.

Suggested reading

Abramowitz, Susan. "A Stalemate on Test-Tube Baby Research." *Hastings Center Report*, February 1984, pp. 5–9. (Politics, not ethics, is the major constraint.)

Annas, George J. "The Baby Broker Boom." *Hastings Center Report*, June 1986, pp. 30–31. (Examines recent court cases involving commercial surrogate motherhood contracts.)

Batchelor, Edward, Jr., ed. *Abortion: The Moral Issues.* New York: Pilgrim Press, 1982.

Blumberg, Grace Ganz. "Legal Issues in Nonsurgical Human Ovum Transfer." *Journal of the American Medical Association*, vol. 251, no. 9 (March 2, 1984), pp. 1178–81.

Callahan, Sidney, and Daniel Callahan. *Abortion: Understanding Differences.* New York: Plenum, 1984.

Elias, Sherman, M.D., and George J. Annas, J.D., M.P.H. "Social Policy Considerations in Noncoital Reproduction." *Journal of the American Medical Association*, vol. 255, no. 1 (January 3, 1986), pp. 62–68.

Hoff, Gerard Alan, and Lawrence J. Schneiderman. "Having Babies at Home: Is it Safe? Is it Ethical?" *Hastings Center Report*, vol. 15, no. 6 (December 1985). (Both home and hospital births entail risks, though hospitals entail a wider range of risks of unknown magnitude; thus, the morality of home births should be decided on a case-by-case basis.)

Jakobovits, Immanuel. *Jewish Medical Ethics.* New York: Bloch, 1975. (Topics covered include artificial insemination, contraception, and abortion.)

Maguire, Marjorie Reiley, and Daniel C. Maguire. *Abortion: A Guide to Making Ethical Choices.* Washington, D.C.: Catholics for a Free Choice, 1983.

Milunsky, Aubrey, M.D. *How to Have the Healthiest Baby You Can.* New York: Simon and Schuster, 1987. (Includes chapters on planning for pregnancy, new methods for infertile couples, prenatal diagnosis of genetic disorders, early pregnancy care, and coping with potential complications during pregnancy, delivery, and newborn period.)

Murray, Thomas H., Ph.D. "Ethical issues in fetal surgery." *American College of Surgeons Bulletin,* vol. 70, no. 6 (June 1985), pp. 6–10.

Robertson, Patricia Anne, M.D., and Peggy Henning Berlin, Ph.D. *The Premature Labor Handbook.* New York: Doubleday, 1986. (Helps women detect signs of premature labor.)

Shaw, Margery W., M.D., J.D., and A. Edward Doudera, J.D., eds. *Defining Human Life: Medical, Legal, and Ethical Implications.* Ann Arbor: AUPHA Press, 1983.

Singer, Peter. "Making Laws on Making Babies." *Hastings Center Report,* August 1985, pp. 5–6. (The government of the Australian state of Victoria has set firm limits on the new reproductive technologies, taking a firm stand against cloning and the creation of animal-human hybrids.)

Walters, William, and Peter Singer, eds. *Test-Tube Babies: A Guide to Moral Questions, Present Techniques and Future Possibilities.* Melbourne: Oxford University Press, 1982.

7 The Baby Doe Dilemma — to Treat or Not to Treat

EACH year, more than 3.5 million infants are born in the United States. Most of these babies are full-term and have no problems. They grow and develop into normal, healthy children. However, 6 to 8 percent of these infants are born prematurely, and others are born with major birth defects.

Modern corrective surgery has given many infants with severe birth defects a chance for new life. Advances in neonatal medicine have markedly improved the chances of survival for many "preemies"—whose odds of living to adulthood from a birthweight of slightly more than a pound would have been nil just ten years ago. Even so, not all babies make it and some are left severely handicapped.

Among the most agonizing dilemmas parents and pediatricians face in this era of high-tech medicine are how aggressively to treat the sick or severely handicapped newborn, when to forgo life-sustaining treatment, and, ultimately, who should decide.

If your son or daughter is a very-low-birth weight (VLBW) infant (less than 1.5 kilograms, or 3.4 pounds) or has a congenital birth defect, it's only natural that you will be under great emotional stress as you face some of the most difficult questions all parents ask: Will my baby live? Will my baby be normal? If not, what kind of life lies ahead for my child? What's the right thing to do now?

The short life of Baby Bryan

Paula and Steve, whose cherished dream of starting a family took shape with Bryan's birth, wrestled with these same questions after their baby was born.

During her pregnancy, Paula thought it strange her baby didn't move much. She had miscarried twice before, but one of those pregnancies had gone twenty-six weeks. Now with only a few more weeks to go until her due date, Paula was worried. Her obstetrician was reassuring. Some babies, she told Paula and Steve, just aren't very active.

From the moment she saw her infant son in the delivery room, however, Paula knew something was wrong. Bryan, born five weeks early, had an unusually small mouth, club feet, and a head that Paula recalls "looked like he was born with a rubber band around it." In the nursery, he cried all the time. "You could not make this baby comfortable," she says. "No one could. He had trouble breathing, didn't suck well, had to be fed with tubes much of the time, and vomited often."

At first, says Paula, the doctors caring for Bryan kept telling her, "He's fine, we'll fix him." Later, the baby's pediatrician and various specialists who saw the child acknowledged that something was wrong, but said they couldn't make an exact diagnosis. Slowly, Bryan gained weight. At last, two weeks after the birth, doctors told the eager parents that they could take their child home to Lake Tahoe, where Steve worked at one of the ski resorts.

The next ten weeks were a nightmare—trying to get a few ounces of milk into a baby who rarely stopped crying, vomited after almost every feeding, and had difficulty breathing as well. When diarrhea added to his problems, Paula began driving her son every other day to see his doctors in Reno, about forty miles away.

At different times during the eighteen weeks of his short life, both sets of grandparents came to help the exhausted parents. "They would walk the floor with this baby," says Paula, "and walk and walk, holding him. The only way he seemed comfortable was when he was hyperextended"—with his back arched—"and that's not normal."

Corrective casts on Bryan's feet needed changing every two weeks, and it was during the trip home from one of these visits to the orthopedic surgeon that the baby stopped breathing. (Later tests would show that he had vomited and apparently aspirated some milk into his lungs.) Doctors had warned Paula and Steve that the baby might suffer momentary cessations of breathing (apnea) and had sent him home on an apnea monitor. They'd also refused to let Bryan leave the nursery until both his parents were trained to administer cardiopulmonary respiration (CPR) to their son.

Paramedics, called to the house, resuscitated Bryan. A Care Flight helicopter transported him to a Reno hospital. He was in coma and never regained consciousness. That night, a consulting neurologist told the anguished parents that he was pessimistic about their infant's prognosis because he had suffered a "severe brain insult." By now, the baby was having repeated seizures, and various tests confirmed brain damage.

"Who are we doing all this for?"

During the next two weeks, Baby Bryan's condition changed little. He remained in coma and had frequent convulsions in spite of medication to try to control them. Repeated attempts to remove Bryan from the respirator failed. Still the orthopedic surgeon continued to change casts on the baby's feet.

When one of the doctors told Paula and Steve the baby would not survive without two surgical procedures—a tracheostomy to aid breathing and a gastrostomy feeding tube inserted through the baby's abdomen—the couple began to ask, "Why? Who are we doing this for? Is all this being done for Bryan, or for us, or for the doctors?"

Night after night, they talked over their concerns. They agreed that if Bryan did not show improvement soon, they should ask to have everything stopped. Paula's mother, a registered nurse, supported their decision. She was the first to say openly that Bryan was *not* going to make it—and to question the value of keeping up such aggressive treatment.

But Paula and Steve were leery of discussing any of this with the doctors and nurses taking care of Bryan. They'd already had an ugly confrontation with the orthopedic surgeon, who had assumed the baby's problems were related to drugs Paula might have taken during her pregnancy. "It wasn't so, and we told him that," Steve says angrily, "but we live at the lake and he just assumed that because I work at a ski resort, it's automatic that we take drugs." The incident had bothered the couple.

Would people think they were bad parents or even immoral for wanting the baby's suffering to stop? The couple felt guilty and afraid to speak up now that one pediatrician was pushing them to consent to even more aggressive and risky therapy to keep their son alive.

"Like it or not, we were into the Baby Doe thing"

One evening after Bryan had been in the hospital two and a half weeks, they saw the "crash cart" for resuscitation next to their son's crib. On the spot, Steve and Paula decided it was time to stop. "We went to the baby's doctor," Paula recalls, "and we said, 'We don't know what you are going to say to us, but we want to know how far we have to take this issue. We're making all this heroic attempt, and who are we doing it for? We need information.'" The doctor was very supportive, and the couple relaxed.

But the Baby Doe controversy was then featured in *Time,*
Newsweek, and every newspaper in the country.[1]

Not only were Paula and Steve not sure what was ethically
right and legally permissible, the baby's doctor wasn't sure
either. With the media airing charges and countercharges of
suspected infant neglect from coast to coast and with a Baby
Doe hotline sitting in the nursery, their anxiety grew worse.

"Our biggest fear was doing something or saying something that would haunt us later on," Paula explains. "We are
Roman Catholics, and we value life a lot. God knows I
wanted the baby to wake up, but he wasn't going to, and we
didn't want him to live in the condition he was in. And my
mother was saying, 'Don't let them push you into doing
something for this baby that isn't necessary.' Like it or not,
we were into the Baby Doe thing," Paula says sadly. "We still
had hope, but we wanted to know what our options were."

Baby Doe and the federal government

In 1982, Baby Doe of Bloomington, Indiana, was born with
Down syndrome and an incomplete esophagus, a life-
threatening obstruction of the upper digestive tract. The
baby's doctors recommended surgery to connect his esophagus and stomach. His parents refused to consent to this
operation, which might have enabled their son to survive.
They believed it wouldn't be in his best interests, since he
would always be severely retarded, and from birth he was
denied food, water, and medical aid.

Baby Doe took his place in history when the hospital took
the case to the Indiana supreme court, which upheld his parents' decision to withhold surgery. The next day, Baby Doe
died. (Today, most doctors and ethicists would agree that surgery should have been performed on this infant despite parental objections, since the operation is relatively simple and
would have permitted him to survive with normal feeding by
mouth.)

Baby Jane Doe was born in 1983 with spina bifida (an incomplete closure of part of the spinal column which often leaves spinal cord and nerves exposed) and an abnormally small head with excess fluid on the brain. Doctors at University Hospital in Stony Brook, New York, believed that without surgery, she might live six months to two years. Surgery to drain the fluid from her brain and close the spinal defect, however, might extend her life as much as twenty years. Her parents, Dan and Linda A., refused to give surgeons permission to operate on their eight-day-old baby girl. Doctors supported their decision.

Alerted by an informer, right-to-life advocate and attorney A. Lawrence Washburn demanded a court review of the decision to forgo surgery. He argued that doctors should be forced to operate on the infant despite her parents' wishes.

At the hearing which followed, attorneys for the hospital and parents, a court-appointed guardian for the child, and State Supreme Court Justice Melvyn Tannenbaum considered the issues. In describing the severity of her problems, Stony Brook physicians painted a bleak picture of Baby Jane Doe's future, but testified that she was not in imminent danger of death. Tannenbaum ordered surgery on her.

On appeal, however, the appellate division of the New York State supreme court upheld the parents' decision to refuse consent for surgery. Not only that, the court was critical of Judge Tannenbaum, who had ordered surgery contrary to the parents' wishes, and of Washburn and the other right-to-life advocates who had taken the case to court in the first place.[2]

But Baby Jane Doe's case didn't end there.

The next day, the Justice Department demanded access to the baby's confidential medical records and sued the hospital for their release. Following several more appeals, the United States Supreme Court refused to intervene and the New York State supreme court ruling in favor of the parents was allowed to stand.

Baby Jane Doe, whose real name is Keri-Lynn, did not die.

According to a 1986 newspaper report on her second birthday, she enjoys playing with her dog and moving about in a walker. Her father believes Keri-Lynn's condition proves he and his wife did *not* "abandon a child to die" when they refused the first operation to close a defect in her spinal cord. (It closed on its own, and when her condition improved at about 5 months, she had surgery to relieve spinal fluid building up in her brain.) Keri-Lynn may be "slightly retarded," he was quoted as saying, "but very little—all her teachers think she's very bright."[3]

Never before had two cases stirred such national debate on the withholding of treatment from handicapped newborns. Doctors, hospitals, medical organizations, advocacy groups for handicapped citizens, right-to-life organizations, attorneys, several agencies of the federal government, and the White House itself became embroiled in the controversy.

"Baby Doe" regulations—Big Brother in the nursery

The so-called Baby Doe rules were the federal government's initial response to this public outcry against allowing babies to starve to death or be deprived of surgery for life-threatening conditions. These regulations (issued under Section 504 of the Rehabilitation Act of 1973) stated that no infant could be denied treatment *solely on the basis of a handicapping condition.*

In effect, they required doctors and hospitals to provide maximum treatment to virtually all infants. Hospitals were also required to display public notices which encouraged the anonymous reporting of violations to federal investigators. Toll-free hotlines were set up in nurseries to make reporting to Washington easy.

The allegation was that many parents, *with* their doctors' support and approval, were denying treatment to their severely handicapped newborns. Not only were parents and physicians being portrayed as child abusers, they were being placed in an adversarial role against the federal government, which saw itself as the guardian of these infants.

But these complaints proved false.

In investigating more than 1,500 hotline reports, the government found only three cases in which infants were allegedly being denied appropriate care.[4] Although the Supreme Court had refused to intervene in the Baby Jane Doe case in New York (noted earlier in this chapter), after many court hearings, it did agree to review the Baby Doe rules promulgated by the Department of Health and Human Services.

In the meantime, Congress passed the Child Abuse Amendments of 1984. The Department of Health and Human Services then issued rules for the implementation of these amendments by state welfare departments.

AMENDED CHILD NEGLECT DEFINITIONS

Many state welfare departments are now adopting the expanded definitions of child abuse and neglect contained in the federal regulations pursuant to the Child Abuse Amendments of 1984 (Public Law 98–457):

MEDICAL NEGLECT   The failure to provide adequate medical care. The term "medical neglect" includes, but is not limited to, the withholding of medically indicated treatment from a disabled infant with a life-threatening condition.

WITHHOLDING OF MEDICALLY INDICATED TREATMENT   The failure to respond to an infant's life-threatening conditions by providing treatment (including nutrition, hydration, and medication) which in the treating physician's reasonable judgment will be likely to be effective in ameliorating or correcting all such conditions. This term does not include the failure to provide treatment (other than appropriate nutrition, hydration, or medication) when in the treating physician's reasonable medical judgment any of the following circumstances apply:
    (i) The infant is chronically and irreversibly comatose;
    (ii) The provision of such treatment would merely:
        1. Prolong dying,

2. Not be effective in ameliorating or correcting ALL of the infant's life-threatening conditions, or

3. Otherwise be futile in terms of the survival of the infant; or

(iii) The provision of such treatment would be virtually futile in terms of the survival of the infant and the treatment itself under such circumstances would be inhumane.

New ruling—support for parents as primary decision-makers

In June 1986, the Supreme Court ruled that the so-called Baby Doe regulations were *not* authorized under Section 504 of the Rehabilitation Act of 1973.[5] The Court agreed with the President's Commission on medical ethics that parents should be the primary decision-makers for their child—provided those decisions are in the best interests of the child.

Furthermore, the Supreme Court emphasized that child protection is a *state responsibility*—and each state has the authority to intervene under its existing laws if parents fail to act in their child's best interests. The federal government was out of the Baby Doe business.

But the debate about the care of the critically ill newborn continues within medical and ethical circles.

Ethical issues in Baby Doe cases

If your baby has a serious problem, there are a number of issues which will affect you, your infant, the baby's doctor, and the hospital.

Your right to decide

You have the constitutional right to privacy, to be left alone, to make decisions for yourself and your family. But there are limits to this right. Through the courts, society prevents you from harming your children or acting in any way that endangers their life or well-being. Child abuse and neglect laws are based on these limits to your freedom and privacy. (Chapter 8 contains a fuller discussion of parental rights.)

Your child's best interests

Every American citizen has the fundamental rights to life, liberty, and the pursuit of happiness. All infants have a right to the protection, nurturing, and care which will enable them to become autonomous adults capable of exercising their rights for themselves.

In considering whether or not to treat a newborn, most experts believe that the *primary* issue is what's in the child's best interests. If his mental and physical handicaps are overwhelming and it would be inhumane to prolong his life, then treatment should be withheld or withdrawn. After all, saving an infant for a life of suffering is hardly a humane and loving act.

Richard McCormick, a theologian at the Kennedy Institute of Ethics, states that "life is a value to be preserved only insofar as it contains some potentiality for human relationships."[6] When this potentiality is totally absent or when it would be subordinated to mere survival, McCormick believes withholding treatment is justified.

Most physicians and ethicists agree it is not in a child's best interests to force futile treatment upon him and to prolong his suffering and dying. For example, when one Stony Brook University Hospital neurologist testified at the Baby Jane Doe court hearing, he described a grim future for her: "Baby Jane would lie in bed, fed by tubes, with sores all over her body, infected bladder and kidneys, pneumonia, seizures, chills, fever, and pain." Not only would she be completely unaware of her surroundings, he said, she would also "experience no joy, no sadness, only pain."[7] Although another expert who testified was not so pessimistic, he agreed the parents had made a reasonable choice in deciding to withhold surgery.

Your best interests

Ethicists recognize that sometimes what is in the infant's best interests can conflict with what is in the best interests of the parents and family as a whole. For instance, your baby's care may be overtaxing your emotional, physical, and financial resources to the point where you or your family are being hurt. You may feel torn between meeting your needs, your baby's needs, and those of other members of your family.

Biomedical expert Carson Strong of the University of Tennessee in Memphis argues that the best interests of the family may be taken into consideration if continued treatment of the infant places a large and unreasonable burden on the family. "In these cases," Strong notes, "the family should be given the opportunity to make the decision whether to go all out for the infant."[8]

Your doctor's duties

Doctors commit themselves to do what is best for their patients, to do no harm, to relieve suffering, and to save life whenever possible. And most consider themselves the infant's advocate. But in caring for sick infants and their parents who may be temporarily quite upset, the physician's obligations and duties sometimes get mixed up. The duty to cure and save life using all available treatments (the so-called technological imperative) may overshadow the duty to care and relieve suffering.

In their book, *The Long Dying of Baby Andrew*, Robert and Peggy Stinson document the short, cruel institutional life their baby underwent as a result of the "heroic" medical efforts to save him. Andrew, born fifteen and a half weeks prematurely, weighed slightly less than two pounds. Almost from the beginning, he seemed to be in a state of painful deterioration. The Stinsons wanted their infant to be allowed to die a natural death. But, they write, Andrew became "hopelessly entrapped in an intensive care unit where the machinery is more sophisticated than the codes of law and ethics governing its use."[9]

While the Stinsons acknowledge that medical research has benefited many premature babies, they question who will set the limits of such research on tiny subjects. And, they ask, if it must continue, can it not be limited to *consenting* families?

Heroic measures

Frequently, the words "ordinary" and "extraordinary" are used in connection with the treatment of infants when they are critically ill.

Many people think these terms refer to the complexity of the proposed treatment or the sophistication of the equipment used. For example, a dialysis machine or respirator seem to be extraordinary; an antibiotic or intravenous (IV) feeding seems to be ordinary. But this is a misinterpretation of the terms as originally used by Pope Pius XII in addressing an international congress of anesthesiologists in 1957.[10]

Pius XII was referring to the *effect* of treatment on the patient. If a treatment would be of benefit, it was considered ordinary and must be used. If it would not benefit the patient and would only be a further burden to him, such treatment was extraordinary and need not be used.

Since then, many courts have reaffirmed the meaning of these terms as Pius XII explained them. For instance, a respirator may indeed be an "ordinary" measure if its use will benefit your child, but "extraordinary" if it merely sustains respiratory function and prolongs his or her dying. The same applies to a feeding tube, an IV, antibiotics, or any other treatment.

In short, if what's being done imposes a heavy burden and

is of little or no benefit to your baby, the treatment would be considered extraordinary. Doctors don't have to provide it; you don't have to accept it on behalf of your infant because it would not be in his or her best interests. Literally, there are instances in which heroic measures do more harm than good.

In making a decision about your infant's treatment, don't be confused by high-tech labels. What's important is whether the treatment will be of help to your baby *without* imposing prolonged or undue pain or suffering.

Right to life versus a life worth living

Before the Baby Doe controversy of the early 1980s, many physicians and surgeons applied "quality of life" judgments in recommending to parents that they consent to the treatment or withholding of treatment to their sick or handicapped newborn. It was usually left to the parents to decide, although doctors sometimes overruled them and obtained court orders to treat the infant.

Several experts hold that the "do no harm" principle requires that the lives of newborns who lack the potential for a minimally acceptable quality of life should not be prolonged. Quality of life, however, means different things to different parents.

A handicapped or potentially retarded infant, for example, may be seen as a tragedy by a family which values intellectual pursuits, education, and success—whether it's in school, sports, the arts, business, the trades, or a profession. Some doctors, nurses, and others who are well educated tend to support these values. These people personalize what it would be like to be mentally retarded, institutionalized, or confined to a wheelchair. In discussing treatment options, they reinforce the parent's worst fears about the infant's future quality of life. But there's a danger when doctors project their own views about life and suffering on others.

Few of us, it's true, would choose to spend our lives in a wheelchair or in an institution for retarded children. But as

University of Wisconsin pediatrician Norman Fost points out, "that does not mean that an infant or child who never knew another life need necessarily be psychologically overwhelmed by the experience."[11]

Fost goes on to say, however, that sometimes there are compelling reasons to withhold treatment and allow a child to die when reasonable grounds exist for concluding that it is in the child's best interests. This is often termed "passive euthanasia" and, less commonly, "benign neglect"—a concept that many doctors and parents find hard to accept as a preferred option to even a minimal life.

Those who support the right-to-life position believe that life is sacred and should be preserved at almost any cost. In their view, to "do no harm" means to prevent the death of all nondying infants—since the ultimate harm is death itself. Here, quality-of-life judgments have no place in the decision to treat or not to treat.

Fair share of resources

When your emotions, energy, and thoughts are focused on your sick infant, raising the issue of costs seems cold and unfeeling. But when you have other children at home, it's important to consider their needs as well. If all your resources are spent treating a *hopelessly* ill child, can you possibly provide adequately for your other children? (For example, in the eighteen weeks Paula and Steve's infant required medical treatment and hospitalization, Bryan's medical and hospital bills surpassed $100,000. To make matters worse, during that same period, Steve lost his job.)

A doctor should treat and do what's best for an infant regardless of cost as long as there is reasonable evidence that continuing treatment will benefit the child. Even when the outcome is uncertain, treatment should continue.

Yet there are times when parents opt to continue vigorous treatment at great cost even after it is clear to all the professionals involved in the child's care that treatment is futile.

Hoping against hope for a miracle, these parents insist that treatment not be stopped. Usually, the baby's doctor will go along with the parent's desires—at least for a little while.

Occasionally, doctors, nurses, or hospital officials may decide to withdraw from the care of such infants. But they can't just abandon the child; they must ensure that other options for care are available from another doctor or at a different hospital, or they must have the consent of a court-appointed guardian to withdraw treatment deemed futile.

What can you expect from your baby's doctor?

If your baby was born prematurely with a very low birth weight or with serious birth defects, or even if your child was born normal but now is critically ill, he or she will undoubtedly be cared for in a neonatal or other intensive care unit.

First, the doctor will do what is necessary to sustain your baby until there's time to fully evaluate the situation and discuss it with you. At the same time, he will evaluate the baby's clinical condition and obtain whatever laboratory tests are necessary to arrive at a diagnosis as quickly as possible.

Typically, when faced with a life-or-death situation, most neonatologists treat the infant aggressively. At this point, doctors are pursing every reasonable diagnostic and therapeutic approach to see what can be done for your baby. You may be asked to give permission for a variety of tests and procedures, such as x-rays, blood tests, spinal tap, CAT scan (a type of computerized x-ray which produces three-dimensional pictures), and EEG (an electroencephalogram or brain-wave test).

You may also be asked to consent to one or more treatment procedures, such as blood transfusions, inserting a chest tube, and possibly putting the infant on a respirator. A number of surgical procedures may also be recommended, depending on the diagnosis and the severity of your baby's condition. For example, an infant with hydrocephalus may need shunts placed in the cavities of the brain to relieve pressure, and a child with spina bifida may require surgery to close the opening in his lower spine.

To parents, these seem like drastic, even horrendous procedures for tiny infants. They are. But when they offer hope of survival or improvement in the baby's condition, the neonatologist, neurologist, and pediatric surgeon view them as standard procedures essential to save an infant's life and/or relieve pain and suffering.

Whether such procedures are mandatory or optional depends on two factors: the nature of the infant's problems and whether these procedures are likely to improve the infant's condition or merely prolong his suffering and dying. From a medical standpoint, you can expect that virtually all doctors will treat an infant when there is doubt about the full nature of the child's condition or the possible benefits of treatment.

Here's how one neonatologist, identified only as Dr. "N," summed up his dual responsibility to parents and child in an April 1984 *Woman's Day* article: "My responsibility as a neonatologist is not just to the parents. First and foremost, I am the baby's doctor. I see myself as the infant's ombudsperson. I try to sense how strongly he or she wants to live. This sense, which nurses share with doctors, goes beyond the flashing numbers on a monitor. It is our feeling about *this* patient, this *baby*, based on our daily experience with infants struggling to survive. I relay that information to the parents."[12]

Communication with your baby's doctor

As soon as your infant is stabilized, you should talk to the neonatologist or other physicians caring for your baby. They should keep you informed about your infant's diagnosis, treatment, condition, and prognosis at every step of the way.

You should have ready access to your baby's doctors and consultants, and, when they are unavailable, to the nurses caring for your infant.

Obviously, some doctors communicate better than others. Some consider it vital to talk to you and explain all they can about your infant's condition. Other physicians don't. Except in an emergency situation, you should *insist* that the doctor answer all your questions so that the consent you're asked to give to treatment for your infant is truly informed.

Most doctors and nursery staffs work hard at maintaining good communication with the family, because they believe parents should participate in all decision-making from the outset. But you'll find some doctors who act paternalistically. They assume the role of decision-maker without adequately involving parents. They screen the amount and kind of information parents receive in the honest belief that they are saving them more pain and suffering.

Still other physicians believe that parents should seldom, if ever, be asked to make a decision, since they are upset and so emotionally involved that they cannot be objective.

Look over the list of questions which follows. Some you will want to ask soon after the baby is born or rehospitalized, if you had already taken the baby home. Other questions are better left for later—after the doctor has had time to fully evaluate your infant and is at the point of recommending treatment. Keep in mind, though, that in a critical situation, you may need answers all at once.

QUESTIONS TO ASK YOUR INFANT'S DOCTOR

Questions to ask early on:

1. What's wrong with my baby?
2. Are you sure of the diagnosis?
3. What are my baby's chances of living?
4. Is my baby suffering or in pain?
5. May I see my baby?

6. Are you suggesting I not see my baby because I'll get upset?
7. What do you think should be done?
8. Can my baby's condition be treated?
9. Will this procedure/treatment help my child?
10. How risky is this procedure/treatment?
11. Will this procedure/treatment just prolong my baby's suffering?
12. What options do we have?
13. Should we get a second or third opinion, or call in consultants?
14. Can you take care of my baby here, or does he have to be moved to another hospital?
15. Do we have to decide right now or do we have time to think it over?
16. Do we have time to talk it over with some other people? (Family members, friends, relatives, etc.)
17. What will all of this cost?

Questions to ask later:

1. What tests have been done on my baby and what are the results?
2. If he lives, will he be normal?
3. How will this affect him?
4. Will he be handicapped or retarded or have a disability?
5. If he has a disability, will it be permanent or temporary?
6. Will he be able to take care of himself?
7. Are there other parents who've been through this that we can talk to?
8. Can you give me any articles, brochures, or other printed material that will help me understand my baby's condition?
9. What should I tell my family, friends, and relatives when they call and say they've heard about the baby?
10. Does the hospital have an infant bioethics committee? Should we consult the committee, or will it automatically review my baby's case?

Your doctor's answers to some of these questions may leave you feeling stunned, confused, and not sure of what to do. The sensitive doctor will realize this and provide the information in such a way that you'll have time to absorb it, think about it, and make a decision based on the realities of your baby's condition.

If your doctor has to leave before you're finished asking questions, or if you're too upset to think about your baby's problems clearly, set a time for another meeting or telephone call before this one ends. You may feel as though you've had the rug pulled out from under you, and you can't bear to hear another word. It's all right to feel that way.

Some parents find that having a friend or family member present in talking to the doctor helps; other mothers and fathers would just as soon be alone when they receive discouraging updates about their infant's condition.

But remember, you need information—even if it comes in bits and pieces—so that you can take part in deciding what's best for your baby and family. Should your infant be treated? Should treatment be stopped? Who should decide? And what if you feel you don't have enough information to decide?

Paul and Marlys Bridge, for instance, felt a tense doctor-parent relationship and poor communication was making it even harder for them to accept *without question* the pediatrician's recommendation that treatment be withheld from their infant son. Born in a Canadian hospital shortly after his mother had undergone emergency exploratory surgery for peritonitis, Christopher had breathing problems and began convulsing. Later, these were diagnosed as symptoms of possible viral encephalitis. Other complications followed; brain damage was extensive.

The long-term outlook for this extremely ill child ran the gamut from severe mental retardation to possible blindness and motor defects extensive enough to make him a quadriplegic. On the fifty-first day of his life and again ten days later, the baby's doctor urged the parents to think about withholding treatment as a possible "treatment" option.

Access to your infant's medical records

Describing their dilemma in a 1981 *Hastings Center Report,* the Bridges detail their frustration in trying to get information about the cause of the baby's problems and his actual condition during the seventy-eight days he lived.

"Aside from one occasion when we were permitted to see a few pages of the hospital records relating to the first two days of Christopher's life," the Bridges write, "we were denied permission to look at his hospital records because this was against 'hospital policy'—an argument that apparently brooks no opposition. We did get detailed verbal updates on our son's condition, but not as many as we would have liked. Our distress was compounded by our awareness that other parents with children similar to Christopher were obtaining access to their children's records with their physician's permission."

As the Bridges point out, in a life-and-death situation, any parent wants to be absolutely sure that whatever treatment option doctors are suggesting is in the child's best interests. "How ironic," they state, "that we were considered privileged enough to take part in discussions concerning the planned termination of our son's life, yet we were insufficiently privileged to check his medical records."[13]

Health professionals, however, often regard the patient or relative who wants to see the medical records as someone who is probably planning to sue the doctor, hospital, or staff —and doctors and hospital attorneys are very nervous about lawsuits. Caution is the byword where patient's charts are concerned; hospital "policy" is the convenient way to say no.

On the other hand, many parents, in the strange environment of a hospital, feel intimidated. They have little awareness of how hospitals function and little information on policies, procedures, and patient rights. Furthermore, they don't want to be considered "pesty" or "pushy" or "overly emotional."

If you feel you're not getting complete information from your infant's physician or want to see the child's medical records, talk to the doctor first. Most physicians will share any and all information about your baby with you. If, as in the Bridges' case, the doctor refuses to let you see the records, ask your attorney to contact the hospital administration. (See Chapter 10 for a fuller discussion of medical records and who owns them.)

But don't be afraid to be "pesty" if you're not getting information you need. It's not only your right as parents, it's also your baby, and your money (or insurance or bank loan) paying for his or her care, and your heartache over the suffering of your child.

Who can best decide?

The President's Commission on medical ethics states that in most cases, the decision-making authority should be left in the hands of parents in consultation with physicians. But there are times when parents simply cannot make an impartial decision.

Doctors, too, can be biased, and they have conflicts of interest among research, teaching, and patient-care concerns. As medical ethicist Robert Weir notes, "Physicians are no better qualified to make sound moral decisions in these cases than parents or other possible proxies.... Specialized medical knowledge does not translate into moral expertise."[14]

This is one reason why infant bioethics committees are being formed in hospitals nationwide.[15] Another is that the federal child abuse regulations strongly recommend the establishment of these committees, especially in hospitals which specialize in high-risk neonatal care. Despite this, many hospitals still do not have working bioethics committees.

214

What to expect from an infant bioethics committee

You should get guidance and information from this committee. But unless you've talked to other parents who have met with infant bioethics committees, you probably won't know what to expect, who will be there, whether you will be judged as parents, what your role will be, how the committee arrives at a decision, or what happens after that.

Who will be present?

Committee membership varies from hospital to hospital. The committee I serve on has three physicians (an internist and two pediatricians, one of whom is also an Episcopal priest), two intensive care nurses, a social worker, and a hospital administrator who is a nun. These seven people make up the core committee. But on occasion, we've asked consultants to join us, such as an attorney and the parent of a disabled child.

American Academy of Pediatrics guidelines suggest that committees include a lay person from the community, an expert in developmental disabilities, and a pastoral counselor, such as a parish priest or minister, a rabbi, or a hospital chaplain. Moreover, many committees are adding professional "ethicists" who can guide the discussion of the moral aspects of the case. Some experts also believe that every committee should have a special advocate to speak for the infant, who, as committees now stand, has no voice.

You have a right to know "who's who" on the committee and what each one's area of expertise is.

Be sure that everyone in the room is introduced to you. These people are becoming a part of your life through this process and may contribute to a decision which will have an enormous impact on your infant, you, and your family. (Paula and Steve, for example, were sure one person in the room—a man wearing a turtleneck sweater when all other doctors had on shirts and ties—was the committee's "resident shrink," there to evaluate them as parents, when, in fact, he was a pediatrician with special training in medical ethics.)

How will the infant bioethics committee become involved?

Most committees will review your baby's case at the request of any member of the hospital staff, whether it comes from a doctor, nurse, social worker, or anyone else involved with your baby's case.

You or a member of your immediate family can also request a review—especially if you believe that heroic measures should be avoided, or life-saving treatment withheld or withdrawn.

Hospital policy may require mandatory review in certain cases, such as Down syndrome or myelomeningocele (a birth defect involving incomplete closure of the spine), when both the attending physician and the parents believe that life-sustaining treatment should be withdrawn or withheld. Generally, bioethics committees do *not* review cases in which the infant's death is imminent, or the child's condition has been previously determined by committee policy to be untreatable.

How does the process start?

Some hospitals publicize the existence of the committee and publicly post the names of its members. You or a member of your family can also request committee review through the hospital social worker, ombudsperson, chaplain, or pastoral counselor. But most parents simply ask their baby's physician to contact the committee. After your request is reviewed, a committee meeting will be called if the issue you've raised is an ethical one.

Don't be surprised if your baby's doctor sees no need for committee review and is not enthusiastic about requesting such a meeting. Many physicians consider infant bioethics committees one more intrusion of others into the doctor-patient relationship and the time-honored way in which decisions have been made by parents and doctor. (I disagree, and my experience has convinced me that when committees are used in a positive way, they can be extremely helpful.) By the same token, you may be upset with your baby's doctor if he or she initiates the review when you don't see the need for it.

In rare instances, the decision may be taken out of your hands and those of your doctor, if a public agency or interested third party strongly feels that your infant is being denied appropriate care (such as in the Baby Jane Doe case) or if hospital policy requires a mandatory review. Withholding treatment from an infant with Down syndrome, for instance, would surely fall into this category.

What will happen at a bioethics committee meeting?

Committee meetings are conducted in a variety of ways, depending on what the issues appear to be and who has initiated the review. It's possible that you won't be involved in the first meeting, or the first several, in which doctors and nurses present the medical details of your infant's condition. Once the committee has a clear understanding of the diagnosis, treatment, and prognosis, you and others will be involved more fully in the discussion.

After all the pertinent facts are brought out, the ethical issues will be clarified and all treatment options (available or proposed) will be thoroughly reviewed. For example, your baby's doctor may say, "I think we should do such and such," but other physicians on the committee may raise additional treatment options. Consultants, nurses, and others involved in your child's care will also have an opportunity to present their views.

But what about you?

Certainly, you will be invited to take part in discussing what's best for your infant. You can expect committee members to be sensitive to your situation and to raise issues they consider important based on their experience with similar cases. They will give strong weight to your views.

If you're asked to wait outside while the committee discusses your infant's case, don't assume the worst. Almost every committee will schedule time to discuss the medical aspects of your baby's diagnosis, treatment, and prognosis. This is part of the fact-gathering stage of decision-making. The committee's responsibility to consider *all* possible alternatives, however, may be misinterpreted by the family as being cold, unfeeling, or even unsupportive of their position. This doesn't mean you'll be excluded from making decisions related to your baby's case.

What is the parent's role?

Your role is to express your views, wishes, and preferences as thoroughly and completely as possible. The same is true of any questions you may have. You don't want the committee second-guessing what's on your mind. The better able you are to speak for yourself, the greater the chances are that you will be comfortable with whatever decision is reached.

Invite to the meeting one or two people who you believe would be of help to you. They may be able to clarify for the committee what's on your mind—especially when you're under great emotional stress or become choked with tears. Many parents are physically and mentally exhausted. They're worried about mounting hospital and doctor bills, the stability of their marriage, how the family may be affected, or how they will cope with a severely handicapped child.

Like Paula and Steve, you may be worried about expressing

your views openly. You may be afraid you'll be judged as emotionally unbalanced or be seen as bad parents—cold, uncaring, or immoral. You may be afraid the committee will recommend that the hospital seek a court-appointed guardian to make decisions for your child.

There are no quick remedies for the anxiety that nearly all parents feel in this situation. But it helps to remember that the committee is not there to find fault or blame anyone. Its job is to see that the best interests of your infant are protected while offering all the support possible to you and those caring for your child.

How are decisions reached?

Usually, the best decision comes when consensus is reached. This is most likely to occur when all views are expressed, medical facts are known, ethical issues are clearly defined, and all conflicts are resolved in a mutually supportive environment. Established hospital policies concerning certain types of infants will make reaching consensus easier. If an infant has a condition which can't be treated effectively, efforts to prolong his or her life may be not only futile but actually harmful.

What if no agreement is reached?

Suppose you and/or the baby's doctor reject the committee's recommendation. You may want to withhold treatment when the physician wants to treat, or vice versa. Perhaps you and your doctor agree on what to do, but you're both opposed by the committee.

To resolve the conflict, you, the physician, or the committee (through the hospital administration) may take the case to a local or district court. The state welfare department can also intervene and seek guardianship of the infant. Until a court rules on the case, every reasonable effort must be made to continue treatment and prevent the baby's condition from becoming worse.[16] The rule of thumb is: *when in doubt, treat.*

All experts agree that in doubtful situations, the infant should be treated—until it is clear that withholding treatment is *justified* under ethical norms and the law. It takes time to decide that an infant is chronically and irreversibly comatose, that the treatment is merely prolonging an inevitable death, that further treatment is futile, or that continuing the treatment under the circumstances would be inhumane.

ACTION PLAN FOR DECISION-MAKING

1. Get all the medical facts about your baby's condition and treatment options and the likely outcome of each.

2. Don't be rushed into making a decision. If a true emergency exists, the decision almost always should be to treat the infant until there is time to consider the alternatives.

3. Be clear about whose needs will be met by the proposed decision—your needs, your infant's, the doctors', the nurses', the hospital's, or those of medical science.

4. Discuss your feelings, anxieties, and all questions you have with your own physician, the baby's doctor, nurses, and specialists caring for your infant. Ask for a second or third opinion if you feel it might help in resolving your dilemma.

5. Talk to others who can assist you in making your decision, such as a minister, rabbi, or priest, or the hospital pastoral counselor or social worker. Other parents who have made a hard choice to withhold treatment and allow their baby to die may provide you with support in making your own decision. Similarly, parents who are raising disabled children can often dispel myths and relieve anxiety about what the future may hold for your handicapped infant.

6. Consider the financial, physical, and emotional impact your decision will have on you and your family.

7. Ask to see your baby if you want to. Some physicians and nurses try to spare parents further emotional pain when their infant is severely deformed and advise against seeing the baby. It's all right to agree, but *you* should be the one to

make that decision. I've found that many parents who imagined the worst are glad they decided to see their infant and even hold him before he died.

8. If your baby's care is reviewed by the hospital's infant bioethics committee, be sure you express your views, concerns, and preferences as fully as possible. Ask a friend, counselor, family member, or other supportive person to go with you.

9. Read all informed consent documents carefully. Don't hesitate to ask questions if you don't understand what you are being asked to agree to. You have a right to get information in words you can understand.

After the decision, then what?

Parents often say it's a great relief to have the difficult decision behind them. That doesn't mean that lingering doubts, second guesses about the decision, or even nagging guilt feelings won't recur for some time after. You will need to work through your feelings. This takes time and often help— whether from a friend, a relative, or a professional counselor.

If the decision was to treat your baby and he or she survives with a major disability, you will have doubts about your ability to care for your baby at home and meet the child's special needs. You may also be worried about his or her future and how you're going to meet all of your child's needs. This is normal. *All* parents of children with disabilities feel this way, especially when they ponder the many hard choices and decisions still ahead of them.

You will need help in obtaining ongoing medical treatment, rehabilitation, and appropriate education as the child grows. You will also need advice in planning the child's future and finding the resources to make the child's life worth living.

Getting on with your life

If your infant dies, you will need time to mourn. Friends and neighbors often don't know how to say they've heard about the baby's death and that they're sorry. They may not call or come to see you, leaving you feeling isolated and alone. The nurses, doctors, and others who were so involved in your baby's care and who took part in the decision-making may also feel the loss—but never say a word to you about it, send a card or note, or go to your baby's funeral. Their life goes on, and they are now caring for and worried about other infants.

Even the bioethics committee, which helped you make the hard choice and supported you at the time, is now out of your life. Some parents feel stranded, abandoned. As one parent put it: "Don't these committees which come into your life when you're in crisis have any obligation *afterward* to reassure you that what you did was all right?"

"I don't think there is any clear-cut end to this kind of situation," Paula says now. "Once the decision is made, you have to get on with your life. We had a funeral. We had Bryan cremated. We are in therapy now, but we are in therapy for a lot of things. We had literally everything, all the stops, pulled on us at once—the baby, Steve's job, and I wasn't working at the time. In terms of one's life, we landed on our head at that point, and it's going to take us time.

"We're still on shaky grounds in terms of our finances, and emotionally. We've sought professional help, and I would say to any parent going through something like this: find somebody you can talk to—somebody who's going to listen and not be judgmental. You have to trust you did the right thing and feel comfortable with your decision, because as time goes on, the doctors, nurses, and ethics committee won't be there to hold your hand. *You* are the one who has to live with the decision for the rest of your life."

A 1985 followup study of twenty families who took part in the decision to withdraw life support from their infants reveals that their grieving patterns differ little from those of other families whose newborns have died. Nor did these twenty families as a group carry a burden of guilt for their participation. "To the contrary," note researchers Edward Walwork and Patricia Ellison, "they tended to accept the responsibility for the decision to withdraw support and to feel that they made the right decision."[17]

But as a couple who may want to have another child someday, there is yet one more decision to make: whether to seek genetic testing and counseling which can provide you with critical data about your chances of having a healthy, normal child in the future. Even if you've decided you never want to become pregnant again, but you already have other children, you might consider such testing for the sake of *their* future babies—your grandchildren.

Is it really a genetic problem?

As a medical specialty, genetic counseling can tell you what the chances are that you will have a child with a genetic defect based on your medical history and a sophisticated knowledge of human genetics (the branch of science dealing with heredity) and "new" or newly defined genetic diseases, which, in theory at least, are nearly infinite. Some of these, such as muscular dystrophy, Huntington's chorea—also known as Woody Guthrie's disease—and some forms of diabetes, may not even show up until a person reaches adolescence or adulthood.

Genetic counseling is not the key to creating perfect human beings every time, but it does provide the family seeking help with realistic information about the nature of the birth defect already manifested in a family member, the risk of its occurring again, and what a recurrence would mean in practical terms for all concerned. In turn, this allows a family or couple to make informed decisions about childbearing with which they can feel comfortable.

To advise you in any *meaningful* way of the risks and probabilities of conceiving a child with a specific genetic defect or disease, geneticists must have enough data to make an accurate diagnosis. Generally, the first step is to obtain a detailed family health history, followed by various tests of blood and body fluids, and more recently, analysis of chromosomes and other genetic material gathered from your cells.

(If your child has just died, you may also be asked to consent to an autopsy to help determine the exact nature of the genetic defect or disorder. While this may seem like one more difficult thing to say yes to, you should give your consent for the sake of any future children you may conceive or those you already have. The information gained could be vital to you, your children, and their children.)

Certainly, the reassuring report geneticists gave Cathie and Brad Van Woert made a world of difference in their decision to have more children after their first child was born with an extremely rare genetic defect.

Shortly after her birth in 1971, Chrissy Van Woert was diagnosed as having Trisomy 18—a fatal genetic defect characterized by profound retardation, failure to thrive, and numerous malformations present at birth. Because 95 percent of children with this condition also have a heart defect, most die within six months and few live more than one year. Chrissy's heart, however, was not affected. She survived for eight years; but during that time, doctors caring for her never once suggested genetic counseling to Cathie and Brad.

It was a physical therapist working with Chrissy who recommended they undergo testing to take the guesswork out of what had caused their daughter's condition. As luck would have it, the local chapter of the March of Dimes Birth Defects Foundation had invited two out-of-town experts to the Van Woerts' hometown to talk about genetic testing and counseling procedures with parents of children in March of

Dimes programs. Brad and Cathie decided to give it a try. The good news came a few weeks later.

After reviewing the family's medical history and completing chromosomal analyses, the doctors told the couple that their chances of having another child with Trisomy 18 were "pretty slim—something like one-half of one percent," recalls Cathie now. "They gave us the statistics, but they never said, you should or you shouldn't become pregnant again. They left it up to us, but the message was, go ahead if you want to."

Since then, the Van Woerts have had two sons and a daughter, all normal and healthy children. During each pregnancy, Cathie underwent amniocentesis to be certain that her fetus did not have the fatal genetic defect. "I wanted to be sure," she says, because never again would she want to bring into the world another child with Trisomy 18.

What causes birth defects?

Birth defects may be inherited or may result from environmental factors—unfavorable "living conditions" for the fetus during its prenatal development. Factors contributing to this environment range from exposure to radiation and potentially dangerous pollutants to poor maternal nutrition, infections (German measles, for instance, or sexually transmitted diseases and infections), alcohol, smoking, "street" drugs, and medicines. Often both heredity and environment contribute to the problem. Sometimes, as in Chrissy Van Woert's case, the defect appears to be a spontaneous genetic "accident" and, fortunately, one not likely to recur.

When a birth defect is inherited (just as we inherit other characteristics, like blue or brown eyes, red or blond hair), the hereditary data are passed from parent to child by genes located on the chromosomes found in body cells. Normal body cells have forty-six chromosomes, except for the reproductive cells—sperm and egg—each of which has only twenty-three chromosomes. At the time of conception, each parent normally contributes twenty-three gene-carrying chromosomes to the hereditary makeup of the child. In short, genes and chromosomes are the body's blueprints for development.

But not all genetic disorders are transmitted the same way. As explained in a March of Dimes booklet on birth defects, in some cases, one affected parent has a single faulty gene which dominates its normal counterpart from the other parent. Each child then has a 50 percent chance of inheriting the faulty gene and the disorder. This is known as *dominant inheritance.* (Achondroplasia, a form of dwarfism, and polydactyly, extra fingers or toes, are two examples of such dominant disorders.) However, there is an equal chance the child will *not* receive the abnormal gene, and thus both he and his children should be free of the defect.

In other genetic disorders, both parents, seemingly normal, carry the same abnormal gene. Each of their children has a 25 percent risk of receiving that gene from both parents. This is known as *recessive inheritance.* Sickle-cell anemia and Tay-Sachs disease are transmitted this way. In still other cases, birth defects result from spontaneous genetic mutations or chromosomal deletions causing the "wrong number" of chromosomes. The resulting disorders are often identified by their chromosome number, e.g., Trisomy 18 or Trisomy 21 (Down syndrome).

Scientists hope that eventually gene therapy will make it possible to treat, and thus cure, many genetic diseases by "editing" a sick gene out of a patient's genetic code and replacing it with a healthy gene—thereby altering the afflicted person's genetic blueprint. Given the approximately three thousand genetic diseases human beings are heir to, the prospect of human gene transplants is rich in medical promise and loaded with ethical controversy.[18] But doctors are also looking at more common health ailments which may result from a chromosome's ability to react to the environment and pass along that data in a particular ethnic or familial gene pool for generations to come.

Right now, however, your best bet lies in having as much information as possible so you can make informed choices about childbearing. But remember, the genetic counselor will *not* tell you what action to take or decision to make.

"People can tell you whatever they want," says Cathie Van Woert, "but you have to be able to live with your own decision and not worry how others feel about it. I don't remember anyone who was really close to me saying you have to do this, or you have to do that—but they were around when we needed them for support. A few pediatricians seemed to have their own (negative) opinions, but you have to consider both sides, too.

"Some people just can't deal with having a child like that in the home or the physical and emotional energy it takes. You don't really think about it until after [the child dies] because you do what you have to do at the time. It is hard on everyone," she says tearfully, "but it makes you a *stronger person.*"

Resources

March of Dimes Birth Defects Foundation
1275 Mamaroneck Avenue
White Plains, NY 10605
(914) 428-7100
Contact: director of public relations

Foundation works to prevent birth defects through support for research in genetics and development of genetic counseling services at many medical centers and their surrounding areas; provides information on prenatal nutrition and related subjects. Write for two free booklets, *Genetic Counseling* and *Birth Defects: Tragedy and Hope.*

National Genetics Foundation, Inc.
555 West 57th Street
New York, NY 10019
(212) 586-5800
Contact: Genetic counselor

Nonprofit clearinghouse for information on hereditary diseases and availability of genetic counseling, testing, screening, and evaluation; offers reviews of genetic family health histories and provides access to genetic services by referrals to medical genetics centers directly or through a physician. Publications include *How Genetic Disease Can Affect Your Family; Can Genetic Counseling Help You?; For the Concerned Couple Planning a Family; Family Health History Scan;* and *Should You Consider Amniocentesis?*

National Center for Education in Maternal and Child Health
38th and R Streets, NW
Washington, DC 20057
(202) 625-8400

Publishes a guide to selected national genetic voluntary organizations ($5) and a directory of comprehensive clinical genetic-service centers (free).

Suggested reading

Bridge, Paul, and Marlys Bridge. "The Brief Life and Death of Christopher Bridge." *Hastings Center Report*, December 1981, pp. 17–19. (A dilemma in decision-making.)

Fletcher, John C. *Coping with Genetic Disorders: A Guide for Clergy and Parents.* San Francisco: Harper and Row, 1982.

Lyon, Jeff. *Playing God in the Nursery.* New York: Norton, 1985.

McCormick, Richard A., S.J. "To Save or Let Die: The Dilemma of Modern Medicine." *Journal of the American Medical Association*, July 8, 1974, p. 174.

Malcolm, Andrew H. "Baby Doe Decision: A Tentative 1st Step in a Profound Issue." *New York Times*, June 11, 1986, p. 16-A. (U.S. Supreme Court's 1986 decision is seen as a major ruling—but only one step in the long and painful development of new policies to govern society in the face of rapidly advancing medical capabilities.)

Moskop, John C., and Rita L. Saldanha. "The Baby Doe Rule: Still a Threat." *Hastings Center Report*, April 1986, pp. 8–14.

"N," Dr., as told to David R. Zimmerman. "Should This Baby Be Kept Alive...Who Can Best Decide?" *Woman's Day*, April 24, 1984, pp. 69–72.

"Prolongation of Life: Allocution to an International Congress of Anesthesiologists" on November 24, 1957, in *The Pope Speaks: The Church Documents Quarterly*, 4:393–98.

Rapp, Rayna. "The Ethics of Choice." *Ms*, April 1984, pp. 97–100. (After amniocentesis, a husband and wife face the toughest decision of their lives.)

Stinson, Robert, and Peggy Stinson. "On the Death of a Baby." *Atlantic Monthly*, July 1979, pp. 46–72.

Strong, Carson. "The Neonatologist's Duty to Patient and Parents." *Hastings Center Report*, August 1984, pp. 10–16.

Van Gelder, Lindsy. "Protect Your Unborn Child." *McCall's*, January 1986, pp. 37–44. (A no-nonsense guide to preventing birth defects and how to find out if you're at risk for hereditary diseases.)

Wallis, Claudia. "The Stormy Legacy of Baby Doe." *Time*, September 2, 1983, p. 58.

8 ❧ Who Speaks for the Child with a Disabling, Life-Threatening, or Terminal Illness?

WHEN 12-year-old Karen Ziegler's Hodgkin's disease was diagnosed in August 1983, her doctors in San Diego recommended conventional therapy of x-ray, surgery, and chemotherapy. When Hodgkin's disease is treated in its early stages, as her disease then was, the five-year survival rate exceeds 90 percent. When it is untreated, death usually occurs within eighteen months to two years, and only the rare child survives for five years without treatment.

But Karen's parents, worried about possible side effects, decided against conventional therapy for her. Instead, the Zieglers took their daughter to the Hoxsey Clinic in Tijuana, Mexico, where she was placed on a special diet and given vitamins and the so-called Hoxsey herb treatment. The California doctor who first diagnosed Karen's disease then reported the Zieglers to the San Diego Welfare Department for child neglect.

By this time, the family had moved to Nevada, where naturopathy was, at the time, legal, and enrolled Karen in a local Reno school. Within a few months, the charges of child neglect caught up with the Zieglers. What happened next resulted in a case the district attorney would later call "ripe for misunderstanding."[1]

"Gestapo tactics"—or child protection?

Fearing the Zieglers might again flee with their daughter, the Washoe County Social Services Department obtained a court order and—without warning—took Karen out of school at 2:00 p.m. on Tuesday, February 14, using what some critics called Gestapo-like tactics.[2] For three days, the girl was kept in a foster home; at no time was she allowed to see or talk to her parents.

On Friday of that week, she was permitted a brief visit with her mother and father following a district court hearing in which the judge refused to return Karen to her parents' custody and ordered further medical evaluation of her condition.

New medical tests showed her disease had progressed to Stage III, involving both her lungs and liver. Again, conventional therapy was recommended. Again, the Zieglers refused to subject their daughter to its risks. The media picked up the story. People watched Karen on television and heard her parents plea for the right to do what they thought best for their child. Letters to the editors followed newspaper headlines like "DA: Return Cancer Victim to Parents," "County Says It's Trying to Protect Cancer Victim," and "Judicial Experts Wrestle with Weighty Issues."

After 10 days of legal battles and more medical testing and public debate, the case was heard in district court. By now, the district attorney had changed his original position (some said politics played a role) and supported the Zieglers' right to decide which treatment would be in Karen's best interest.[3] He used as legal precedent the New York case of 8-year-old

Joseph Hofbauer. (In 1978, the New York court of appeals decided *not* to interfere with Joseph's parents' decision to have their son's Hodgkin's disease treated with laetrile, nutrition, and metabolic therapy by a physician licensed in New York.)

Who speaks for the child?

District Court Judge Richard Minor returned Karen to her family. He did not order her to undergo therapy. But in his ruling, he said to the Zieglers: "You are facing an awesome decision to subject Karen to the unpleasant, painful, and possibly crippling effects of radiation and chemotherapy...or you may see her die. I would advise you to let your doctor tell you when the time has come...to change treatment to keep Karen alive. I certainly tell you that I am not qualified to make that decision and frankly, I don't think you are either...."[4]

Within sixteen months, Karen was dead. Three days before she died, the attorney who earlier had represented the Zieglers' right to make treatment decisions for their daughter resigned from the case and asked the court to intervene in Karen's care to save her life. It was too late.

In *Who Speaks for the Child?* psychiatrist Willard Gaylin, who coedited the book with Ruth Macklin, acknowledges that no issue presents as anguished a conflict as that of proxy consent.

"If we examine those values that have a high priority in our present culture," Gaylin says, "certainly we would list life itself; the family; health...certain aspects of autonomy, dignity and privacy. The problems of proxy consent in terms of the child ask us to balance these respected rights against each other.... there is no conclusion that is worthy of adopting that *will* not lead to distress." But Gaylin cautions that whatever conclusions are reached must always be tentative, continually reexamined, and "receptive to immediate modification."[5]

That, of course, did not happen in Karen's case, which illustrates the strong feelings that such treatment dilemmas often generate. Many judges would not have agreed with the decision in the Ziegler case, even in states where laetrile and naturopathy are legal. Neither would bioethicists line up wholeheartedly behind the decision. Many also believe that the New York court of appeals decision in the Hofbauer case was wrong.[6]

In both instances, the Hofbauer and Ziegler parents told the court they would consider conventional treatment if the alternative therapies were not effective in arresting their child's disease. In arguing the Nevada case, the district attorney never mentioned the fact that Joseph died at age 10 in the Bahamas because his parents—despite their promise to the court two years earlier—continued to deny their child conventional treatment to the end.

If your child is diagnosed as having a life-threatening illness or a condition that is severely disabling—physically or mentally—you will be asked to make some of the most difficult decisions a parent ever has to make.[7] You'll need to consider what kind of treatment, if any, is best for your child, where to go for expert opinions and recommended treatment, how to pay for it all, and what to tell your child as well as family, friends, and relatives.

Most likely, at this point, you'll feel numb, scared, sad, and worried about making medical decisions for your child, and concerned about the impact those decisions will have on your family. (If your child can understand what it means to be seriously ill or disabled, then he or she should be included in making decisions. Even if your doctor is reluctant to do so, encourage your child to participate. Many experts believe children as young as 6 years are able to understand what it means to be seriously ill and to die.)

Three important things to remember:

- You must have complete and *up-to-date* information to make good medical and ethical decisions for your child and family. (Proper diagnosis calls for a careful evaluation of your child's medical history, physical examination, x-rays, and blood and other laboratory tests.)

- You can use the same legal and ethical reasoning put forth by the courts or bioethical experts in cases similar to yours to help you and your family in making hard choices and arguing your own position—whatever it is.

- You are not alone. There are experts, organizations, and self-help groups that can help you make those stressful decisions and be supportive along the way. (See Resources section at the end of this chapter and Appendix J.)

It's natural to hope your child's life-threatening illness or disability will go away by itself or improve without treatment. Certainly this dream tops every parent's wish list. While it's rare that this happens, it's not unheard of in medicine. In fact, it's one of the questions you'll want your child's doctor to answer for you. What are the chances this disease will go away by itself *without any treatment?* You have a right to know.

Waiting can be disastrous

But if you suspect your child's mental or physical development is delayed, or that he has a learning disability or shows signs of severe emotional disturbance, don't wait. As one mother whose daughter is mentally retarded puts it: "Parents should realize that the word *wait* is disaster."[8]

Don't be put off by your doctor's reassurance that "he'll outgrow it" or "she's just a little slow for her age—she'll catch up." I've seen too many cases of unnecessary delays in getting infants and children appropriate help. Irving Dickman writes in *One Miracle at a Time,* "Early intervention won't make every child born with a disability progress 'normally,' but delaying such help is an almost certain guarantee that the disabled boy or girl will fall further behind needlessly."[9]

The first step is to get all the information you can from

your child's doctor. And don't hesitate to get second opinions from consultants who are experts in child development, neurology, and genetics. Some doctors are better than others in communicating bad news and explaining what's happened to your child. Almost always, when parents first learn their child is seriously ill or has a disability, they are in a state of shock and disbelief.

"I can't believe it—are you sure?" they ask. Feelings of anger and guilt often follow. "Why *my* child? Was it the wrong diet? An infection? Something we did or didn't do?"

As you work through the stages of shock and realize that indeed your child has a serious illness or disability, you should try to learn as much as possible about the disorder and its probable outcome. Here is a basic list of questions you'll need answers to. Being unaware of them may give you a false sense of security and may seriously affect your ability to make the *right* decision for your child.

QUESTIONS TO ASK YOUR CHILD'S DOCTOR

About the illness or condition:

1. What is this condition/disease?
2. How will it affect my child?
3. How serious is it?
4. How is the diagnosis made?
5. Are you sure of the diagnosis?
6. Should the test(s) be repeated? Sent to another lab?
7. Shouldn't we get a second opinion?
8. Will my child be in pain?
9. Will my child die?
10. How long will my child live?
11. What disabilities will my child have? (Will he or she be deaf, blind, mentally retarded, confined to a wheelchair?)
12. How will my child's growth and development be affected?
13. What kind of life will my child be able to live? Will my child live a *normal* life until he or she dies?

About assessing your child's development:

1. Is my child normal?
2. Why isn't he or she doing what others the same age are doing?
3. Where can I take my child for a complete evaluation?
4. Should my child be in an early intervention or infant stimulation program?
5. Is it likely my child will be physically or mentally disabled?
6. Is my child too young to test? (If you get a "yes" to this question, look for another doctor. No child is ever too young to evaluate!)
7. What tests will be done? Are they painful or risky?
8. Who does the testing? (Your child may be seen by a number of specialists, such as psychologists, physical therapists, speech pathologists, audiologists, etc.)
9. Who pays for the diagnostic evaluation—insurance, the government, or I?

About your child and family:

1. What's the best way to discuss the disease (or condition) and treatment with my child?
2. What should I tell family, friends, and relatives?
3. Can my child understand what's going on?
4. Is my child able to make his or her *own* decision about treatment?
5. How soon must we decide what to do? Is it an emergency?
6. What effect will my child's illness (or condition) and treatment have on the rest of the family?
7. What effect will stress or other illnesses have on my child and the disease or condition?

About those who can help:

1. Are there other families with similar problems whom we can talk to?
2. What self-help groups are in our area?
3. Are there groups or organizations that help families like ours to meet hospital bills and other costs?

Four treatment options

Depending on your child's condition and its prognosis, your values, and what doctors have recommended, you have four options open to you in medically treating your child: conventional treatment, experimental treatment, alternative treatment—or no treatment at all. Most of the rest of this chapter examines the pros and cons of each.

Conventional therapy

Think of conventional treatment as state-of-the-art therapy. In other words, it's the best treatment that modern medicine now has to offer for a given disorder. It's the most accepted method of treating the illness based on scientific evidence, experience of experts in the field, the best cure or survival rates, and broad medical experience with treating hundreds and often thousands of similar cases. While it may be far from perfect, it's considered the best we've got today.

When talking with parents of children with cancer, I explain what terms like "remission," "survival rates," "cure," "palliative care," and "medical neglect" mean. For example:

· *A five-year survival rate* is based on the percentage of children alive five years after the diagnosis of cancer was confirmed.

- *Remission* refers to the temporary abatement of a disease or an easing of the symptoms to such a degree that the usual physical signs and x-ray or laboratory evidence of the disease are gone or no longer discernible.
- *Cure* is a word many doctors hesitate to use in talking about cancers, preferring instead to talk of "survival advantage." However, there are many instances in which cancer is *truly cured*, and by that is meant that the body is restored to a sound or healthy condition through the permanent removal of all evidence of the disease.
- *Supportive (palliative) care* is designed to relieve the symptoms or effects of a disease or condition, but not to cure it.
- *Medical neglect* is the withholding or withdrawing of acceptable treatment for life-threatening situations but also may include denial of appropriate diagnostic tests for the child.

I say to parents, "What I am recommending appears to be the best available treatment. It's what's recommended at the major medical centers around the country where many children such as yours are treated. If it were my child, I would follow such recommendations for conventional therapy."

It's rare, at least at the onset of a life-threatening illness, for parents to decide against treatment. However, don't make your decision until you have asked the following questions of your child's doctor and other knowledgeable people, and received answers you're comfortable with.

Questions about conventional treatment

1. What's involved in the conventional method of treatment?
2. How long does such treatment take?
3. What are the reasons for surgery or radiation or chemotherapy?
4. What are the benefits? the risks?
5. What are the chances for cure or remission?
6. Are there side effects? How serious are they?

7. How long will these side effects last? When will they go away?
8. How many patients have you treated with this condition?
9. Can treatment be carried out on an outpatient basis or must my child be hospitalized?
10. Should I take my child to a large medical center that specializes in such treatment?
11. How much does it cost?

Experimental treatment

Although it sounds risky, experimental therapy can be the way to go when there is no adequate conventional therapy or when the experts disagree about the best treatment for the illness.

Look at it this way. Many of today's conventional therapies were yesterday's medical experiments. There are few diseases for which the ultimate treatment has been determined. That's why physicians and scientists are constantly searching for new and better ways to treat most every disease. Your child may be the one who benefits from today's experimental therapy destined to become the accepted treatment in the future. You should ask the same questions of a doctor treating your child by experimental methods that you would ask of the doctor treating your child conventionally.

The "Baby Fae" transplant

Consider the celebrated case of Baby Fae, the anonymous five-pound infant who made history by living for more than a week with an animal-heart transplant. She had been born with a congenital defect known as hypoplastic left heart syndrome, in which the left side of the heart is much less developed than the right, and from which she almost died on the sixth day of life.

239

A week later, Dr. Leonard Bailey of Loma Linda University Medical Center replaced her defective organ with the heart of a young female baboon, because, according to hospital officials, no compatible human heart was available for transplant. (Bailey would later admit he never tried to find a human donor before performing the baboon transplant and didn't seek a human heart "replacement" until one week after the surgery.)[10]

Baby Fae died twenty days later from kidney failure and other complications related to her body's rejection of the transplanted organ. By then, the bold baboon-to-human heart swap had stirred medical controversy—with supporters hailing it as a breakthrough transplant in newborns and critics arguing the time for organ transplants which cross species (xenographs) had not yet come. Although a few animal-to-human transplants had been performed on adults, all had failed.

Troubling ethical issues

Medical and ethical experts focused on the timing of the transplant, the publicity surrounding it, and questions related to the giving of informed consent by Baby Fae's mother. Did she know what her baby was getting into? Was it proper for the infant to be used as a human subject when the scientific basis for such an experiment was minimal? Were alternative surgical procedures fully considered? Should such an experiment be done on a child until proved successful in an adult first?

Defending his position in an *American Medical News* interview, Dr. Bailey maintained that such debate is a "luxury" for the surgeon who's dealing with the dying baby and must act.[11] Many surgeons support Bailey. They point out that in the United States each year some three hundred to five hundred infants are born with the same fatal condition as Baby Fae. And the only alternatives doctors can offer are a human heart transplant (and there are only a handful of donor organs available each year) and surgery to gain time until a donor heart is available, such as the Norwood procedure, which has a 50 percent mortality rate.

Although the likelihood of your child's ever needing this type of surgery is almost nil, it's helpful to look at what critics claimed were "shortcomings" in the Baby Fae consent process, because the potential for similar problems exists every time a parent is asked to consent to an experimental treatment for his or her child.

Flaws in the Baby Fae consent procedure

In its review of the Baby Fae case, the National Institutes of Health (NIH) concluded that "the parents were given an appropriate and thorough explanation of the alternatives available, the risks and benefits of the procedure and the experimental nature of the transplant." The NIH investigators were also convinced that this information had been presented in an "atmosphere which allowed the parents an opportunity to carefully consider, without coercion or undue influence, whether to give permission for the transplant."[12]

However, the review team noted three "shortcomings" in the informed consent procedure the surgeons used:

First, there was no "explanation as to whether compensation and medical treatment was available if injury occurred, and if so, what they consisted of, or where further information could be obtained."

Second, expected benefits of the procedure "appeared to have been overstated—the document had stated specifically that 'long-term survival' is an expected possibility with no further explanation" and, indeed, with no scientific evidence to support such optimism.

Finally, NIH visitors noted that the research procedure followed by the surgical team did not include the possibility of searching for a human donor organ, or performing a human heart transplant either at Loma Linda Hospital or another medical center if a donor organ had become available. The consent document simply stated, "Since sizematched human hearts are not available we recommend the use of an immature primate donor heart."

In a *Journal of the American Medical Association* editorial commenting on the case several months later, two experts acknowledged Bailey's "remarkable experiment" and noted that in the future xenographs might be suitable as "short-term support for the circulation of a newborn with fatal congenital heart disease until a human donor can be found."[13]

Baby Moses—a different story

In late 1985, critics of Dr. Bailey's baboon-heart transplant in Baby Fae applauded his newborn-to-newborn heart transplant, which made an infant known as Baby Moses the longest-living survivor of such surgery. Few details are known, but apparently the world's third infant-heart recipient was born with the same fatal defect as Baby Fae and underwent a donor heart transplant when only four days old. Six weeks later, his delighted parents took their son home in good condition, with no signs of infection or rejection of his new heart.

Both Baby Fae and Moses were involved in experimental procedures. But as ethicists point out, the problem in Baby Fae's case was volunteering an infant in an experiment that lacked sufficient justification—especially since animal hearts had been shown to have a high potential to be rejected in adults. The odds of a good prognosis for Baby Moses were much greater because several hundred adult human heart transplants had already succeeded.

But Baby Moses's successful transplant sharply focuses our attention on the acute shortage of infant heart donors—and the plight of similar babies, most of whom will die unless they receive new hearts. Lucky timing saved Baby Moses. If no human donor heart is available, however, parents face a difficult question: Is it *fair* to our baby to try to "buy" time however we can?

Nationally syndicated columnist Ellen Goodman would answer no: "Those who cannot give consent should be the last, not the first, people we use for experiments."[14] And I agree.

But I also believe there may be some valid reasons for entering your child in a research program as long as there is sound experimental evidence in animals and in adult human beings that the proposed treatment has a reasonable chance of benefiting your infant or child.

What to look for in giving consent

If your child has a fatal or severely disabling illness or condition, and it's recommended you participate in a research program which is so new there is not yet enough data to evaluate the true risks and benefits in humans, go into it with your eyes open. (See Chapter 3 for guidelines for evaluating a research program.)

Remember, there's a big difference between a *therapeutic* procedure or treatment and an *experimental* one. The therapeutic procedure has been thoroughly tested over time—first in animals, then in humans. It has been critically reviewed by independent groups and researchers, and found to be of more value than other recommended treatments, no treatment at all, or a placebo.

The experimental procedure, of course, is unproven. Risks often seem to outweigh potential benefits. Should your child be entered into an experimental program which may not save his life or help him directly, but may help *other children* in the future? And if your child is capable of participating in this type of decision, how does he or she feel about taking part in an experimental procedure which may be of little or no personal benefit?

In deciding whether experimental therapy is right for your child, you'll need information about programs, costs and who's eligible for such treatment.

Questions to ask about experimental treatment for your child

1. What new research methods are available for treating my child's condition?

2. Why should my child participate in this research program?

3. Will there be any benefit to *my* child, or is this primarily a research project to obtain new information which might help *other* children in the future?

4. What are the risks to my child? Will he or she die sooner, or be in more pain or discomfort?

5. Will we be free to withdraw our child from the research program at any time that either we or our child wants out? (If the answer is "no," don't enter your child in the experimental program!)

6. Do some researchers have more experience than others in using this experimental approach?

7. How can we contact these researchers for a second opinion and advice on whether to put our child in an experimental program?

8. Will taking part in the program require travel to another medical center? Will we have to live away from home or move to a new area?

9. Who pays for the care of my child in this experimental program—the government, a foundation, the researchers, or our insurance company? Do we pay anything?

Some parents feel new medical procedures and experimental approaches are worth a try if the results of conventional therapy aren't good. Other parents refuse to put their children in experimental treatment programs and stick with conventional therapy to the end. Still other parents decide that if their only hope is an experimental program, they would rather treat their child with diet, herbs, and other alternative methods, even if it means going to a foreign country to obtain them.

Alternative treatment

Although there may be a number of conventional and experimental treatments to choose from in treating your child, you may have reasons for not wanting to subject your child to any of them. You don't want to reject *all* treatment. Neither do you want to expose your child to conventional treatment because of its risks or to experimental programs because the benefits haven't been proven.

You've heard about alternative therapies—especially in cancer cases—such as naturalistic healing, prayer, acupuncture, laetrile,[15] herbal medicines, diet, coffee enemas, and other therapies which often are played up in the media. You may want your child to try these methods first, or to combine them with conventional therapies later on. You should be aware, however, that the *time factor is extremely important—especially in treating children with cancer*. If you wait too long to begin accepted therapy, you may jeopardize your child's chances of a cure—or even of arresting the course of the disease.

Questions to ask your doctors about alternative therapies

1. What alternative methods of treatment are available?
2. What are the benefits and risks of these methods?
3. What are the chances of cure or remission if we choose one of these methods?
4. Will one enhance or inhibit the benefits of the other?
5. Will you continue to see my child even if we seek alternative treatment elsewhere?
6. Will you refer us to an expert in alternative treatment methods?

You'll find it's the rare physician who will encourage you to even consider alternative therapies for your child. However, it's not unusual for patients with cancer or their families, under pressure from well-meaning friends, relatives, or coworkers, to try any and every cure—to seek out unorthodox cancer treatments. An M. D. Anderson Cancer Center study found that 39 percent of children with cancer had "tried," considered, or received recommendations to try unproven remedies.[16]

Most doctors would argue that the option for alternative treatment shouldn't even be presented in a book like this because of the possible harmful side effects of unproven methods. But I believe that parents have the right to know what's involved if they choose to forgo recommended conventional treatment for their child and decide instead to try an alternative method, as did the families of Karen Ziegler and Joseph Hofbauer, whose stories begin this chapter.

Basic ethical issues at stake

Some basic ethical issues are involved in cases like the Zieglers' and Hofbauers'. You may be faced with the same issues, which range from medical neglect of children and the right of the state to intervene in parental decisions to criteria for determining when minor children are competent to speak for themselves and who has the final say in deciding what's in a child's best interests if he or she is not competent to choose.

It is possible that you as the child's parent may *not* have the final say. It has happened before in cases where society, through the court system, has determined that a parent's health-related decision was harmful to the child, or potentially harmful. Here's what you should know to protect your interests and those of your child.

Your rights as a parent

History, culture, and much case law and opinion support the fundamental American tradition of recognizing parents' rights and responsibility to make health care decisions for their children. Almost always, and with few exceptions, the family's right to privacy—as guaranteed by the Fourteenth Amendment—should not be violated. This notion of parental autonomy goes back to Roman times when the *paterfamilias* exercised absolute authority over members of his household.

Through the centuries, however, the law has recognized limits to *total* parental authority.

When a parent's decision doesn't seem to be in the child's best interest, society objects and attempts to intervene. Child abuse and neglect laws in all fifty states are based on the notion that there are times when parents' decisions and actions are harmful to their children.

Where does that leave you when you're a well-meaning, loving, conscientious parent who believes your decision is the best for your child? Who else understands your child better than you do?

First of all, the U.S. Supreme Court in *Prince* v. *Massachusetts* (1944) stated that "parents are free to become martyrs themselves but it does not follow they are free...to make martyrs of their children."[17]

For example, in the famous 1974 Jehovah's Witness case *In re Pogue*, District of Columbia Superior Court Judge Murphy made the distinction between being an adult and being a child when it comes to medical choices.[18] He declined to order a blood transfusion for a mother who was dying, but did order it for her infant—despite the mother's refusal on religious grounds to consent to blood transfusions for either herself or her child. In doing so, the judge allowed the woman to make a decision for herself, but not for her baby.

When states should—and should not— intervene

Most experts agree the state has a right to intervene and to overrule a parent's decision not to treat his child when the following criteria, proposed by Yale professor Joseph Goldstein, are met: (1) the medical profession agrees on the most appropriate treatment for the child; (2) to deny the recommended treatment means death for the child; and (3) the expected outcome of that treatment is what society agrees to be right for any child—a chance for normal healthy growth toward adulthood, or a life worth living.[19]

On the contrary, most experts contend the state has no right to intrude on parental decision-making when: (1) there is no proven medical treatment for the child's condition; (2) when parents are confronted with conflicting medical advice as to the best treatment; and (3) when there is very low probability that such treatment will allow the child to live a life worth living or to grow to normal adulthood.

Clearly, risk-benefit analysis plays an important role in the way doctors arrive at recommended treatment. The courts and biomedical ethicists use a similar analysis in deciding whether or not to support parents' health care decisions for their children—especially if a parent refuses recommended treatment in a life-threatening situation.

Before it gets to that point and hefty legal fees, you need to know how medical risks are weighed in relation to potential benefits of treatment—or no treatment at all. You need to know when the state or an ethics committee is likely to support your decision or step in to overrule it and order therapy for your child. You don't always *have* the right to decide.

The following chart* gives examples of common situations in which a parent's right to make a medical decision for a child is either supported or overruled.

Evidence is that...	Right of parent to decide is...
there is significant controversy about what treatment is in child's best interest.	supported and upheld.

*Adapted from Joseph Goldstein, "Medical Care for the Child at Risk," in Willard Gaylin and Ruth Macklin, eds., *Who Speaks for the Child: The Problems of Proxy Consent* (New York: Plenum, 1982).

the treatment means life for the child, even with moderate discomfort, pain or disability.	overruled if parent decides against treatment.
benefits and risks of treatment are balanced.	usually supported and upheld.
state law permits the proposed treatment.	supported and upheld.
state law prohibits the proposed treatment.	overruled and treatment prohibited.
proposed treatment is worthless, dangerous,unproven, or experimental.	sometimes overruled, depending on strength of expert testimony.

A second look at the Karen Ziegler case

Using these examples and Goldstein's criteria for state intervention, I think Karen Ziegler's case was bungled. I believe the case was clouded by so many emotional issues that her best interests were *not* served—either medically *or* ethically —despite the well-meaning judge, district attorney, welfare department, doctors, lawyers, and her own parents. Here's why.

First of all, the court could have ordered Karen examined by medical experts while she remained at home and in school. All it would have taken was a court order requiring the family to remain in the county. This would have eliminated the public outcry over the "kidnapping" of Karen by the welfare department and violation of her rights.

(From the start, if Karen had been under the care of a licensed physician, homeopath, or naturopath in Nevada, and if originally she had been taking laetrile, which she began later on, the district attorney wouldn't have instituted action against the Zieglers for medical child neglect. Simply put, he wouldn't have had a case. Laetrile is legal in the state, as are acupuncture and homeopathy. The Hoxsey treatment is illegal in Nevada as is naturopathy which was repealed by the Nevada state legislature in 1987.)

With Karen in her own home, pressure would have been off the judge to make a quick decision. More time for proper legal, medical, and ethical research would have uncovered details of the Hofbauer case and other similar ones, such as the Chad Greene and Phillip Becker cases, where treatment *was* ordered by the court.[20] Expert testimony from regional and national authorities in bioethics and in the treatment of Hodgkin's disease in children would have helped the court in assessing the benefits and risks of conventional versus alternative therapies.

As it was, neither Judge Minor nor the district attorney knew young Joseph Hofbauer had died while undergoing alternative therapy. Using the Hofbauer case as a precedent for supporting the Zieglers' decision to treat Karen with the Hoxsey tonic seems to have been an error.

The issue of Karen's right to decide for herself as a potentially competent minor was never explored. Psychologists, psychiatrists, and the judge could have talked to her to determine if she met—even minimally—the criteria for competency. Although Karen's attorney pleaded with Judge Minor to allow her to testify, he declined, claiming he already knew what she would say and that he was "most reluctant to subject a 12-year-old to the trauma."[21]

The only way anyone knew what Karen was thinking was through her mother's statements regarding Karen's wishes for alternative therapy and a comment Karen made to the press that she didn't want surgery and preferred her usual treatment because it didn't have side effects. I think Karen deserved a chance to speak on her own behalf.

What it boils down to is that the public furor over "kidnapping" the girl from school clouded the issues of what would be best for her. In the rush to return Karen to her parents (which everyone agreed was top priority), the court cut short its inquiry into apparent risks and benefits of various therapies. If expert testimony had been sought, and if the emotional fervor over parental rights had been kept in perspective, then I think the medical evidence would have tipped the balance in favor of ordering conventional treatment.

No doubt about it, if Karen were our daughter, we would have wanted her back home at once just as the Zieglers wanted Karen returned to them. But statistically, with a 90 percent five-year-survival rate in her favor, we'd have opted to treat her with conventional therapy.

We'd want our daughter to have every chance to grow up a normal healthy adult. We'd understand her fear of possible side effects; we'd be scared of them ourselves. But we'd help our child understand the importance of taking those risks in *this* case for the greater benefit of life and a life worth living. If, however, our daughter was judged competent to make her own medical decision—and her choice was *not* to undergo such therapy—we would still try to persuade her otherwise; but ultimately, we would respect her decision.

Karen Ziegler continued to undergo treatment at a naturopathic center in Reno and at a holistic medical center in Tijuana, Mexico. Cancer specialists familiar with the girl's case predicted that without conventional treatment, the disease would be fatal. Karen died at San Diego's Children's Hospital from an intestinal hemorrhage on Christmas Day, 1984—sixteen months after her illness was diagnosed as Hodgkin's disease. In a tearful newspaper interview, her mother said Karen had grown so weary of her family's struggle over her unorthodox cancer therapy that "she lost the will to live."[22]

"The real tragedy [of people seeking unproven treatment] is dealing with cancers that are curable—like Karen's," says Dr. John Shields, the oncologist who examined her and testified at the court hearing in favor of chemotherapy and radiation. "These patients waste precious time, and then, when their cancer is advanced, they go to the hospital and we end up having to take care of them when there's no longer anything anyone can do."[23]

HOW TO SPOT POSSIBLE HEALTH FRAUD AND QUACKERY

Here are guidelines for spotting health fraud compiled by Emory University history professor James Harvey Young, who has studied and written about the field for more than thirty years:

1. Exploitation of fear
2. Promise of painless treatment and good results
3. Claims of a miraculous scientific breakthrough
4. Simpleton science: disease has but one cause, and one treatment is all that is needed to fight it. For example, bad nutrition causes all disease; good nutrition cures it.
5. The "Galileo ploy": like Galileo, we cult gurus are misunderstood by blind scientists, but are destined to be heroes to future generations
6. The conspiracy theory, also known as "The establishment is out to get us"
7. The moving target: shifts in theory to adjust to circumstances. Laetrile went from drug to "vitamin," from cure to palliative to preventive, from low to high dosages, from working alone to never working alone, from one chemical formula to another, and so forth. "B-15" ("pangamate") is any chemical or combination of chemicals the seller chooses to put in the bottle.
8. Reliance on anecdotes and testimonials. They don't separate fact from fiction, or cause and effect from coincidence.
9. Distortion of the idea of "freedom." By distorting "freedom of informed choice" to "freedom of choice," snake-oil salesmen acquire freedom to defraud, and their victims can lose their money, their health, and their lives.
10. Large sums of money

Adapted from guidelines presented at an American Association for the Advancement of Science panel on laetrile. The complete version is found in Gerald E. Markle and James C. Peterson, eds., *Politics, Science and Cancer: The Laetrile Phenomenon* (Boulder, Colo.: Westview, 1980).

Health fraud and quackery

No parent wants to jeopardize his or her child's chances of a cure. But when the child's life is at stake and the pressure is on to "do something" and not leave a stone unturned, it may be tempting to try the unproven treatment—either in addition to or instead of the treatment your child's doctor recommends.

Not all alternative treatments are harmful. But many are —either because they are inherently dangerous (e.g., highly toxic drugs) or because they promise cures they cannot deliver, cost a fortune, and distract patients from getting proper care. Health quackery is big business, and typically such fraud relies on several common elements which you can quickly learn to spot, using the accompanying list of tips.

Your child's right to decide

Many physicians, parents, and attorneys feel that a "child is just a child" and is unable to understand the consequences of his or her decisions when it comes to health care.

Consider the case of 12-year-old "Peter F." Physicians at a university medical center had examined the Little League catcher and recommended amputation of his leg because of bone cancer. But Peter, whose dream was to become a professional baseball player, begged his parents and doctors to let him keep his leg.

Traditionally, parents make all such medical decisions for children like Peter based on the doctor's advice. But today attitudes of both doctors and parents are changing—and children's *assent* to treatment or nontreatment is sought more and more often, especially from children who have life-threatening illnesses. (Although it is a less rigorous concept than informed consent, psychologist Lois Weithorn explains that *assent* requires that the child appreciate the nature, extent, and probable consequences of undergoing a treatment or participating in a study.)[24]

In Peter's case, his parents supported his wishes. They agreed to experimental treatment which included chemotherapy and surgery to remove the tumor and replace lost bone with transplants. They didn't rule out amputation at a later date, but told doctors their son deserved a chance at less radical therapy first.

A study from Oklahoma Children's Memorial Hospital showed that children older than 5 years with cancer "comprehended the finality of death and were able to make rational decisions about continuing their cancer therapy. Most children who selected supportive (not curative) care tolerated the knowledge of their impending death... and severe depression and behavioral problems were rare."[25]

Although you may find it hard to think of your 9- or 10-year-old as competent to take part in decision-making, many experts agree that such participation enhances communication in the family and improves the ability of the child to cope with serious illness.

When is a child competent to make medical decisions?

No one knows for sure when a child is competent to make medical decisions for himself or herself. But there are guidelines. The key is to evaluate each child individually, since children vary widely in their emotional and intellectual development and their ability to think logically.

Generally speaking, there are four conditions which must be met for a child to be deemed competent: the abilities to understand, to reason, to communicate, and to give voluntary consent.[26]

Understanding. According to the late Swiss psychologist Jean Piaget and other developmental psychologists, children between the ages of 7 and 10 can begin to differentiate between themselves and others and to look at the causes of illness as external to their own body. At about 11 years, Pia-

254

get claimed, children begin to understand not only the nature of different treatments but also that there may be multiple causes for an illness. They begin to understand risks and benefits and to sort out options. They become aware that their own thoughts and feelings can affect body functions.[27]

In other words, understanding in this context includes an ability to form concepts, the capacity for intelligence, and some knowledge or information about the situation or illness. The severely retarded child, for example, is not competent to make important health decisions by the very nature of his limited intelligence.

Reasoning. No one agrees on the age at which the ability to reason begins. But psychologists say children between 9 and 14 begin to think and express themselves logically and rationally and can begin to understand and express their treatment preferences and look at relevant treatment options.

According to Sanford Leiken, a pediatric oncologist at Children's Hospital in Washington, D.C., children less than 10 years of age usually are not competent to make their own medical decisions. New York psychiatrist Willard Gaylin, an expert in patients' rights, further spells out some of these limits: "The child is not competent either because he has not reached the age of communication or . . . his perception of his world and his place in it, or his grasp of the problems and their implications is too limited."[28]

Communicating. To be considered competent to give informed consent, a child must be able to express his thoughts and desires in a way which others can understand. Obviously, the child who hasn't reached the age of developing expressive language or who is unconscious or severely retarded is totally incompetent.

Volunteering. To give informed consent freely, a child must be free of coercion and pressure and understand what he or she is being asked to do and why, based on the child's perception of what's right for him or her—and not for someone else. This is hard to do for most children. Studies indicate that before the age of 14, most children are unlikely to assert themselves against authority figures such as doctors or parents.

Minors 14 years or older are more likely to believe they are in control of their health or illness outcomes. "Therefore," says Dr. Leiken, "it would appear unlikely that a minor under 14 years of age, particularly one who is ill, will dissent in the presence of parents who have already agreed to a proposed treatment."[29]

Children mature at different rates and different ages. Some are quite capable at young ages to actively take part in medical decision-making and give *assent* to treatment. Studies show that children as young as 6 who have been in cancer treatment programs can participate actively in the decision to continue that therapy or to stop it. Certainly these children are among the world's most sophisticated young patients.

When you and your child are faced with a diagnostic or treatment dilemma—especially when the disease is potentially life-threatening—make every effort to include your child in the decision-making process. In most instances, you and your child will decide on some form of treatment.

But there are many times when caring, comforting, and relief of pain are the best and *only* treatment.

No treatment—let nature take its course

In some medical situations, the parents of a child have the option of saying, "I don't want my child treated at all. I'm going to take him home and let nature take its course. If he dies, so be it—it's God's will, nature's way."

This is an approach parents frequently take when the child's case appears hopeless and there's nothing more modern medicine can offer the child, no reasonable experimental drug or treatment, only palliative care geared to making the child comfortable for as much time as he or she has left.

In addition, some parents choose to reject any or all medical treatment for their child on religious grounds regardless of the alleged benefits the treatment may have for the child. For example, they may prefer to try prayer, meditation, visualization or other forms of faith healing. Jehovah's Witnesses generally reject blood transfusions for themselves and their children, and Christian Scientists often reject all medical treatment.

In such instances, parents may subject themselves to state intervention on the basis of medical neglect of their children when it can be shown that the benefits of conventional medical therapy far outweigh the risks of not treating the child. Two landmark cases which have set the precedents for medical neglect of children on religious grounds are *Prince* v. *Massachusetts* and *In re Pogue* as discussed on page 247.

Children's hospices—help when you most need it

Children who are dying need a place to die that's warm, caring, and comfortable, and where their medical needs can be met. And most parents of dying children want to be involved in their child's care and have some control over it. In a hospital setting, doctors are in control; in your own home, you are.

Your child's doctor may suggest that you take him home and let him do as much as he wants to do or feels like doing. Or you may bring up the subject yourself. Many times, it's the child who says, "No more of this—I want to go home."

The idea of caring for your child at home, however, may be frightening. You don't want to let your child down, but the "what ifs" that could happen—ranging from hemorrhaging to choking or worse—are problems you aren't prepared to deal with. Take heart. If your community doesn't already have a hospice program for children, Children's Hospice International (CHI), a clearinghouse for such information, can put you in touch with the kind of professional support and volunteer help you need.

"Hospices," explains CHI executive director Ann Dailey, "can provide that place. The goal isn't to have a home death for everyone, but rather to improve the quality of the remaining life with as few of the trappings of hospital care as possible and help the relatives deal with the impending death. A hospice isn't for everyone, but for those who use them, the benefits are tremendous."

Currently there are nearly 1,500 hospice programs in the United States; however, a recent survey showed only about three hundred are willing to admit children.[30] "Some of these programs are housed in hospitals and others in separate facilities," explains Dailey. "But since hospice is basically a *concept of care*, it can actually take place anywhere—whether it's in a Ronald McDonald House or the intensive care unit or your own home." (The more than sixty Ronald McDonald Houses around the country provide temporary homes near major medical centers and hospitals for parents of children who are undergoing treatment.)

In a hospice setting, for example, you provide all your child's essential day-to-day care, which is geared toward comfort rather than cure. Although ideally your child's doctor should remain involved in this care, not all do.

But helping you every step of the way is a hospice team, which may include, but isn't limited to, a consulting doctor, an in-home nurse, a social worker, clergy, and often various therapists and specially trained volunteers—who run errands, do housework, baby-sit siblings, or spell parents so they can get some badly needed sleep. "Emphasis," Dailey says, "is on those kinds of things which can free up the family so they can spend as much time as possible with their child."

For some families, a highlight of this time is a trip to Disneyland, special out-of-season graduation ceremonies, a day at the beach, or box seats at a special sports or artistic event arranged through the Make-a-Wish Foundation or other non-profit groups listed at the end of this chapter, whose purpose is granting wishes for children who are terminally ill.

Should children be told?

Today, there is strong evidence—not only in theory but in practice—that families who try to protect dying children from knowing they're dying rarely serve the child's best interests. This conspiracy of silence, however well-meaning, often puts nurses, relatives, and others who spend the most time with the patient, especially in their lonely moments, on the spot.

"Nobody's talking to me"

Consider what happened late one night when a 10-year-old we'll call Julie asked Linda Hicks, her favorite nurse, if she was dying. "I was really close to her," explains Linda. "This was not just a matter of giving her shots. She was like a little friend, and often I'd stay after work to read to her."

About a week earlier, however, Julie's doctor had told the hospital staff and her parents that her cancer was out of control and he didn't think she would live much longer. Julie's parents stated clearly that they didn't want their daughter to know how serious her condition was.

Although the doctor disagreed with this approach and did his best to talk them out of it, the parents insisted. Reluctantly, he wrote orders in Julie's chart that under *no* circumstances should she be told she was dying.

That same night, Linda remembers, Julie was feeling miserable and couldn't sleep. "I offered to read to her, but after a page or two, I noticed she was crying. I gathered her into my arms and asked what was wrong. Julie told me, 'Nobody's talking to me, but you're my friend. Linda, am I dying?'"

Under orders not to discuss it with the child, Linda felt trapped. Telling a lie or withholding the truth from the child whose cancer was far advanced seemed neither ethical nor kind. Linda did the only thing she felt she could. "I held her in my arms, hugged her, and cried with her. Then she asked again, 'Am I dying?' and I said, 'Honey, we're doing all we can for you, and you're not getting any better.'"

Telling only as much as the child wants to know

Many physicians agree with Episcopal minister and pediatrician Burton Dudding when he says he would seriously consider withdrawing from a case in which parents asked him not to tell a child he or she was dying when he felt it was in the child's best interests to know. "I would tell the parents that I couldn't provide the kind of care their child needed unless I had the freedom to respond to the child's questions."

But being honest with children *doesn't* mean overloading them with more than they want to know.

"Initially," Dudding says, "you want children to mobilize all the psychic energy they can to fight the disease. I'd still answer questions as truthfully as I possibly could, dealing with the situation on a week-by-week or month-by-month basis—depending on the child's condition—but I believe it's important to hold out hope until death is imminent."

Experts agree it's imperative to be a good listener so you can find out what children really want to know.

The problem is that none of us has had concrete experience with death; we don't know the answers. We feel insecure, and when we're anxious, we tend to use words and euphemisms like "He's off to a long sleep." The next thing you know the child is petrified of bedtime and wakes up with night terrors—and you can hardly blame him.

"Go slowly," Dudding advises, "and don't try to hide your own feelings while you're talking about death. Encourage your child to put into words what he's feeling or frightened about. A simple 'Would you like to tell me about it?' or 'You can write it down [or draw a picture, or tape-record it] so we'll have it later' is often all it takes. Leave it open-ended. If your child wants to talk again later, he'll let you know."[31]

The whole point is to be sensitive to what the child wants to know—or *doesn't* want to know—and tailor your response accordingly.

Children's "unfinished business"

Even children have what Elisabeth Kübler-Ross calls "unfinished business" which they have a right to complete before they die. Some want to give away their toys or favorite possessions; others want a say in planning their funeral. Older children may want to donate their organs or make out a will. Here, in part, is what one mother wrote to nationally syndicated columnist Ann Landers:

> Our only child died of bone cancer two years ago. He was 15. He had his leg amputated above the knee and then had three operations to remove tumors from his lungs. He went through extensive chemotherapy and never once complained. What a terrific fighter he was!
>
> He knew from the beginning that his illness might be fatal. When the doctors told us there was no hope, our son was sitting right with us. On the trip home we talked openly about death. He planned his own funeral—what he wanted to wear, the music he wanted played, and who should be the pall-bearers.
>
> He asked to die at home—no tubes, no artificial life supports. Of course, we respected his wishes. The last week of his life he told us to whom we should give his favorite possessions. We wrote everything down. The day before he died he thanked us for not babying him and for being honest throughout his illness....

In response, Ann Landers said in part, "A terminally ill patient almost always knows the truth and doesn't need to be told. It is best to talk openly about the situation. Cry together, laugh together—share it all."[32]

Parents, however, shouldn't feel that they have to do this all by themselves.

Help in breaking sad news

In 1982, Susan and Roland Cotes welcomed the help of a nurse in explaining to their 5-year-old daughter why she hadn't received a liver transplant that might have saved her life. Renee had waited six months for a donor organ to become available. Public appeals for a donor, including national news broadcasts, a *People* article, and a television appearance by Renee had put the New England family in the media limelight. Now the news was devastating.

For when the University of Pittsburgh transplant team began the surgery, they found cancer had spread to Renee's diaphragm and would have consumed the healthy liver as well, making her unsuitable for the transplant. Because donor organs are so scarce, a backup recipient is always on call. In this case, the liver intended for Renee went to a 5-year-old from Wyoming.

When Boston Children's Hospital head nurse Pat Rutherford heard what had happened, she flew to Pittsburgh to be with the family and help in breaking the sad news to Renee. She knew the child well and, before Renee had left for Pittsburgh, had helped in the preoperative teaching typically given a child facing surgery. Having heard Renee say on television that she wanted the operation and "if I don't [have it] I'm going to die," the nurse and Renee's parents had even talked to her about death during the teaching sessions.

First, the nurse talked to Renee's parents. "I discussed with them that it was important for her to know the truth." The Coteses agreed their daughter needed to know, but didn't feel capable of sharing that because they were so devastated themselves. "So I told her. It was very difficult," says Rutherford, "because at some level, I think Renee understood that she might die and really didn't want to talk about her situation. Because I was the bearer of bad news, she was very angry at me and pushed me away. But I feel that Renee's ability to share her feelings openly, even though they were negative, was very healthy."

In retrospect, says the nurse, she's glad she was the one who told Renee, "because *whoever* carries the message may get a lot of anger. And if it had been Renee's parents, that would have been even more devastating at a time when they were letting go and grieving a lot for their daughter."

Renee died six weeks later.

Knowing what to expect

All experts agree that there's no blanket rule that covers all situations. In each case, what and how you tell a child he's going to die has to be individualized to meet that child's needs. In some cases a nurse, doctor, or other professional person may be the one best able to discuss dying with the child. But many times, the parents can and should be the ones who tell—because their children trust them.

A consultant (such as a psychologist, psychiatric nurse, physician, or social worker) or even a team of care-givers, explains Rutherford, can help prepare parents, and siblings as well, to anticipate what the process is and deal with the reactions which may result from such stressful news. "I think," she says, "whoever is going to be carrying that message—the parents or health care professional—needs to know the possible consequences of being the deliverer of that message, and it may not always be anger. It could be an unwillingness to listen to you or even total denial."

Today, most parents are advised to discuss their child's questions about the future and the possibility of death when the child asks or gives clues to what he or she is thinking about. If the child is older, the subject may arise when he or she learns of the diagnosis. Frequently, a relapse triggers such questions; they generally don't pop up in times of remission, when everyone seems grateful for the "breather."

In short, open communication—at the child's request—

can lead to mutual support among family members. However, researchers have discovered that a *forced* openness which comes too soon for some families can be destructive. The added stress may cause "inappropriate coping behavior"—family members may cause one another more pain and may be less able to make wise decisions than before.[33]

Forgoing further treatment

Your child's medical needs may preclude his or her ever leaving the hospital. The child may be unconscious or in coma. Although a miracle would be the answer to your prayers, a miracle may be unlikely in this case. You may be wondering if it's now time to stop treatment and let your child die in peace.

You may hesitate to bring up the topic for fear you'll be judged a bad or unfeeling parent. But today, more and more people are questioning just how long treatment should be continued when it seems to be getting nowhere. In short, if you're worried and wondering, don't sit around waiting for the doctor to bring up the issue. Ask.

If you would like a friend to be with you when you talk to the doctor, by all means ask him or her to be there with you. But if you're too upset to communicate effectively, ask the doctor to discuss the details of your child's care with a family spokesperson of your choosing. Some doctors will talk to family members in the waiting room; others will find a quiet room or office where you can discuss your child's condition. If the waiting room is filled with visitors who are "all ears," ask if there is some other place you can talk.

Questions to ask when your child is unconscious

1. What is my child's condition now?
2. Is my child brain-dead?
3. Is my child in permanent coma or will he or she wake up?
4. When will you know? How long do we have to wait to find out?
5. Should we get a second opinion?
6. Would new methods of treating children in coma work in my child's case?[34]
7. If not, will my child be in a persistent vegetative state like Karen Quinlan? How long could he or she last that way?
8. Should a "Do not resuscitate" (DNR) order be written in my child's chart?
9. Should we withhold all treatment?
10. Should we stop everything and just let my child die peacefully?
11. Does that include withdrawing IVs and/or feeding tube?
12. Are there other people I could talk to about this?
13. Should we consult with the hospital's bioethics committee?
14. If I want to be with my child until the very end, can I stay by his or her side when life supports or other treatments are removed?
15. What might I expect at that point?
16. Will we be able to donate my child's organs?

In those states with brain-death statutes, the physician is not obligated to continue treating a child declared brain-dead. (See Chapters 5 and 9 for a fuller explanation of brain death.) All life-support systems will then be removed.

Some parents wish to be with their child during the process of removing the IVs, respirator, and other monitoring equipment. Others prefer not to be present but want to see and hold their child immediately afterward for a short period of quiet time together. You have the right to say goodbye in privacy and in your own way—and this is also true if your child's organs are removed for transplant.

The deep sense of loss

Losing a child can be shattering to parents and hard to accept. In terms of stress in a family's life and effects on a marriage and on surviving brothers and sisters, it can be devastating. Yet support and understanding can help to ease the pain and stress.[35]

During this time, many parents find it helpful to network with other parents whose children suffer from similar illnesses or conditions. (Several groups are listed in the Resources section at the end of this chapter.) In addition, many hospitals now have bereavement clinics, and some psychologists specialize in grief counseling.

However, if during your child's illness you were part of a parents' support group, you may feel it's now time to quit, just as Janet Ryser did after the deaths of two of her sons from cystic fibrosis. Although she had helped start the cystic fibrosis organization in her area, she says, "At the end, I didn't want to forget the boys—but I did want to forget the disease."

Resources

You owe it to your child to get the best medical advice. Consider getting a second and possibly a third medical opinion. Contact a medical school in your area or a major medical or research center for advice on whom to see or talk to. These organizations can refer you to experts in the field of your child's illness or condition.

In your own community, there may already be a network of families whose children have similar medical problems and who know where the experts are, which health care professionals work well with young children, or who is good in dealing with teenagers. To locate such groups, check the Yellow Pages of your telephone directory, contact the self-help clearinghouse in your state if there is one, or ask your child's doctor and nurses, as well as your neighbors and friends. Word of mouth from informed people is one of the best recommendations you can get.

Here is a partial list of self-help and special-interest groups, many of which produce newsletters, cassettes and various publications:

National toll-free numbers:

American Kidney Fund, (800) 638-8299
Cancer Information Service, (800) 422-6237
Cystic Fibrosis Foundation, (800) 342-2681
HeartLife, (800) 241-6993
Juvenile Diabetes Foundation, (800) 223-1138
National Down Syndrome Society, (800) 221-4602
Spina Bifida Association Hotline, (800) 621-3141
Spinal Cord Injury Hotline, (800) 526-3456

Advisory and support organizations:

National Information Center for Handicapped Children and Youth
P.O. Box 1492
Washington, DC 20013
(703) 522-3332
Toni Haas, director

Provides free information concerning educational rights and special services to parents, educators, care-givers, and advocates of children with physical, mental, and emotional handicaps. Ask to be placed on mailing list and receive free publications.

The Candlelighters Childhood Cancer Foundation
2025 Eye St., NW, Suite 1011
Washington, DC 20006
(202) 659-5136
Grace Powers Monaco, board chairperson

International network of self-help groups for parents of children who have cancer.

Ronald McDonald Houses
c/o Golan-Harris Communications
500 N. Michigan Avenue
Chicago, IL 60611
(312) 836-7100
Person to contact: International Ronald McDonald House Coordinator

Nonprofit temporary homes away from home for families of children receiving treatment at nearby hospitals.

Children's Hospice International (CHI)
1101 King Street, Suite 131
Alexandria, VA 22314
(703) 684-0330 or 684-0331
Ann A. Dailey, executive director

Nonprofit clearinghouse for information and education in children's hospice care, which coordinates support systems for families of seriously ill children or those who have encountered sudden loss of a child through accident or violence.

National Self-Help Clearinghouse (NSHC)
City University of New York Graduate School and University
    Center
33 West 42nd Street, Room 1227
New York, NY 10036
(212) 840-1259
Frank Riessman, associate director

General clearinghouse of information and referral service concerning self-help groups.

The Compassionate Friends
National Headquarters
P.O. Box 3696
Oak Brook, IL 60522
(312) 323-5010
Therese Goodrich, executive director

Self-help group for bereaved family and siblings, providing information, empathy, and support.

Organizations dedicated to granting wishes of chronically and terminally ill children:

Make-a-Wish Foundation of America
4601 North 16th Street, Suite 206
Phoenix, AR 85016
(602) 234-0960
Linda Dozeretz, executive director

Operation Liftoff
1171 Kings Avenue
Bensalem, PA 19020
(215) 639-1586
Ernest Bischoff, national chairman

Starlight Foundation
9021 Melrose Avenue, Suite 204
Los Angeles, CA 90069
(213) 205-0631
Lois Sapadin, executive director

Suggested reading

Brozan, Nadine. "The Last Days of Ill Children: Best at Home?" *New York Times*, October 14, 1985, p. 87.

Chambers, Marcia. "Tough Transplant Questions Raised by 'Baby Jesse' Case." *New York Times*, June 15, 1986, p. 1.

Cohen, Daniel. "Children's Hospices: Easing Early Deaths." *Esquire*, May 1985, p. 76.

Dickman, Irving, with Dr. Sol Gordon. *One Miracle at a Time: How to Get Help for Your Disabled Child.* New York: Simon and Schuster, 1985. (Parents share experiences and ways to overcome man-made and system-made problems in getting help.)

Fost, Norman C., M.D., M.P.H. "Ethical Issues in the Care of Handicapped, Chronically Ill, and Dying Children." *Pediatrics in Review*, vol. 6, no. 10 (April 1985), p. 291 + .

Gaylin, Jody. "When a Child Dies." *Parents*, February 1985, p. 80.

Gaylin, Willard, and Ruth Macklin, eds. *Who Speaks for the Child: The Problems of Proxy Consent.* New York: Plenum Press,

1982. (Covers the rights of children and parents, family privacy, and autonomy as well as human independence, consent, competency of minors, and the best interests of the child.)

Grollman, Earl A., ed. *Explaining Death to Children*. Boston: Beacon Press, 1967. (See prologue; explains what *not* to tell children.)

Holder, A.R. "Parents, Courts and Refusal of Treatment." *Journal of Pediatrics*, vol. 103, no. 4 (October 1983), pp. 515–21.

Jones, Monica Loose. *Home Care for the Chronically Ill or Disabled Child: A Manual and Source Book for Parents and Professionals*. New York: Harper & Row, 1985. (Available at bookstores or contact: Harper & Row Publishers, Inc., Attn: R. Brengel, 10 E. 53rd Street, New York, NY 10022.)

Kushner, Harold S. *When Bad Things Happen to Good People*. New York: Schocken, 1981. (Offers a compassionate and humane approach to dealing with questions of suffering and life and death in a way which affirms humanity and inspires peace of mind.)

Leikin, Sanford, M.D. "Minors' Assent or Dissent to Medical Treatment." *Journal of Pediatrics*, vol. 102, no. 2 (February 1983).

Nierenberg, Judith, R.N., M.A., and Florence Janovic. *The Hospital Experience*, rev. ed. New York: Berkley, 1985. (See "When the Patient Is a Child: How Parents Can Help," pp. 42–48.)

For children:

Buscaglia, Leo, Ph.D. *The Fall of Freddie the Leaf*. New York: Charles B. Slack, 1982.

Rofes, Eric, ed. *The Kids Book About Death and Dying*. New York: Little, Brown, 1986. (Researched and written by 11-to-14-year-old students who also recommend other books about death and dying; covers topics such as euthanasia, organ donation, autopsy, emotions, and how children feel about the death of a friend, pet, parent, or their own life-threatening illness. However, section on brain death needs updating.)

White, E.B. *Charlotte's Web*. New York: Harper & Row, 1952.

Books for children available from Children's Hospice International (CHI):

Dodge, Nancy C. *Thumpy's Story—A Story of Love and Grief* (shared by Thumpy, the Bunny; English and Spanish editions;

$6); *Thumpy's Story* (coloring book, $5); and *Sharing with Thumpy—My Story of Love and Grief* (workbook, $9). Postage and handling extra.

Kübler-Ross, Elisabeth, M.D. *Letter to a Child with Cancer*. (Answers to questions asked by a 9-year-old boy dying from leukemia; $3; $2.75 to CHI members.)

9 Making Life-and-Death Decisions for Another Adult

HOSPITALS are in the business of saving lives and "doing things" for patients.

In an emergency or where there is doubt about the medical outcome, patients are treated. Unless orders are written to the contrary, doctors and nurses work vigorously to restore heart, lung, kidney, and other vital organ functions when any of these has failed. In such settings, ethical problems center on whether to start or stop life-saving measures and who should decide.

Experts agree, and the laws on privacy and informed consent are clear, that a competent person has full authority over his or her body and what will be done to it.

Problems arise when a patient is unconscious or, if conscious, is unable to make health care decisions for himself or herself. In such cases, family members, if available, are usually asked to consent to treatment for a relative whom they are caring for at home or who is already in a hospital, hospice, or nursing home.

Factors to weigh

If doctors have asked you to take part in making a decision to start, stop, or continue life-sustaining treatment for a relative or friend, you'll need to consider the following:

Is there a legal guardian? You may be the legal guardian for your relative's estate, property, or bank account. You may be executor of someone's will. But none of these necessarily gives you the authority to make *medical* decisions for that person. In most states, a family member or friend has no legal right to consent to medical treatment for another adult—although doctors often think they do and, in practice, usually turn to relatives for advice and consent to treat or not to treat. Unless a court has appointed you the guardian or "conservator" of an adult patient with specific authority to make health care decisions, you have no legal right to make such decisions for that person.

Is there a Durable Power of Attorney for Health Care Decisions? Many states now recognize the right of any patient to designate an attorney-in-fact to make health care decisions for the patient if he or she is unable to do so. This document can be quite general or very detailed, specifying everything from the right to consent to or refuse treatment to complete withdrawal of all life-support systems. You need to know whether an attorney-in-fact has been designated and if such a document is still in effect. If so, that person should be contacted at once.

Is there a Directive to Physicians/Living Will? A Living Will (sometimes called "Directives" or "Instructions to Physicians") permits patients to document their wishes regarding the type of life-saving treatment they do or don't want. Thirty-six states and the District of Columbia now have a

Natural Death Act which permits the carrying out of the Living Will. Thirty-one of these states make it legally binding upon the physician to either comply with the patient's directive or transfer the patient to another physician willing to do so. However, only twelve states penalize physicians who fail to do so.

Even if you or the doctor disagree with the directives in the Living Will, don't dismiss it lightly. It's an important record of the patient's wishes.

But what happens if you haven't seen your relative in years or if you don't know if he or she has executed legal documents? That's the position a man I'll call Bill Flowers found himself in a few years ago.

"I'm being asked to play God and I don't know what to do."

On Thanksgiving Day a few years ago, Bill Flowers telephoned me from a nearby hospital. "You don't know who I am, but a nurse at the hospital told me you're on the ethics committee and could give me some advice."

The day before, he explained, a doctor had called his home in Florida to say his father had suffered a stroke the week before and had been in coma ever since. Bill Flowers, who had never felt close to his father and hadn't seen him since his parents had divorced fifteen years earlier, was now being asked to decide whether his father's doctors should continue treating the 72-year-old man or write a "no-code" order if his heart should stop. (For a full explanation of "code" and "no code" orders, see Chapter 4.)

"I flew into town today," he told me, "and understand that Dad's kidneys, which had shut down, are now working again. My mother is dead and there are no other family members to talk this over with. Here I'm being asked to play God and I'm not sure what to do. What really worries me is that if Dad's kidneys are making a comeback, maybe he's still got a chance."

Bill Flowers didn't want his father to suffer if there was no hope of recovery, but neither did he want to be "guilty of Dad's death."

First of all, I reassured him that no decision had to be made overnight. He had time to think about it. But making the decision would be easier, I told him, if he could find and talk to some of his father's friends, neighbors, or even coworkers who could say whether his father had ever expressed his wishes about medical care in such circumstances. Hospitals, I explained, are in the business of preserving life if possible. His father would be resuscitated if his heart or lungs failed, unless his doctor wrote a specific no-code order.

What Bill Flowers needed most at this point was a clear picture of his father's medical condition and some idea of what his father's wishes might be. Only then could he share in decision-making with the doctor and feel he'd done the right thing. You will need the same information if you are asked to be a guardian for a friend or relative, or asked to help decide if medical treatment should be continued, withheld, or withdrawn. These are questions which I suggested he ask the doctor:

Questions to ask the doctor

1. What happened? How serious is his condition?
2. Why is he unconscious? (For example, lack of oxygen to the brain, bleeding, stroke, shock, drug overdose, or increased pressure on or in the brain.)
3. Is he in any pain?
4. Is he in coma? Is the coma irreversible?
5. Is he brain-dead or likely to be soon? When will you know?
6. Is he likely to regain consciousness? How long will that take—weeks, months? Will he wake up completely?
7. Will he be permanently unconscious? Will he enter the persistent vegetative state? When will you know?
8. How long does he need to be on the respirator? Can he live without it?

9. If his heart stops, should he be resuscitated?

10. If he gets an infection, should he be treated with antibiotics?

11. If he doesn't begin to eat or drink, should he be continued on IV or tube feedings?

12. If he lives, will he be in pain? Will he be able to do anything for himself, or will he need special care of some kind?

13. If he lives, will he be aware of his surroundings? Will he be able to communicate with us in some way?

14. If he lives, will he be able to make decisions for himself, or will he need a guardian?

15. What do you suggest at this point? Should we get other opinions and talk to additional specialists?

These questions relate to the patient's medical condition, prognosis, and quality of life if he or she survives. But you will need other important information as well.

Did the patient ever talk to you or anyone else about what he or she would want done in this situation? What do you and others remember about those conversations? How specific was the patient about his or her wishes? You may have to scout around for this information among family members, friends, relatives, coworkers, the patient's attorney, minister, or doctors who have cared for the patient in the past. You may need to talk to a home health care worker if the patient has been cared for at home, or to a nursing home administrator if he or she has been living in an extended care facility of some kind.

After you have the facts about the medical condition of your relative or friend, and some evidence that the patient did or didn't express his or her wishes, the next step is to consult with family members if they're available and with the patient's doctor to decide what to do.

If your relative or friend has a legal guardian, has left a Durable Power of Attorney for Health Care Decisions, or has signed a Directive to Physicians or a Living Will, you should share this information at once with the patient's doctors. (For a more detailed discussion of the Living Will and Durable Power of Attorney, see Chapter 4.)

TERMS YOU SHOULD KNOW

COMA   An imprecise term generally referring to total lack of responsiveness to the environment, inability to be aroused, no purposeful activity or sign of mental activity. The patient's eyes are usually closed. Brain death is the most severe form of coma. But in many other cases the coma is not permanent. Some patients awaken but are left in the persistent vegetative state (see below). Others wake up completely with few or no apparent aftereffects. The eventual level of recovery is often related to the cause of the coma and the patient's age. (The young person in coma from drug overdose, for example, has a better chance of recovery than does an 80-year-old person who has suffered a severe brain hemorrhage.)

BRAIN DEATH   Irreversible cessation of all functions of the entire brain, including the brain stem, which controls automatic body functions, such as heartbeat and breathing. It is the deepest form of coma, and a respirator is essential to maintain heart and lung functions. Survival on life-support systems beyond a few days is rare, but may continue for four to six weeks. Most state laws recognize this condition as one of two accepted definitions of death. (See UDDA definition below.)

UNIFORM DETERMINATION OF DEATH ACT (UDDA)   An individual who has sustained either (1) irreversible cessation of circulation and respiratory functions or (2) irreversible cessation of all functions of the entire brain, including the brain stem, is dead. A determination of death must be made in accordance with accepted medical standards.

PERSISTENT VEGETATIVE STATE   Permanent loss of consciousness. The brain stem is intact and functioning, but there has been irreversible cessation of higher cortical or cerebral functions, such as awareness of the surroundings and ability to think, reason, and experience pleasure and pain. The patient is not in coma. He has sleep-wake cycles, but when awake, he has no conscious interaction with the environment. It is a state of the most profound dementia. After the initial need for respirator support, the patient may survive for months or years, as did Karen Quinlan, provided the patient is fed and given other general medical and nursing care.

EXTRAORDINARY MEANS   "Heroic" or extraordinary efforts to keep a dying patient alive when there is no reasonable medical evidence the treatment will benefit the patient and may, in fact, only burden him. It's important to remember that the terms "ordinary" and "extraordinary" do *not* refer to the technology, equipment (ventilator, IV, dialysis, feeding tube), or drugs used, but rather to their effect on the patient. This means determining whether or not the benefits of the proposed treatment are in proportion to the burdens imposed on the patient.

Track records of values and wishes— written or spoken

If, however, your relative never wrote anything down, but did express his or her wishes strongly to you, friends, or others, then this "track record" of beliefs and values should also be clearly stated to the doctor so that it can be given the highest priority in making decisions on the patient's behalf.

Write down your recollection of what the patient told you, date and sign it before witnesses, and give it to the physician for inclusion in the patient's medical record. Be sure you keep a photocopy for your own files. Many courts have considered this type of verbal and written testimony from friends and relatives in settling disputes over whether to withdraw life supports from a patient.

The case of Brother Fox

Brother Fox, for example, was an 83-year-old member of a Roman Catholic teaching order in Long Island, New York. When his heart stopped while he was being operated on for a hernia, efforts to resuscitate him left the former teacher permanently unconscious, and he slipped into a persistent vegetative state. Father Eichner, his religious superior, requested that the respirator be disconnected. When hospital officials and doctors refused, he asked a court to appoint him Brother Fox's guardian with authority to make the same request.

At the hearing, fellow teachers and members of his religious order testified that Brother Fox had often taken part in discussions about the Karen Quinlan case and agreed with the decision to remove her from the ventilator. He had stated that he would not want any of that "extraordinary business" done to him.

Based on these previously expressed wishes, the court appointed Father Eichner guardian with the authority to request removal of the ventilator. In his ruling, the judge stated that if Brother Fox were competent, he would be entitled to exercise his constitutional right of privacy and ask to have the respirator removed. The ruling was upheld by the New York court of appeals, the state's highest court, but by then, Brother Fox had already died.[1]

Unlike Brother Fox, most people don't talk about their own death. They don't leave written or verbal "track records." They haven't *clearly* said in straightforward terms what, if any, treatment they would want for themselves if they were ever incapable of making their own health care choices.

In these cases, doctors often look to the family as decision-makers and the principle of "substituted judgment" comes into play.

Substituted judgment in decision-making

The substituted judgment standard holds that the health care decision should reflect, as closely as possible, what the patient would have wanted if competent to speak for him or herself. (Of course, this does not apply in making decisions for infants, young children, or severely retarded persons who are incapable of expressing values, goals, or preferences.)

The President's Commission on medical ethics has recommended this approach, stating that, usually, close family members are most concerned about the patient, most knowledgeable about his or her values and wishes, and in the best position to know what he or she would have wanted. For these reasons, the President's Commission states that "a family member ought usually to be designated as surrogate to make such decisions for an incapacitated patient in consultation with the doctor and other health care professionals."[2]

Consider what happened to a man I'll call Kevin McCarthy, the brother of a Dominican nun who is a friend of mine.

"We wanted to believe he'd be well again."

Sister Moira's 33-year-old brother Kevin was a handsome, unmarried deputy district attorney from California, who went to New York City for a friend's wedding. Mugged late one night, he fell, striking his head on the pavement.

Witnesses' cries brought police running to the scene. An ambulance rushed him in semicoma to Lenox Hill Hospital, where he was admitted to the intensive care unit on a respirator. Hospital officials called family members on the West Coast to tell them what had happened. His parents left at once for New York; Sister Moira and a younger brother flew to the city the next day. The McCarthys, together with friends in town for the wedding, kept a week-long vigil at the hospital.

"We wanted to believe he'd be well again," says Sister Moira, "and we spent time planning his recovery—it gave us something to do." They looked into rehabilitation facilities he might need later and asked themselves various questions: How much care would the family be able to give if he lived? Would they all be able to share the responsibility? What aunt or cousin could come and help out?

"We had A-number-one care and tremendous support from the nurses, the hospital chaplain, the doctors—and that made it so much easier day by day," recalls Sister Moira. But by the fourth day, reality had set in. Kevin was never going to get better, and the family accepted the fact he was dying. "My father," she says, "was ready to pull the plug before any of us, but the physicians were still being cautious."

The McCarthys wanted information; they kept up a steady barrage of questions even though the doctors often had no answers for them. "Finally," the nun says, "the family told Kevin's doctor, 'We really want to consider taking him off the ventilator. We're not sure what the law is here in New York, but we want to find out what it is; and if he's going to die, we want to speed up the process. We don't want to prolong his death.'"

(In New York, as a result of a 1981 decision, *In re John Storar*, unless there is clear and convincing evidence that the patient had previously expressed his or her wishes when competent to do so, a physician cannot legally withdraw life support without court review.)

But when Sister Moira asked the doctor point-blank if he thought her brother would recover, the physician didn't say a word. However, his look, she says, told her no. "Looking back now, I think he wanted a few more days so Kevin could go naturally. But we as a family had decided it was time to stop. We were a close-knit Irish family who knew each other well, shared the same values and loved each other a lot," she says, adding tearfully, "So when my father said, 'Kevin never would want to live that way,' we all agreed." However, before life supports could be removed, Kevin died.

Substituted judgment, however, is at best an *assumption* about the patient's wishes. Because of this uncertainty, many courts have required an independent review within the hospital or judicial review leading to appointment of a guardian to make specific health care decisions.

That's what happened in the case of Karen Quinlan, who, says George J. Annas, professor of health law at Boston University School of Medicine, "has become a symbol and part of our language."[3]

Karen Quinlan—the landmark "right to die" case

In June 1985, Karen Quinlan died after more than ten years in a coma presumably caused by a drug overdose, and nine years after her parents won the right from the New Jersey supreme court to remove her shrunken body from a life-supporting respirator. By then, millions of people knew of her famous right-to-die legal case, which had made media headlines for a decade and been the topic of a book, *Karen Ann*, and a film, *In the Matter of Karen Ann Quinlan*.

Karen, born Mary Anne Monahan, had been adopted at 4 weeks of age by the Quinlans, who renamed her and raised her in their New Jersey home in a strict Roman Catholic tradition. An average and popular student, Karen seemed to have little trouble until spring 1975, when she had some difficulty finding and holding jobs, and moved in with friends.

One night in April, she apparently consumed drugs and alcohol and suddenly stopped breathing. Her companions tried mouth-to-mouth resuscitation and then took her to a hospital, where she was placed on a respirator. She never regained consciousness. Although she was in an irreversible coma, doctors did not consider her terminally ill.

After three months with no hope of recovery, the Quinlans asked Karen's doctors to remove the respirator. When her physicians refused, Karen's parents, supported not only by their parish priest but also by the Catholic bishops of New Jersey, took their case to court, requesting permission for their daughter to die "with grace and dignity." Never before had a United States court granted the right to die—and the conflict made front-page news around the world.

At stake, according to the Quinlans' lawyer, was Karen's constitutional right to die based on freedom of religion and the right to privacy. It would be cruel and unusual punishment, he argued, to keep her alive "after the dignity, beauty, promise, and meaning of earthly life had vanished."

But Karen's court-appointed guardian maintained that her parents had no right to request what for all practical purposes, he said, was euthanasia. And the attorney for the doctors stated that no court could know whether Karen might still recover. When the judge ruled against the Quinlans, they appealed to the state supreme court. In a landmark decision, the higher court reinstated Karen's father as her guardian and recognized his right to decide what was in his daughter's best interest based on her right to privacy.[4]

But there was one other legacy of the Karen Quinlan case. Ethics committees, which up to that point were little known and seldom used in hospitals, were suddenly thrust into the limelight. The New Jersey supreme court had required that Karen's doctors, together with her guardian and family, consult with a hospital ethics committee or similar group. If they agreed that there was no expectation she would recover from coma, life-support systems could be removed "without criminal or civil liability" to anyone involved in the decision.

The ethics committee had come of age.

Making choices based on "best interests"

Like Karen Quinlan's father, you may find yourself forced to make a health care decision for someone else based on the "best interests" principle. In these situations, you cannot use your own personal views of what's best for the patient.

Rather, as surrogate decision-maker, you must take into consideration what the President's Commission calls "more objective societally shared criteria."[5] These are expressed through various members of society—not only doctors, but also nurses, ministers, social workers, attorneys, administrators, and the public at large. The patient's welfare is paramount, and the deciding factor is what is in the patient's best interests.

A hospital ethics committee serves to express the views of

our pluralistic society and can help you and the doctor in considering such factors as the following:

· The relief of suffering
· Restoring or preserving body functions
· The quality as well as the length of life which may result

Take, for example, the case of "Jane Phillips," a comatose 67-year-old woman whose family was divided over what was in her best interests. Two daughters agreed with Jane's doctor that the burdens of continuing life-support systems and kidney dialysis offered no benefit and were merely prolonging their mother's dying. A sister of the patient, however, was not convinced that "all that should be done had been done."

Because the family was struggling to come to the right decision, they asked to meet with the hospital's ethics committee. After reviewing the case, the committee agreed with Jane's physician and daughters that all treatment could be stopped, since there was no chance of preserving or restoring normal functioning for Mrs. Phillips.

However, they also suggested that the aunt, who had not seen her sister in ten days, visit Jane in the intensive care unit to see for herself the futility of continuing any further therapy. The doctors agreed not to withdraw life-support systems until the sister could satisfy herself that further treatment was of no benefit. While her sister was visiting, and before life-support systems were withdrawn, Jane Phillips died.

Later the sister confided to her nieces, "Hard as it was, when I saw Jane like that, I knew it was time to let her go—it was all right to stop treating her."

If you're trying to decide what's in the best interests of someone who is incompetent to make decisions, for whatever reason, the task may be awesome and frightening. Down deep you may worry that your decision might *not* be, in fact, the same choice that friend or relative would have made. And.

making matters worse can be the additional pressure from various aunts, uncles, cousins, or friends who question whether it's right to "take away the breath of life" or "cut off food and water."

To feed or not to feed

Since the Karen Quinlan case ten years ago, turning off a ventilator that is forcing air into a patient's lungs and keeping him alive is no longer unusual. Nor is discontinuing kidney dialysis for comatose or terminally ill patients. Many competent patients, in fact, make that choice for themselves.

Now, however, the focus of ethical debate has shifted from disconnecting respirators and writing "no code" orders to whether it is ever morally permissible to stop nutrition and fluids.

Since 1983, seven highly publicized cases have begun to shape the law in California, Massachusetts, and New Jersey, thereby setting legal precedents which will affect other cases sure to follow.[6] And in May 1986, the American Medical Association's Council on Ethical and Judicial Affairs issued bold new guidelines for doctors in dealing with a family's request to end all treatment involving nutrition and hydration. (See Appendix H.)

According to Dr. Nancy Dickey, who chaired the AMA council, "It's not unethical to discontinue all means of life-prolonging medical treatment...including medication and artificially or technologically supplied respiration, nutrition or hydration—even if death is not imminent but the patient's coma is beyond doubt irreversible."[7]

The legal issue of withholding nutrition first came to public attention when two doctors at the Kaiser Hospital in Long Beach, California, were accused of murder and later found innocent. At the family's request, Drs. Barber and Nejdl had removed not only the respirator but also the intravenous feeding tubes from Clarence Herbert, who had suffered irreversible brain damage when his heart stopped after routine surgery.

At this point, you may be asking yourself: Is there a difference between a ventilator and IV fluids? Is there a basic difference between providing patients with air through their lungs and water through their veins?

In the *Barber and Nejdl* case, the California court rejected such a distinction. It emphasized that IV feedings are no different from any other life-sustaining mechanism, such as a respirator, and no physician has an obligation to continue any treatment if it proves ineffective or futile or the burden of continuing it is too heavy.[8]

But aren't food and water essential to the basic *comfort* of a person?

Food and water—comfort or treatment?

Most religious traditions admonish us to "feed the hungry," to "give a cup of water in my name," to "comfort the afflicted." Indeed, food and water seem so much a part of caring, comfort, and nurturing that it's hard to think of them as medical treatments.

But John Paris, a Jesuit priest and expert in medical ethics, believes that artificially provided nutrition and fluids through nasogastric or gastrostomy tubes or IV lines "are medical treatments and should be assessed like any other treatments on the basis of their efficacy and benefit to the patient."[9] And the American Medical Association agrees.

Those opposed to this view hold that food and water provide comfort to the patient and withdrawing them would be cruel and inhumane, resulting in the patient's "starving to death." This would be true if the patient were conscious, could experience pain and discomfort, or wanted to be nourished. But patients in the persistent vegetative state, around whom these debates arise, have permanent loss of consciousness, are unaware of their surroundings, and can experience neither pain nor pleasure. Thus, food and water provide no benefit or comfort to such patients—other than prolonging their physical existence.

In the United States today, there are some ten thousand persons living in the persistent vegetative state, many of whom were the young, healthy victims of trauma. Although many die within days or weeks, some live for years, like Karen Quinlan. The longest case on record is that of Elaine Esposito, a six-year-old who never regained consciousness following an appendectomy in the mid-1940s and survived for more than thirty-seven years.

Paul Brophy and Nancy Jobes— feeding-tube dilemmas

A former emergency medical technician, 48-year-old Paul Brophy had been in the persistent vegetative state for three years. When his wife requested that a feeding tube be removed, his physician refused, claiming, "That would be killing him." A probate judge agreed.

Mrs. Brophy—supported by their five children and his seven brothers and sisters and 91-year-old mother, as well as the parish priest—testified that before his stroke from a ruptured aneurysm, her husband had said of Karen Quinlan, "No way do I want to live like that."[10] Despite this and other testimony, the judge ruled against "removing or clamping" the gastrostomy tube. On appeal, however, the Massachusetts supreme court upheld the hospital's right to resist Mrs. Brophy's request that her husband not be fed, but authorized her to move her husband to a facility that would honor her wishes. In its September 1986 ruling, the court stated that artificial nutrition was a form of medication that could be rejected and thus the feeding tube could be removed. This was done a month later and Paul Brophy died of pneumonia within eight days.

In a similar case in New Jersey, John Jobes, together with his wife's parents and siblings, ran into a thicket of legal and medical roadblocks in his attempts to have a feeding tube removed from his comatose wife, Nancy, 31, who for six years had been cared for in a nursing home. "There is no quality of life," *Time* magazine quoted him as saying in March 1986, "and Nancy would not want to be in this state."[11]

A month later, a New Jersey judge ruled that the feeding tube could be disconnected from the woman "in a persistent vegetative state with no prospect of improvement" and said her husband, John Jobes, would be the suitable person to disconnect the tube if the nursing home's appeal to a higher court failed.[12]

On appeal, the New Jersey Supreme Court overruled the nursing home and upheld John Jobes' right to remove the feeding tube. This was done and Nancy Jobes died in August 1987.

Feeding tubes have no rights—only people do. And medical treatments, once started, do not take on a life of their own. Some argue that doctors are not obliged to begin treatment, but once they do, treatment cannot be stopped, because to do so would cause the death of the patient.

But John Paris, who frequently testifies in quality-of-life cases, says that "this approach removes human moral judgment as a factor in the analysis; it reduces the patient to a mere cog in the machine and the machine takes over."[13]

The "Claire Conroy Pattern"

A case which set broad right-to-die guidelines for situations in which a patient is severely demented but neither terminally ill nor in the persistent vegetative state is that of Claire

288

Conroy, who at age 79 entered a nursing home in 1979. Four years later, she was unable to move from a semifetal position and was diagnosed to be in a state of progressive senile dementia. In addition, she suffered from heart disease, hypertension, diabetes, a gangrenous leg, eye problems, and an inability to control her bowels, speak, or swallow.

When her nephew requested that the feeding tube be removed, the nursing home refused, and the case went to court. Before final arguments in the case were heard, Claire Conroy died, her nasogastric tube still in place.

In what has become known as the "Claire Conroy pattern," the New Jersey supreme court ruled that although the patient was not terminal or in a comatose state, artificial feeding—like any other medical treatment—could be stopped if one of three conditions was met.[14]

First, employing a "subjective test," it should be absolutely clear that the patient wanted to avoid or stop such treatment; a signed Living Will would be one such example. Lacking such a clear directive, life-sustaining treatment could also be withdrawn or withheld if either of two "best interests" tests (a "limited objective" or a "pure objective" test) is met satisfactorily.

In both of these "tests," said the court, "the decision-maker would have to be satisfied that the burdens of the patient's continued life with the treatment outweigh the benefits of that life for him." The only difference between the two is that in applying the first test (the limited objective test), the guardian would attempt to deduce what the patient would have decided for himself based on trustworthy evidence, whereas in the "pure" objective test, the guardian would attempt to make the decision without resorting to what the patient would have wanted.

The court was clear that this three-pronged test for withholding or withdrawing treatment was specifically directed at extended care facilities where cases like Claire Conroy's are most likely to pose dilemmas for care-givers and family alike. Such situations occur in thousands of hospitals and nursing homes from coast to coast, where an estimated 80 percent of deaths occur and many patients spend their final days surrounded by a mass of tubes, monitors, and other life-support equipment.

Public opinion polls have consistently shown that most Americans support the patient's right to die with dignity. They also fear and oppose the intrusion of life-support technology into one of life's most private moments.[15]

My mother was one of these people. She never wanted to be attached to tubes at the end of her life and wanted to die at home.

A strong, healthy, active woman, she worked all of her life —first on a farm in Sparta, Illinois, later as a registered nurse in Missouri and New York. Widowed at age 46, she managed to raise seven children, of whom I was the youngest.

Shortly after her 82nd birthday, however, we noticed a change. This confident and capable woman was becoming confused and "accident-prone." Worried about her safety, her landlord was loath to renew the lease on her apartment; he felt she could no longer live on her own.

My mother, of course, was determined she'd never "be a burden to anyone." But after a particularly frightening dizzy spell, she agreed to move in with family members living on the East Coast. Within eighteen months, their patience and ability to cope had run out. Hoping her problems were treatable and reversible, I brought her to my home and had her evaluated by experts in gerontology. Despite their best efforts, it was clear that her mental deterioration was irreversible and she would need to spend the rest of her days in a protected environment.

I became her guardian.

The nursing home

Following a stroke, my mother was admitted to a nursing home which was not our first choice, but was the only one with an available bed. Much to our delight, my mother was placed in a room with an alert, gentle, caring woman whom my mother began calling "Mother" at once.

I'll call her Sara Clarke. A former nurse, she was 72 and was paralyzed from the neck down. She relied on attendants for everything—from daily care to reading letters from her only daughter, who was frequently traveling. My mother, by then 84, rarely knew who we were, where she was, or even when to call the aides for help. Because she was so frail and had fallen several times at home trying to get to the bathroom by herself, her doctor had ordered a light restraint around her waist to keep her from falling from her wheel-chair or bed.

Often when we'd visit, we'd find my mother leaning way out of her bed so she could hold her new "mother's" hand. Mrs. Clarke kept an eye on her new charge, calling for help when my mother was perilously close to falling out of bed.

One night, it happened. Mrs. Clarke told us later she screamed for help for twenty minutes before anyone came. My mother was taken to the hospital for x-rays. There were no broken bones, only bruises. She'd fallen; it was an acci-dent. We talked to the nursing home's administrator, and she assured us it wouldn't happen again.

The next time, my mother fell from the toilet. Again, Sara Clarke tried to summon help for several minutes. When an aide finally came, she stood my mother up and was annoyed when she cried out in pain. X-rays this time showed a broken hip, and my mother was hospitalized. Temporarily, she was safe—but what about later?

"Don't tell them I told you."

We went back to the nursing home. The administrator wasn't in. The head nurse said she didn't have time to talk. Aides who previously would smile and greet us now turned away. We went to see Mrs. Clarke.

"Don't tell them I told you anything," she told us, "because I'm afraid they'll take it out on me somehow, and I need them. But your mother's not getting the care you think she is. I can't do any more for her. I see her falling; I call for help. I worry about her—but she's going to keep falling if you bring her back, because on the weekends, this place is understaffed and people forget to tie her into her bed. She fell off the toilet because she was left there all alone. And if you're wondering why nobody's talking to you, it's because they've been told not to."

My wife and I were furious that my mother was receiving such poor care, and we realized we were now "the enemy" as far as the nursing home's administrator was concerned. Without referring to Sara Clarke, we tried to discuss the problem with the administrator. We even considered suing the nursing home, but ultimately decided against it, even though an aide confirmed all that Mrs. Clarke had told us.

But neither woman was willing to testify publicly—the aide for fear of losing her job and Sara Clarke for fear she'd be deprived of the nursing care she could not do without.

We moved my mother to a new and much better nursing home. Shortly after, the first facility was sold. New management improved the nursing care.

Within the year, Sara Clarke died. So, too, did my mother —without ever being readmitted to a hospital and burdened with IVs, feeding tubes, or last-minute efforts to resuscitate her. She didn't die at home, it's true. But my mother did die in peace and with dignity as my wife and I held her hands and whispered to her that she was free to go to the heaven she so believed in.

Respecting the person who was

Placing a parent in a nursing home is certainly one of the most difficult "life" decisions we ever make for another person.

Anyone who has ever struggled with the decision to place a

parent, spouse, or relative in an extended care facility of some kind knows how hard it is to maintain a balance between beneficence (seeking for him or her a greater balance of goods over harms) and the person's right to make his or her own choices.

Clearly, my mother was incapable of making any decisions for herself those last few years of her life. Efforts to help her maintain her autonomy through simple choices like what dress to wear or what piece of jewelry to wear with it were meaning less and less to her as time went on. She was in "another world."

But the majority of America's senior citizens are very much in touch with the real world. They're competent and autonomous—handling their own affairs, traveling, looking out for their own interests, and making their own health care decisions.

Of the 29 million Americans who today are over 65, approximately 5 percent live in institutions, and, contrary to popular myth, only about 2.5 percent of the elderly population will become senile in their old age because of Alzheimer's disease or other conditions. (And according to the National Council on the Aging, of the 1.5 million people in nursing homes today over age 65, about half have Alzheimer's disease.)[16]

If your parent or relative falls into this small percentage of people who are incompetent, you will see some heartbreaking changes in the person and may have to make some difficult decisions for him or her. If a very close and loving relationship has existed between you, you may feel no cost should be spared and "nothing is too much."

On the other hand, if there's little love lost between you, even minimal emotional, physical, or financial support may seem a great burden or drain on your time, energy, and financial and emotional reserves. And if affluent families often find the burden of economic care a hardship, what about those much less well off?

In a *Hastings Center Report* article titled "What Do Children Owe Elderly Parents?" Daniel Callahan examines the legal, moral, and social aspects of this question and how great a sacrifice "honoring one's elderly parents" ought to entail. With the prospect of increasing competition among generations for society's limited resources, he argues for public policy that will promote—not corrupt—family bonds.[17]

What are your ethical obligations?

At the outset, you must recognize that several conflicting principles come into play in caring for an elderly person who is dependent on you for help. You may wish to help your loved ones, do good for them, and prevent harm from coming to them. But in so doing, you may be aware that your elderly relative has different ideas about his or her own needs.

If you're going to respect that autonomy, even in a limited way, you must appreciate the uniqueness of his or her values and the often imaginative and inventive ways that the elderly person uses in attempting to hold on to even the slightest semblance of self-determination. (In my mother's case, for example, her roommate, Sara Clarke, who was totally paralyzed and dependent on others for virtually everything she needed, still vigorously fought "the system" whenever she felt it was oppressing someone else.)

In addition, you may have filial responsibilities and duties. These may include financial and emotional support as well as helping your elderly parent to find *meaning* in his or her new existence. Yet justice, on the other hand, may require that you meet significant obligations to your own spouse, children, and other family members, whose needs must be balanced against those of the elderly person.

Pros and cons of nursing homes

In May 1985, the Senate Select Committee on Aging released a grim report regarding the nation's fifteen thousand nursing homes—11 percent of which, it claimed, were grossly substandard. "We've warehoused tens of thousands of our oldest, sickest citizens, and the federal government isn't doing anything about it," newspaper reports quoted panel chairman Senator John Heinz of Pennsylvania as saying. "We must act to strengthen inspections, enforce penalties, and put the care of patients first."[18]

Most of us don't need a Senate report to make us acutely aware of some of the negative aspects of extended care facilities, such as typical odors, significant change in life-style and with it a loss of privacy, control, and autonomy, and, sometimes, lack of emotional support. No doubt improvements are needed, and the sooner they come, the better.

Less often, however, do we hear of the positive aspects of extended care facilities and nursing homes. These include security and protection, balanced meals served on a regular basis, stimulation through seeing and socializing with other people, and often entertainment and arts or educational programs of one kind or another, as well as round-the-clock coverage for health problems and help in coping with them.

Although your loved one may have said many times that he or she "would never want to go into a nursing home" and you may even have promised it would never happen, a study by Aloen Townsend of the Rose Institute in Cleveland, Ohio, indicated that 90 percent of the families she studied found no other alternative to a nursing home when their loved one became severely incapacitated.[19]

Our family was also one that had no other alternative. The decision to put my mother in a nursing home was not made lightly. And our experience in moving her from one facility to another also taught us much about what to look for in selecting a nursing home. But before you go the nursing home route, check out *all* the other alternatives open to you, such as home health care and visiting nurse programs, homemaker services, and small-group living arrangements in sheltered and supervised environments, to name but a few.

Choosing a nursing home with care

In selecting a nursing home or extended care facility for a family member, choose carefully—keeping in mind not only the level of care your relative needs, but also the policies and guidelines by which the facility is run. (Skilled nursing facilities—SNFs—offer care similar to that in hospitals, including twenty-four-hour nursing services and vigorous therapy programs; intermediate care homes provide nursing services and group activities, holiday programs, and outings for residents who can't live alone but don't require round-the-clock care.)

Unfortunately, since many good homes are filled 100 percent of the time and have long waiting lists, more often than not the deciding factor is simply the availability of a bed. If the facility is far away, it is hard for families and friends to visit.

For suggestions on how families can work together more effectively in dealing with the problems of their aging relatives to reach solutions acceptable to everyone, consult "The Family Task Force" in *You and Your Aging Parent* by Barbara Silverstone and Helen Kandel Hyman (New York: Pantheon, 1982). This invaluable book also includes information on handling legal and financial matters when relatives can no longer manage on their own.

Two free publications from the American Health Care Association (see Resources section at end of chapter) are helpful in making the hard decisions regarding nursing home placement: *Facts in Brief on Long-Term Care* and *Thinking About a Nursing Home*. Doing your homework first can spare you and your loved one a lot of grief later.

But don't ignore that intuitive feeling that tells you "this place just isn't right" for your parent or spouse. Here are some pointers to help you find the most suitable facility available:

Ask people whose opinion you respect which are the best facilities in your area. Ask them why they rate these places so highly. Check out the information you receive with someone whose family member is a resident of the home. Is he or she satisfied with the quality of care? Are families encouraged to visit or take relatives on outings or home for the day?

Visit potential nursing homes or care settings. Compare what you see with your state's regulations for such facilities. (Remember, however, that meeting state, county, or city licensing rules and regulations establishes *minimum* standards and is not a guarantee of quality.) Even if your relative has enough money to cover monthly rates, which may easily be $1,800 to $2,400 or more, check on the home's eligibility for Medicare, Medicaid, and other third-party payments.

Ask for a tour of the facility. Insist on seeing the type of room or suite your relative would live in. Investigate safety features. Make sure bathroom and sleeping areas are sanitary, comfortable, and equipped with safety features, such as window screens, grip bars, and emergency light or call bell. Visit the laundry and kitchen. Look into food preparation and storage spaces. Are dining and sitting areas clean, secure, and spacious enough? Does the home provide special diets? Stay for a meal and judge the food for yourself.

Interview the administrator and key staff members in person to get a sense of their values. Do they appear to be qualified professionals who are caring and knowledgeable? Are staff members encouraged to upgrade their skills and attend educational programs, seminars, or workshops in gerontology and other related fields? (A facility which provides continuing education credits or covers fees for staff to attend such workshops is indeed committed to improving the quality of care its patients receive.) What is the ratio of aides to patients? Ask for a copy of the facility's Mission Statement (what the institution stands for, its goals and objectives) as well as the Nursing Home Bill of Rights, which stresses the patient's rights to visits, to handle his or her own financial affairs and mail, wear his or her own clothing, etc. (See Appendix E for excerpts from the Bill of Rights.) Be sure to ask if residents are given a choice of roommates and how often they're changed around. This is important—not only when roommates are incompatible and should be separated, but also when a special relationship develops and two friends should not be arbitrarily separated.

Be clear about fees, house rules, visiting hours, programs, and any amenities which might be available. If there is a beauty salon on the premises, for example, you may wish to make a standing appointment for your relative. Is there a shuttle bus to take people to town, church, doctor's offices, or the senior citizen center? Are there facilities for physical, occupational, and/or recreational therapy? Find out if these services require extra fees. Inquire about any limits on the amount and type of personal belongings permitted (furniture, memorabilia, decorations, clothing). Are families encouraged to decorate the patient's room to make it as homey as possible? If your relative requires a walker or wheelchair, will it be supplied or must you buy one of your own? Remember, you should have access to the facility twenty-four hours a day; for security reasons, however, you may have to make special arrangements for evening, late-night, or early-morning visits.

Check out the nursing services. Are care-givers prepared to handle common emergencies? Do patients have long waits before their needs are attended to? Is the nursing station orderly and efficient, with patient records, supplies, and medication stored appropriately? Are aides, orderlies, and other care-givers supervised by a trained and experienced nurse? Is there a registered nurse on duty on every shift? Is a doctor on call?

Observe the aides, cooks, laundry help, and business office staff. Do they appear to be "down" and sullen people who hate their jobs? Or do they seem to be warm, friendly, and caring in their treatment of residents? Listen for the tone of voice; look for a smile. It doesn't take long to get a feel for the way staff interact with one another and with patients. But don't let your own negative feelings about a nursing home get in the way of your ability to assess the situation accurately.

Find out if there is an ombudsman who represents patients' rights and interests—someone whom you can contact to express your concerns or complaints. Some facilities also have residents' councils or family advocacy committees to identify problem areas and work with staff to upgrade services. All states have an ombudsman for the institutionalized elderly who has considerable say in the supervision of nursing home quality. In New Jersey, for example, the state ombudsman must review decisions to remove life-support systems from patients.

Inquire about the "ethics" of the facility and specific policies, e.g., "Do not resuscitate," "Do not hospitalize," "Do not call emergency," and "Support care only." (Support care means oral feeding, bathing, skin and mouth care, and keeping the patient in clean and comfortable surroundings.) One nursing home administrator suggests the questions to ask are: If my parent's doctor writes a "Do not resuscitate" (or "Support care only") order, is it within your facility's ethic to respect the doctor's order? How are these orders implemented, and is there a review process, such as an institutional ethics committee? Are sedatives and other drugs used to control behavior? If so, who decides when they will be used?

Make sure you know who your relative's primary-care doctor will be in the nursing home. Will it be his long-time family physician or the last specialist who referred him to the facility? Or will a new doctor under contract with or employed by the facility take over your relative's care? How often does this doctor visit patients in this facility? If a new doctor is taking over, talk to him and be clear about his values and goals in caring for your parent or spouse. (See Chapter 2.) For example, what is his attitude toward the use of narcotics and other addictive drugs to relieve pain in the chronically or terminally ill patient? What about tube feeding, withdrawing life-support systems, or writing "Do not resuscitate" orders? Will you be involved in such decisions?

Anxiety and guilt

One other point. Entering a nursing home is often a stressful and bewildering experience for the patient. Families, too, can suffer from guilt feelings or, in some cases, feelings of anger that the patient "failed" to respond to treatment which might have kept him or her out of such a facility in the first place.

The challenge, of course, is to balance the patient's need for privacy, self-determination, and some degree of control over his or her life against your obligation—and that of the nursing home—to do what's in his or her best interests. You may wish to spare your loved one anxiety and emotional upset about going to a nursing home. You may be tempted to gloss over the truth to avoid an unpleasant scene or family squabble.

But take a tip from Sylvia Smith, assistant administrator of Sierra Health Care Center in northern Nevada: "Be honest from the beginning. Even if you think your loved one won't understand, tell the truth. I've had patients arrive here furious because they were told at the hospital that they were going home, and they ended up in a nursing home. Or they were told they were only going to stay for a week—and it's actually for long-term placement."

Having a choice—the key to happiness

A 1985 survey of 455 nursing home residents in fifteen cities, conducted by the National Citizens' Coalition for Nursing Home Reform, found that their first concern was with attitude, quality, and size of staff in the home. Next was the size and privacy of rooms. Again and again, however, residents stressed that the key to their happiness was *having a choice* —whether the decision is on food to be eaten, when to get up or go to bed, or the choice of a personal care attendant and physician.[20]

But when patients are dying, they're often no longer concerned about choices related to the *physical* self. Instead, they are involved in reorienting their values—putting their children first, or, perhaps, nieces and nephews. At this point, says ethicist David Thomasma, who has studied dying cancer patients, they tend to leave decision-making to their doctors, because these patients see their bodies as having, in a sense, betrayed them. Thomasma explains, "It's as though they're saying to themselves, 'The doctor can do whatever he wants with the body, it doesn't matter. I'm dying—the body is not part of me anymore. I'm in another world, and part of that *other world experience* is reorganizing my values.'"[21]

Even if you don't agree with these values—or with new priorities your loved one has assigned to them—don't forget that for each of us, rethinking our values is an important part of being faithful to ourselves.

Resources

American Health Care Association
1200 15th Street, NW
Washington, DC 20025
(202) 833-2050

The nation's largest federation of nursing homes and long-term health care facilities for the aged and the convalescent person. Seeks to provide leadership in promoting high standards of professional operation and administration of such facilities and to ensure quality care for patients and residents in safe surroundings on a basis of fair payment for services. Write for free single copies of *Facts in Brief on Long-Term Care* and *Thinking About a Nursing Home.*

Administration on Aging
Department of Health and Human Resources
Washington, DC 20201

The major administrative body in the federal government concerned with aging, AOA works on local levels through state offices and more than five hundred Area Offices on Aging.

The National Council on the Aging, Inc.
1828 L Street, NW
Washington, DC 20036
(202) 223-6250

A nonprofit, membership organization of professionals, organizations, and the concerned public, NCOA runs a Media Resource Center, sponsors a variety of programs, maintains the nation's largest and most complete library devoted to aging, and publishes books and pamphlets. Publications list available.

Friends and Relatives of Institutionalized Aged, Inc.
440 East 26th Street
New York, NY 10010
(212) 481-4422
Randy Blom, coordinator

A private nonprofit consumer group. Publishes *A Consumer's Guide to Nursing Home Care in New York State* ($25.), which explains alternatives to nursing home care for less seriously impaired relatives, then provides a step-by-step guide on how to place a relative in a nursing home, with particular emphasis on a nursing home resident's rights and New York rules and regulations. Lists public and private nursing homes as well as certified home health agencies, enriched housing programs, adult homes, hospice programs, ombudsman services, advocacy groups, and legal services. Provides free single copies of *Consumer's Guide to Improved Nursing Home Care: The Use of Restraints in New York State*, which explains what physical and medical restraints are, when they are or are not appropriate, and the rights of residents, under state regulations, to challenge the physician's decision to use restraints.

State Nursing Home Ombudsman Programs

The purpose of these programs is to improve the quality of life for nursing home residents by receiving and resolving complaints, monitoring the state health department's regulation of nursing homes, studying the need for additional laws to protect nursing home residents, etc. If you need help with a nursing home problem and are not sure where to turn, consult the telephone directory for your State Division of Aging Services, under whose jurisdiction most nursing home ombudsmen work. In those cases where separate offices are maintained, you will be referred to the proper location.

Alzheimer's Disease and Related Disorders Association
70 East Lake Street
Chicago, IL 60601
(312) 853-3060

A privately funded national voluntary health organization with more than five hundred support groups and over 140 chapters and affiliates nationwide. Supports research, provides family support through local chapters and support groups, stimulates education and public awareness of Alzheimer's disease, and advocates legislation which responds to needs of patients and their families at all levels of government. Maintains twenty-four-hour hotline: (800) 3621-0379; in Illinois, (800) 572-6037. Write for list of publications.

Suggested reading

Annas, George J. "Transferring the Ethical Hot Potato." *Hastings Center Report*, February 1987, pp. 20–21. (Legal discussion of the William Bartling, Elizabeth Bouvia, and Paul Brophy cases.)

Brown, Robert N., with Clifford D. Allo, Alan D. Freeman, and Gordon W. Netzorg. *The Rights of Older Persons: The Basic ACLU Guide to an Older Person's Rights*. New York: Avon, 1979. (Part II covers nursing homes, Medicare, and Medicaid; Part III deals with guardianship and civil commitment and rights to refuse medical treatment.)

Callahan, Daniel. "What Do Children Owe Elderly Parents?" *Hastings Center Report*, April 1985, pp. 32–37.

Committee on Psychiatry and the Community. *A Family Affair: Helping Families Cope with Mental Illness*. New York: Brunner/Mazel Publishers, 1987. (Available in bookstores and from the publisher, 19 Union Square West, New York, NY 10003, $10 plus $1 for postage and handling.) Reports on experiences of family members in dealing with mentally ill relatives, and what they need in order to continue in their heroic task.

Doudera, A. Edward, J.D., and J. Douglas Peters, J.D., eds. *Legal and Ethical Aspects of Treating Critically and Terminally Ill Patients*. Ann Arbor, Mich.: AUPHA Press, 1982. (Parts I and II cover major topics discussed in this chapter.)

Lo, Bernard, M.D., and Laurie Dornbrand, M.D. "Guiding the Hand That Feeds: Caring for the Demented Elderly." *New England Journal of Medicine*, vol. 311, no. 6 (August 9, 1984), pp. 402–4.

Katzman, Robert, M.D. "Alzheimer's Disease." *New England Journal of Medicine*, vol. 314, no. 5 (April 10, 1986), pp. 964–71. (An excellent review of what we know and still don't know about this single most common cause of dementia. The article refers to a widely used instructional manual—"The 36-Hour Day"—as a useful book for families.)

Lynn, Joanne, and James F. Childress. "Must Patients Always Be Given Food and Water?" *Hastings Center Report*, October 1983, pp. 17–21.

Ostling, Richard N. "Is It Wrong to Cut Off Feeding?" *Time*, February 23, 1987, p. 71.

Paris, John J., S.J., Ph.D., and Frank E. Reardon, J.D. "Court Responses to Withholding or Withdrawing Artificial Nutrition and Fluids." *Journal of the American Medical Association*, vol. 253, no. 15 (April 19, 1985), pp. 2243–45.

President's Commission for the Study of Ethical Problems in Medicine and Biomedical and Behavioral Research. *Deciding to Forego Life-Sustaining Treatment.* Washington, D.C.: U.S. Government Printing Office, 1983.

Rosenfeld, Isadore, M.D. "Never Stop Hoping—It May Not Be Alzheimer's Disease." *Woman's Day,* March 4, 1986, p. 46.

Silverstone, Barbara, and Helen Kandel Hyman. *You and Your Aging Parent: The Modern Family's Guide to Emotional, Physical, and Financial Problems.* New York: Pantheon, 1982.

Steinbrook, Robert, M.D., and Bernard Lo, M.D. "Decision Making for Incompetent Patients by Designated Proxy: California's New Law." *New England Journal of Medicine,* vol. 314, no. 24, June 14, 1984, pp. 1598–1601.

Wallis, Claudia. "To Feed or Not to Feed?" *Time,* March 31, 1986, p. 60.

Wanzer, Sidney H., M.D., *et al.* "The Physician's Responsibility Toward Hopelessly Ill Patients." *New England Journal of Medicine,* vol. 310, no. 15 (April 12, 1984), pp. 955–59.

10 From Malpractice to Billing Fraud— Getting Action When You've Been Wronged

WHEN "Susan Goodman" rushed her 7-year-old daughter to the family doctor, she suspected Danielle had broken her collarbone or pulled a shoulder muscle in a fall from her tree house. An x-ray indicated the second-grader had actually fractured her sternum, or breastbone. But to be sure of the diagnosis, the doctor suggested that Susan might want an orthopedic surgeon, who was sharing the same office, to see her daughter, too. She agreed, but says she was appalled at what happened next.

"The doctor came in, looked at the x-ray, looked at Danielle, moved her shoulders a little bit, and said, 'It's a fractured sternum bone, there's nothing you can do for it, and don't let her do anything.' He said she'd be all right, told me to call if there were any problems, and left the room. I walked outside and the nurse said to me, 'That will be three hundred and seventy-five dollars—and the doctor wants to be paid right away.' It absolutely floored me," says Susan, who didn't have such a sum in her purse and refused to write a check for it.

Even though the Goodmans carry health insurance which covers accidents like Danielle's, Susan couldn't believe her ears. "Don't you think that's pretty high for five minutes of his time?" she asked the nurse. Her answer: "Well, that's what Blue Cross and Blue Shield pay for a fractured sternum bone." Susan took the bill home, paid it, and later was reimbursed by her insurance company.

Susan Goodman and her husband, David, are willing to pay for good medical care. They keep up their health insurance premiums, because they know major surgery or a prolonged illness could bankrupt them. But, like many Americans, they balk at the excessive fees charged by some doctors, dentists, and lawyers. In fact, in an earlier attempt to obtain Susan's medical records from a New York City physician, they had hesitated to engage an attorney's help because they feared the cost of such legal proceedings.

The Goodmans are not "suit-happy" people who take pleasure in suing a doctor. They are the first to admit that modern medicine can work some special miracles. Two of their three daughters were conceived only after the couple consulted a prominent infertility specialist who, with his brother (also a doctor), was pioneering fertility techniques in the mid-1960s.

No help in getting medical records

The doctors, Cyril C. Marcus and his identical twin Stewart Lee Marcus, were on the staff of Cornell University Medical School and its affiliate, New York Hospital; few people could tell them apart. "They were genius guys," David Goodman says now, "but at the time, I was never really sure I was dealing with the twin who was *our* doctor—which was bizarre."

As it turned out, the Marcus brothers not only covered each other's medical practice, they *covered up* for each other as well.

In July 1975, both brothers were found dead—apparent victims of a drug-related suicide pact. As reported in the *New York Times*, Cyril's drug habit had begun perhaps two years earlier; Stewart's, within only a few months of his death.[1] Both doctors performed gynecological surgery and made medical decisions on several occasions during the time they were regularly taking barbiturates.

Although many health professionals apparently knew the brothers' mental health was deteriorating, few attempts were made either to help the brothers deal with their addiction or to protect their patients from malpractice. (Not until two weeks before their deaths did New York Hospital revoke their hospital privileges.)

Luckily, Susan Goodman didn't have any medical complications during either of her deliveries or during a six-hour operation in 1967 when Cyril Marcus performed surgery to open her fallopian tubes, which were blocked by scar tissue and adhesions formed in her childhood after she was hit by a bus.

By 1971, however, she was growing increasingly apprehensive each time she went for a visit. Her doctor, once a well-groomed perfectionist, was now unkempt and difficult to get along with. So was his twin. Their office was dirty where once it had been spotless; the doctors couldn't seem to keep their nurses. The nurse they finally had not only seemed strange, but was "nasty" to patients, Susan recalls. No longer feeling confident in Cyril Marcus's abilities and finding that he was canceling appointments on her repeatedly, she decided to switch to a gynecologist in Westchester County, where she lived.

Getting her medical records, however, proved to be a four-year struggle.

Susan's letters to Cyril Marcus and numerous calls to his office requesting that he forward her records to her new doctor were fruitless. Her letters to the New York State Education Department, Division of Professional Conduct, reporting Marcus's inaction and asking for help in obtaining her records went unanswered.

An appeal for help to the New York County Medical Society brought the response that the society was unable to obtain the records. Furthermore, Susan says that the society admitted that it "had set up at least two or three appointments to meet with Marcus and he didn't show up. When he did appear, the doctor denied knowing Susan or anything about the case." Later a secretary confided to her that committee members were not even sure the twin they met with was Cyril—Susan's doctor.

Shortly after the Marcus brothers died, another physician took over their practice, located her medical records, and forwarded them at once. "I am very angry and feel I have been very scarred as a result of that experience," Susan says now, adding, "I just don't trust doctors the way I used to."

Like the Goodmans, who have experienced three of the most common problems patients run into in dealing with the health care system, many patients and their families have had their eyes opened. They trusted their doctors and believed they were ethical in the way they practiced medicine. What doctors did on their own time was their own business; but whatever it was, it shouldn't interfere with the doctor-patient relationship.

Americans today are wiser and more wary. They're better educated and medically more sophisticated. They're less willing to accept their doctor's word for everything and more likely to seek out second opinions. Frequently, they recognize or intuitively sense that a physician, nurse, or other health practitioner is incompetent, impaired, or engaging in unethical practices—and they want to do something about it. Increasingly, they're willing to blow the whistle on such health professionals.

They're also filing three times as many medical malpractice claims as they did ten years ago, and they're winning record settlements.[2] According to *Megatrends* author John Naisbitt, the average malpractice jury verdict award is $1 million—triple the average in 1980.[3]

But, notes Alexander M. Capron, former executive director of the President's Commission on medical ethics, "only a small number of physicians are responsible for the worst sorts of claims. Only 10 percent of all malpractice claims come to trial—and the defendants (physicians/hospitals) win in most cases."[4] In addition, most large jury awards are reduced either by the trial judge or, later, on appeal.

Is there a real problem with doctors?

Before going any further, I want to say I believe American and Canadian doctors are the best-trained and best-equipped in the world. Most are honest, conscientious, ethical, and hard-working men and women. They care about their patients and do their best to help them get better, feel better, cope better.

But I've also served for eight years on the Nevada State Board of Medical Examiners—the body which sets practice standards, and licenses and disciplines physicians who practice in the state—and I've seen the other side. As board secretary, my job was to screen complaints against doctors, carry out investigations to see if the cases warranted further action, and, if so, present the facts to the full board at a hearing. These cases ran the gamut from sexual abuse of patients to drug and alcohol addiction, gross negligence in performing surgery, falsifying credentials, and Medicare fraud.

I believe that the medical profession should weed out its own "bad apples." But I also know that this can't be done without patients' help. Unfortunately, doctors are reluctant to get involved. In 1983, only 4 percent of the 819 complaints received by the New York Disciplinary Board were filed by physicians.[5] In Nevada, only three of the one hundred complaints received by my board in 1984 came from doctors.

Yet Ralph Nader's Health Research Group estimates that

as many as two hundred thousand Americans are injured or killed in hospitals each year as a result of negligent care. According to a *New York Times* article, Dr. Arnold S. Relman, editor of the *New England Journal of Medicine,* believes that at least twenty thousand grossly incompetent or negligent doctors continue to practice in this country—and that figure may actually be twice as high.[6]

"Few physicians relish the idea of being a policeman, and fewer still are willing to assume that role by initiating a formal complaint against an errant colleague," Relman says in a medical journal editorial. "Yet their obligation is clear and they avoid it at the risk of serious damage to the standing of their profession."[7]

Reasons to blow the whistle

If you feel you have a complaint about your doctor, this chapter will help you know where to go for help, how to present and document your case, and what results you can expect.

Basically, there are three reasons why you may feel you need to blow the whistle on your doctor, a nurse, or a clinic or hospital where you or a family member has been a patient: (1) you've *been* wronged or harmed in some way and you want to do something about it; (2) you're afraid you *will be* wronged or harmed and want to prevent it; and (3) you've been harmed and *don't want someone else to go through the same bad experience*—whether it's fiscal, physical or emotional.

In short, people blow the whistle because of a mix of anger, pain, self-interest, and altruism. At times, when it seems a patient should take action against a doctor, the person doesn't. Consider what happened to "Jim," a West Coast media celebrity who told his story to doctors attending a 1986 bioethics conference.[8]

Violation of confidentiality

Jim, who is in his early 50s, had spent twelve years developing a highly successful and, as he puts it, "high-energy and
jet-set" type of food business. Beginning as a chef and gour-
met cook, he switched next to designing restaurants and the
food they served, then catering huge parties, and finally producing his own television show. His name and face were well
known; his major private clients were doctors who would
hire him to cater parties, cook for them on travels, and the
like. Jim's schedule took him to major cities from coast to
coast several times a month.

But he also did an enormous amount of charity work. One
of his favorite benefits was a Doctors' Wives Auxiliary which
every year put on an enormously popular cooking demonstration as a fund raiser. Since he was well known in TV, Jim
always took part in it.

Some time in 1984, however, his frenetic pace began to
catch up with him. He often felt tired and low on energy.
When suddenly he began experiencing night sweats, fever,
and weight loss, his doctor hospitalized him for tests which
later would prove positive for AIDS (acquired immune deficiency syndrome).

But his symptoms soon disappeared and he felt quite well
again. When Jim checked with his doctor about returning to
work, he was told it would be all right as long as he observed
the same precautions he had always taken when working in
restaurants and handling food.

About a month later, Jim's employers (whom he had not
told about his illness) informed him they had been at a cocktail party where a nurse from another hospital had told them
about his having AIDS. Was it true, they wanted to know. Jim
said it was, knowing that once word got around he could no
longer continue his work in restaurants.

"Up to that point, I had always believed in medical confidentiality," he says, "but I began to discover quickly that there are no secrets. Not when there are technicians doing all sorts of tests, clerks handling records, and nurses from one hospital talking to nurses at another. Nurses who would think nothing of casually mentioning my having AIDS at a party!"

But what happened a few months later wiped out Jim's career overnight.

Jim had been undergoing chemotherapy, but feeling quite well with no side effects. A few weeks before the annual Doctors' Wives Auxiliary benefit, he received a telephone call from the president of the group. The woman "very nicely explained to me that they had been told I had AIDS, did not want me to take part because they disapproved of my lifestyle, and if I attempted to appear or cook in public or work in public at all, they would expose me." It's a threat, he says, which has been used against him many times.

Jim explained that he would not be cooking *for* anyone— no one else would be eating the food or even touching it; he was simply going to do a food demonstration. The woman repeated her warning: "If you ever again work in public or appear in public, we will expose you." Jim was horrified to learn that this stance had been agreed upon in a large committee meeting where his name had been casually bandied about. What hurt him most, however, is that he knows who told the woman he has AIDS—his own physician!

Jim's oncologist had revealed it to his wife, the auxiliary's president. Furious, Jim confronted this man later. "How can you take my money to keep me alive when your wife has just destroyed my career?" The doctor's response: "I can't tell my wife what to do."

Jim says he is afraid to appear on television now and he doesn't think he could develop another line of work with that Doctors' Wives Auxiliary threat hanging over his head. Summing it all up, he says, "Confidentiality is very important, because as your confidentiality leaves, isolation enters. It's stripped me of everything—everything I worked for. It's taken every bit of self-respect I had; it's literally wiped me out. Fighting the medical bills and fighting the social part makes fighting the disease that much harder."

Legal limits to doctor-patient confidentiality

Jim had every reason to believe his privacy and confidentiality would be respected by all the physicians treating him and that none would discuss his condition with a spouse.[9] Since the time of Hippocrates, the doctor-patient relationship has generally been held to be confidential, unless the patient wishes it to be otherwise, and, legally, a patient can sue the doctor or hospital for disclosing information about him or her without permission.

According to AMA president Dr. John J. Coury, Jr., medical ethics and the threat of legal action keep doctors from disclosing the presence of a risk of AIDS in an individual, even when the physician's silence may result in the patient's partner's being infected or in the birth of an AIDS-infected infant. "We have been urging all people who have had multiple partners to voluntarily tell those partners," said Coury in an Associated Press report, adding, "under patient confidentiality, we can't tell."[10]

This is true of *all* sexually transmitted diseases. But physicians strongly urge all patients who have these diseases to voluntarily inform their sexual partners of the potential risk to their health.

There are rare times when the law requires a doctor to breach patient confidentiality, such as reporting a communicable disease, child abuse, or a threat of serious bodily harm to a specific person (as in the landmark Tarasoff case).[11] Even though AIDS is a communicable disease reportable by law, that report should only go to the health department, *not* to the physician's spouse.

When I asked Jim why he didn't sue the doctor or report

his unprofessional conduct to the county medical society or state medical licensing and disciplinary board, he said, "The hell with that—I'm telling my story directly, but anonymously, to doctors and lay people at meetings like this. I'm making a plea for compassion and for protection of privacy—not just for the person with AIDS but for each and every patient."

Jim also felt there was no point in starting legal action, as he might not live long enough to see a court case through to the end. So he's chosen to speak out as a way to make others aware of his experience and what can happen when a patient's confidentiality is violated.

When the doctor-patient contract is broken

All doctor-patient relationships are based on a contract. It may be *explicit* (a written or oral agreement, such as "I've asked you to take care of me and you have agreed") or *implicit* (as in an emergency when you are taken unconscious to a hospital and treated by the doctor on duty).

As a patient, you trust that your doctor is competent to care for you and will fulfill his or her responsibility to do what is in your best interest. You trust your welfare will be your doctor's foremost concern, that you will not be harmed or killed, that your life and health will be preserved, your suffering relieved, and your privacy protected.

If your physician harms you, lies to you, or betrays your trust, then the bond between you is destroyed. From an ethical point of view, your doctor has *violated your rights and broken a contract with you.* When this happens, you will feel angry, disappointed, let down. "I've been taken," you may say, or "My doctor betrayed me" or "Now what do I do?" You may also feel that you've been manipulated or that your body space has been violated—and you're powerless to do anything about it.

315

But you're not powerless; you can do something.

Depending on the circumstances, you or a family member have at least ten different ways to blow the whistle on a health professional or facility.

Will blowing the whistle do any good?

Certainly you have a right to compensation when you can prove you've been injured because of a doctor's negligence. For years, though, people have said, "Why bother—it won't get me anywhere," or "Doctors protect each other, so what's the use?"

Today, however, it's worth your while to blow the whistle and voice your complaint.

A whole new attitude toward disciplining incompetent and unethical doctors is sweeping the country at all levels of the health care system.[12] There's a growing movement to weed out the bad doctor and clean up the profession. One reason is economics, but certainly enlightened self-interest plays a big role. Not only is it good for the patient, it's good for the profession.

Since 1980, state medical boards have become much more active in *formally* disciplining the bad doctor.[13] But that's only part of the picture.

"Keep in mind," says Dale Breaden of the Federation of State Medical Boards of the United States, "that for every formal action, as many as ten to twenty *informal* encounters take place between disciplinary boards and physicians." (For example, when confronted by the board in an informal meeting, a physician with a drinking problem may agree to seek treatment; another doctor writing inappropriate prescriptions for dangerous or useless drugs may agree to stop—but this isn't always the case.)

Further impetus comes from soaring malpractice insurance premiums doctors must pay, from the so-called "doctor glut" resulting in increased competition for patients and their health care dollars, and recent legal decisions holding doctors and hospitals liable for allowing substandard practices to continue. Even in the private office setting, doctors are being forced to become their brother's keeper. As a result of recent court rulings, a doctor who knows his or her partner is incompetent and does nothing about it can be held liable as well.

Despite these changes, doctors still have a long way to go in cleaning up their profession, and the public is getting into the act. An increasing number of lay persons now serve as members of state licensing boards, hospital boards of trustees, and health systems agencies. Many of these operate under so-called "sunshine" or open meeting laws, requiring that most of their activities, including disciplinary proceedings, be carried out in public view.

How to get action

Are you dissatisfied with the care you or a family member is receiving in the doctor's office or hospital? Are the fees you've been charged exorbitant? Have you been charged for services you didn't receive? Are existing laws and regulations making it harder to get better health care for yourself or a family member? Depending on the nature of the problem, here are several ways to do something about it:

***Talk over the problem with your doctor
—he or she may not be aware that there
is a problem.***

Talking face to face with your doctor about a problem isn't easy, but open communication is often the quickest route to a solution. For example, you might say, "Doctor, you didn't tell me the side effects of that drug," or "I think you charged me too much for this procedure," or "I'm concerned I can't get in touch with you at night and on weekends," or "Why won't you send my records to Dr. So-and-so?"

Though it's not the way to solve every problem, the value of open discussion is that sometimes what you thought was a problem can be quickly cleared up. You may find in talking to your doctor that he or she was acting in good faith with no intent to harm you in any way.

"Frequently when people call the medical board to complain," says one state board executive secretary, "we find that it's a problem of communication, rather than one requiring disciplinary action. We suggest they call and talk it over with their doctor."

Fee disputes, for instance, are best handled this way. You'll also find doctors react quickly to a call or letter informing them that you will be forced to contact your lawyer if your medical records are not forwarded to your new physician as you've requested. Even if you don't actually plan to go the legal route, the mere suggestion of an attorney's involvement usually gets prompt action. Doctors don't want to be sued.

Contrary to what you might think, you don't own your medical record. It's not your property. The information is yours—but the degree of access you have to your records depends upon where you live.

Currently, sixteen states allow patients unrestricted access to their medical records.[14] Laws in fifteen other states vary: some allow patients to have access to hospital records but not doctors' records; most states permit only "restricted access," which means patients can get their records through an attorney or if they can prove "good cause." In every state, however, patients, or their authorized representatives, have the right to obtain copies of their medical records through a court order. They also have the right to have their records released with their permission to another physician or health care facility.

If you have trouble obtaining release of your records, ask your lawyer or the state board of medical examiners to contact the doctor or the hospital. That plus a written release signed by you is usually all that's needed to free up a record that's been tied up. However, expect to pay a reasonable copying fee, which in some states is set by law. (For other sources of help, see Resources section at the end of this chapter.)

When it comes to confronting your doctor about professional behavior, including possible alcohol- or drug-related problems, don't be surprised if you are rebuffed. Most physicians will ignore or rebuff a patient who tries to discuss the doctor's apparent drinking or drug problem.

Of course, there's always a risk in direct confrontation. Your doctor may end the relationship and tell you to find another physician. Frankly, you may be better off to do so.

Discuss the problem with the hospital, clinic, or nursing home ombudsman and/ or administrator.

Given today's competitive health care market, hospitals are much more receptive to your complaints about their doctors and nurses than they were in the past. Hospital administrators not only want to protect patients from harm, they want to protect the hospital as well. It's in their best interests to intervene quickly and avoid lawsuits. Satisfied patients are the key to a hospital's financial success.

Not only that, hospitals can respond to complaints faster than state licensing boards or the courts, with their crowded calendars and lengthy due-process proceedings.

If you're a patient in the hospital and want to register a complaint, talk to the nursing supervisor, the hospital social worker, or the ombudsman if there is one. Ask whomever you consult to take your complaint to the proper authority; ask for a meeting to discuss the problem. If you've already left the hospital, send a certified letter with your complaint to the chief of the medical staff *and* to the administrator of the hospital or other health care facility in which the alleged misconduct or problem occurred.

Most hospitals renew a doctor's privileges annually after a review of his or her past performance and any complaints received about the doctor. The hospital governing board, on recommendation of the chief of the medical staff, can suspend or limit a doctor's practice within that facility. For serious misconduct, it can expel the doctor from the hospital staff.

The governing board can also require that the doctor's practice be monitored and that he or she take part in continuing medical education and upgrade specific skills in order to maintain privileges to treat patients within the hospital. Such sanctions may open the doctor to review by other hospitals in the same community or prevent the doctor from obtaining hospital privileges in another city.

However, without hospital privileges, the doctor can *still practice in an office*—a fact you should keep in mind if you decide to file your complaint *only* with the hospital.

Make a written complaint to the appropriate state medical licensing and professional conduct board.

Physicians practice medicine in each of the fifty states by virtue of a license granted by the state through its licensing board. In most states, the governor appoints a group of lay people and doctors to act as a board to license and discipline doctors. (The same is true for dentists, nurses, and all other health professionals.)

You can make a complaint—it must be in writing—to the state board of medical examiners or the equivalent licensing agency in your state. (In California, for example, this would be the California Board of Medical Quality Assurance. In New York, it's the State Board of Education. To find out who licenses and disciplines physicians in your state, call your county or state medical association, listed in the telephone directory.)

State laws vary regarding grounds for disciplining a licensed physician or other health professional.[15] According to Robert C. Derbyshire, M.D., a former president of the Federation of State Medical Boards, which represents licensing agencies, the ten most common grounds for disciplining doctors are:[16]

Medicare/Medicaid fraud
Controlled-substance violations, including narcotics
Impairment due to alcohol
Gross malpractice
Professional incompetence
Unprofessional conduct
Conviction of a felony
Failure to maintain adequate records
Lack of or inadequate informed consent
Sexual activity with patient

These are serious offenses. Although there's always a chance your complaint may be dismissed as having no grounds for action under a state board's statute, if action *is* warranted, then a quasi-judicial process begins. This includes the presentation of charges and evidence, cross-examination, and defense. In most states, the process is public and subject to appeal through the courts.

But due process takes time.

Even though you believe what happened to you is awful and the doctor (or nurse, therapist, or other health professional) is obviously in the wrong, it's unlikely your complaint will get fast action—*unless* it raises the strong possibility that the doctor poses an immediate threat to the public health, safety, or welfare. In that case, the doctor's license can be suspended at once pending a hearing.

If the physician is found guilty, the board can impose a number of sanctions, singly or in combination. Among these are revocation or suspension of the doctor's medical license, probation, fines, reprimands, censure and letters of concern, and stipulated agreements placing limits and conditions on the physician's license to practice.

For example, one Nevada doctor found guilty of prescribing

321

drugs for a known addict was placed on probation for five years and denied prescription-writing privileges for specific drugs. The rest of his practice was not affected. Another physician indicted for alleged sexual abuse of children while examining them in his office was immediately suspended from seeing any patient under the age of 18 pending results of criminal prosecution.

Until recently, doctors who had been disciplined in one state would quickly move to another and set up practice, hoping their record wouldn't catch up with them. But now, a central registry maintained by the Federation of State Medical Boards limits the opportunities for a doctor who has been disciplined to jump from one state to another and start practicing all over again.

Send a written complaint to the county, state, and professional societies to which your doctor belongs.

Most, but not all, physicians are members of their county and state medical associations. They may also belong to national groups, such as the American Medical Association and one of many specialty societies (the American College of Surgeons, the American College of Physicians, the American Academy of Pediatrics, the American Academy of Family Physicians, etc.).

(To find out if your doctor is a member of a local or state group, call the state or county medical society. For membership in the American Medical Association or specialty societies, consult the *American Medical Directory* and/or the *Directory of Medical Specialists*, found in the reference section of all hospital and medical school libraries and many public libraries.)

These memberships are a matter of pride and a sign of a doctor's good standing in the professional community. Reporting your complaint in writing to any of these societies enables the organization to review the doctor's conduct and take appropriate action. Ask for a written acknowledgment of the group's findings and any sanctions imposed on the doctor.

County, state, national, and specialty medical societies can censure a physician and expel him or her from membership. Although this results in professional embarrassment and may affect the doctor's standing among peers and cut down on patient referrals, this action has *no legal impact* and is not made public.

Notify your health/medical insurance company or other third-party payer such as Medicare and/or Medicaid.

If you think you've been overcharged or your insurance billings are incorrect or that you've been billed for medical services you haven't received, immediately contact your doctor or hospital to correct any inadvertent clerical or computer error. If you aren't satisfied or you become convinced that the erroneous billings are *intentional*, report the problem to your health insurance company, to the state insurance commissioner, or to the third-party payer handling Medicare or Medicaid payments in your community.

Although Susan Goodman, in the case described early in this chapter, was surprised by the fee charged by the surgeon who diagnosed her daughter's chest injury, the amount was within guidelines set by Blue Cross/Blue Shield. That wasn't so in the case of a 74-year-old woman I'll call Alice Jones.

When Mrs. Jones saw her bill for skin surgery to remove a small growth from her lower eyelid, she was horrified. She had been in the doctor's office less than half an hour, but the bill totaled more than $2,000. Since her daughter worked at a Medicare office in town, Alice showed her the charges. Suspecting that the bill was padded, her daughter quietly looked into the matter.

Billing fraud is serious business. The doctor who pads a bill runs the risk of incurring legal sanctions, such as criminal prosecution for fraud and civil suit for repayment of fees received through fraudulent claims. In addition, the board of medical examiners can discipline a physician for unprofessional conduct. When Alice Jones's surgeon was found guilty of billing fraud, he was prohibited from further participation in Medicare programs.

This type of fraud is less likely to occur today because of more intense monitoring of all Medicare billings by the government and recently-established professional review organizations (PROs) in each state, but still, it pays to check all your medical bills carefully. Be sure you've received all the services you're being charged for. If charges seem too high, ask why.

If you believe your doctor is violating any state or federal law, submitting false insurance or Medicare/Medicaid claims, or prescribing, selling, or distributing controlled substances inappropriately, contact the appropriate state or federal agency (for example, the U.S. Drug Enforcement Administration, the state pharmacy board, the federal or state Medicare office, or the state welfare department).

Discuss the problem with your attorney —you may have reason to file suit against your doctor or health facility.

You can't expect doctors to be infallible. Accidents occur, and perfect results cannot be guaranteed. If, however, you've been injured or harmed by the treatment you've received from your doctor as a result of his negligence or incompetence, consult an attorney about suing your doctor for malpractice.

Malpractice is a *legal* concept based upon accepted standards of practice nationwide. As explained by attorney and physician Donald J. Flaster in a 1983 *New Woman* article on medical malpractice and negligence, malpractice "refers to certain types of misconduct or improper performance of professional duties by the physician (or other professional), for which he or she becomes legally liable to compensate a person who is the victim of the wrongful act."[17]

The malpractice process is one of peer review in which judgments are made on the basis of expert medical testimony concerning the specifics of *the care you received*—and not a general evaluation of the doctor's competence. In other words, you don't sue a doctor because you think "he's bad." You sue because of specific acts done or not done to you.

(In a case still pending, for instance, Patti and Sam Frustaci have filed a $3.2 million malpractice suit against their doctor, Jaroslav Marik, and the Tyler Medical Clinic in Los Angeles, claiming that she received too high a dose of the fertility drug Pergonal and that its effects were not monitored properly by ultrasound.[18] Marik has stated that Patti Frustaci was negligent in failing to obtain the ultrasound he recommended. Patti, whose own health was endangered by the twenty-eight-week pregnancy, gave birth prematurely to septuplets in May 1985. Only three infants survived, and in the first year of life, expenses for their medical care exceeded $1 million.)

In some states, the medical and legal professions jointly conduct *screening panels* prior to the filing of such suits. The panel will advise you, your lawyer, *and* your doctor whether there is a resonable basis for your complaint and the filing of a suit.

If you win your case, you may be entitled to damages. But you should be aware that your doctor can file a countersuit if your action was taken without a reasonable basis. Furthermore, some state laws provide for penalties *against you and your attorney* for filing a suit contrary to the advice of the panel, should you ultimately lose the case in court. This is one way state legislatures are trying to limit the filing of frivolous suits and clogging of court calendars.

Doctors, too, are trying to reduce the spiraling number of malpractice suits against them. Harvard Medical School physicians recently developed that institution's first mandatory standards for monitoring patients under anesthesia in hopes of preventing deaths or other mistakes. According to a report issued by the group, of the twenty million patients in the United States who receive anesthesia during operations each year, about two thousand or more die of causes "primarily attributable to anesthesia"—deaths that are thought to be "preventable."

"Physicians traditionally have resisted standards of practice which prescribe specific details of their day-to-day conduct of medical care," writes Dr. John H. Eichhorn, who with five colleagues published the report in the *Journal of the American Medical Association*.[19] The report contends that by adopting specific, required standards, doctors nationwide could not only improve their patient care but also cut down on malpractice cases.

In Los Angeles, the newly established Physician's Alert Screening Service enables a doctor to review a prospective patient's litigation history before accepting the person as a patient.[20] In turn, the Los Angeles Trial Lawyers Association has initiated a hotline service providing patients with information on the number of times a doctor has been sued for malpractice.

It's important to remember that neither a suit against a physician nor an out-of-court settlement necessarily means that the doctor was incompetent or guilty of wrongdoing. Insurance companies frequently settle out of court as a less expensive alternative to a lengthy court battle, and one study of 23,545 claims revealed that 74 percent were settled without indemnity.[21] In short, despite the huge malpractice dollar awards that make newspaper headlines, the odds are that you won't win the same.

Contact the district attorney's office if you believe criminal charges are warranted.

Fraud, misrepresentation of professional qualifications, falsification of records, practicing without a license, false advertising, and many other offenses which constitute criminal behavior should be reported to your local district attorney for investigation and possible prosecution.

You should also contact the district attorney if you believe a statute has been violated (such as the failure of a health professional to report child abuse) or if a crime has been committed, e.g., participation in active euthanasia, assisting in a patient's suicide, or the *unlawful* withholding or withdrawal of treatment.

In a 1982 case which attracted national attention, the Los Angeles district attorney filed charges of murder against two physicians, Neil L. Barber and Robert J. Nejdl.[22] An intensive care nurse had accused them of illegally removing all life-support systems and deliberately starving 55-year-old Clarence Herbert, who remained in coma for eleven days following a postoperative cardiopulmonary arrest. Convinced his condition was hopeless, the doctors had acted at the request of Herbert's wife and eight children, who did not want his death prolonged. Following several lower-court decisions, charges were dropped when a California appellate panel ruled that the doctors had not acted unlawfully.

Your local district attorney, the state attorney general, or the United States attorney may act in similar cases when a doctor's conduct allegedly violates any state or federal statute. If found guilty, the doctor could be fined, placed on probation, or sentenced to prison.

For example, when a young Nevada doctor was found guilty of writing prescriptions for controlled substances and trading them for street drugs, not only was he convicted of a felony, but his license to practice medicine was revoked by the state disciplinary board. Besides receiving a jail term, the doctor had to participate in a special drug and alcohol abuse program geared to health professionals.

Contact the physician's aid committee of your local hospital or county medical society if you suspect your doctor has a drinking or drug problem.

It's estimated that from 10 to 15 percent of the nation's 400,000 doctors are impaired at some time during their career because of drug or alcohol abuse.[23] Others are impaired because of mental illness and senility. The American Medical Association concedes that 4 to 5 percent of physicians may be incompetent. (National nursing organizations admit that the two most common reasons for disciplining nurses are alcohol abuse and drug diversion—the personal use and selling of drugs prescribed for patients.)[24]

"When impaired physicians arrive in an altered state of consciousness at their job, it is usually very late in the disease and the rest of their lives are already in turmoil," says G. Douglas Talbott, M.D., director of the highly successful Georgia Impaired Physicians Program. "Symptoms are apparent last at the office or the hospital."[25]

CLUES THAT YOUR DOCTOR MAY BE IMPAIRED

Your doctor is a loner; has no hospital privileges; doesn't stay active in medical circles or take part in continuing education programs. He or she is isolated from friends and peers, unreliable and unpredictable in community or social activities, and withdrawn from community affairs, leisure activities, and hobbies which had interested him or her before.

Your doctor tells lies; shows radical personality changes or uncharacteristic and unpredictable behavior, such as wide mood swings, altered states of consciousness, slurred speech, poor personal hygiene or deterioration in clothing and dressing habits, inappropriate spending, embarrassing behavior at clubs or parties, or hostile, deceitful, or unreasonable behavior toward patients and staff.

Your doctor repeatedly misses appointments; is accident-prone; is frequently ill or hospitalized; is away from the office without explanation or call-forwarding system. In an emergency, you can't get hold of your doctor or else he or she is slow to respond.

Your doctor has family problems, which may include unexplained absences from home, fights, child abuse, extramarital affairs, strange sexual behavior, or geographical separation or divorce proceedings by spouse. Your doctor's family may cover up or make excuses for the doctor's behavior, and the doctor's children may be involved in abnormal, antisocial, and/or illegal behavior.

Your doctor is picked up for driving under the influence (DUI).

Your doctor shows signs of decreasing quality of performance in caring for patients; makes hospital rounds late or shows inappropriate, abnormal behavior during rounds; writes inappropriate orders or overprescribes medications. Office and/or hospital staff are receiving patients' complaints about the doctor's behavior and he or she is involved in malpractice suits and legal sanctions against the hospital.

Adapted from a chart titled "Clues to Alcoholism or Drug Addiction in Six Areas of a Physician's Life," in G. Douglass Talbott, M.D., and Earl B. Benson, M.D., "Impaired Physicians: The Dilemma of Identification," *Postgraduate Medicine*, vol. 68, no. 6 (December 1980).

For years, this problem was kept in the closet. The so-called conspiracy of silence protected doctors and nurses from public scrutiny.[26]

When the Marcus brothers died of severe barbiturate withdrawal symptoms in 1975, for example, a *New York Times* editorial stated: "What is most amazing is that nobody reported their condition or tried to do anything about it, though their deterioration and aberrant behavior must have been plain to numerous colleagues and other health workers. The New York County Medical Society knew something was amiss because patients complained of insurance forms not filled out and records not transferred to other doctors. But the society's investigation was superficial; it never came close to revealing that both men were so much under the influence of barbiturates that their lives—as well as those of their patients—were endangered."[27]

Today, however, not only does the problem of the impaired health professional get media attention, but more important, the medical and nursing professions are actively trying to do something about it.

If you suspect a nurse is impaired, call his or her hospital supervisor, the state board of nursing, or the state nursing association, many of which have peer assistance committees. Since most nurses are employed by hospitals or other health care facilities, the quickest way to get action is through the nursing supervisor. Once alerted, nursing and pharmacy administrators can monitor drug use within the hospital by nursing unit and shift.

If you think a doctor is impaired, for whatever reason, and want him or her to get professional help without being punished, call your county or state medical association or the chief of staff at the hospital where your doctor is a staff member. In some states you can report your concern anonymously. In others, you must identify yourself, but you can ask to have your report investigated confidentially.

When a physician's aid committee gets involved, members will confront the doctor and try to intervene in a positive and helpful way. They will insist that the doctor seek medical and psychiatric care. Also required is active participation in Alcoholics Anonymous or other drug self-help and support-group programs, such as Narcotics Anonymous or the "Caduceus Clubs" whose members are all health professionals with alcohol and/or drug problems.

The intention is to assist the doctor to deal with the problem while remaining professionally active. Physician's aid committees work cooperatively with state licensing boards to rehabilitate impaired doctors before their licenses and livelihoods are placed in jeopardy. (Nursing association peer assistance committees work in similar fashion.)

When you contact the committee, ask the chairperson to let you know the outcome of the group's action. Occasionally, no action can be taken against the doctor, despite the best efforts of his or her family, colleagues, and the committee.

In one case I know of, a father reported that he had seen his doctor son using cocaine at home. He had also seen him drunk more than a few times and, afraid the young doctor was heading for serious trouble, wanted the physician's aid committee to do something before it was too late. Yet two independent investigations failed to come up with enough evidence for the committee to act. The father was angry and frustrated that "the system" could not "do something"—a complaint that is often heard by those who serve on disciplinary boards or impaired-physician committees.

Don't forget, the courts view a doctor's license as a fundamental property right. It is essential to his or her livelihood and not easily revoked. In most states, the law requires "clear and convincing" evidence before a board can revoke a license.

Go public—take your story to the media.

If you are frustrated and feel you're getting nowhere, the media can often get results. Investigative reporting and the articles, editorials, and op-ed pieces that follow it can identify problems in the way the health care system in your community deals with medical incompetence, malpractice, and unethical conduct. These become the impetus for legislative action and professional change. (You'll find pointers on working with the media in Appendix I.)

Besides going to the media, there are other effective methods of getting public attention, among them forming concerned citizen groups; gathering signatures on petitions for change; and speaking at meetings—as "Jim" does to let people know what can happen when a patient's confidentiality is violated.

The public appeal route can be especially helpful when you are getting the runaround by health care professionals or when you suspect there is coverup, evasion, or stonewalling.

If a change in regulations or laws is needed, lobby for legislative change wherever appropriate—city hall, your state capital, or the U.S. Congress.

*Finally, inform yourself fully and contact
self-help, support, and consumer groups
—there's clout in numbers, and "squeaky
wheels" get action where a single voice
may not.*

Remember, none of these options for action is mutually exclusive. You want to target your complaint to the right group, but nothing says you can't report simultaneously to several different agencies. Reporting to the state licensing board, for example, does not rule out sending the same complaint to the district attorney, the hospital chief of staff, or the county medical society, or from taking any other appeal route, such as discussing your problem with the hospital ombudsperson or taking your story to the media.

Making sure you want to take action

You may be angry, hurt, dissatisfied, or frustrated because of the treatment you or someone you care about has received. You want something done about it. But before you go any further, give careful thought to the following questions, which can help you look realistically at the situation, your chances of proving your case, and what you may be letting yourself in for along the way.

Why are you doing this?

Be clear about your motivation, since it's sure to be challenged by the physician you're accusing and his or her defense attorneys—if not by your own friends, relatives, and coworkers. Others may imply that you're acting because of a grudge or personal vendetta against the doctor or a desire to "make a buck."

In a 1985 American Medical Association survey, 30 percent said that people suing doctors were "usually justified in bringing suit." However, 44 percent said these people were "just looking for an easy way to make money."[28] If you've got an ax to grind or you're looking for easy money and these motivations are exposed, you can be sure that they will weaken your case. On the other hand, a sincere desire to protect other patients from similar harm, to punish wrongdoing, and to obtain redress of grievance will make your case stronger.

Do you have the necessary evidence and documentation to support your complaint?

To back up your complaint, you'll need medical records in which the facts of your case are recorded. Are these available? Are people willing to testify or submit affidavits about the alleged wrongful acts? Are doctors and/or other health professionals willing to testify on your behalf and against a colleague?

After reviewing their complaints, I've frequently had to tell patients that the board could not proceed with a disciplinary action without more evidence, documentation, and witnesses. One of these patients, for example, was a woman who was accusing a doctor of sexual advances but had no witnesses and, naturally, no record of the incident. All the board had to go on was her word against his, so all we could do was file her report for further reference.[29] But that didn't rule out her going to the district attorney and/or her lawyer if she was willing to testify in court against her doctor—action she decided against.

Even if you aren't sure you have enough to go on or your complaint seems "slight" or, perhaps, trivial, there is an important reason why you should make a report to the medical board anyway. (This applies to *any complaint*, whether it's sexual harassment, verbal abuse, exorbitant fees, an inadequate or inappropriate examination, or anything else.) Often, when one person's complaint is added to several other complaints about the same physician, a pattern of bizarre, inappropriate, or unprofessional behavior emerges. The board can then act on the complaints as a whole and investigate the doctor.

What do you want to result from your action?

Do you want the physician to be fined? Disciplined? Taken out of practice? Do you want redress of grievance? Or do you hope that the nurse, physician, or dentist with a drinking or drug problem will get professional help? Are you trying to prevent injury to other patients and keep them from going through what you did?

Most people want to see other patients protected and the doctor disciplined. A spouse, parent, or colleague usually wants the doctor to get in a treatment or rehabilitation program for the problem so that he or she can remain in practice. Still others want compensation for injury they've incurred—and they deserve it.

For instance, in a clinic for handicapped children, I take care of a four-year-old boy with severe cerebral palsy and mental retardation—the results of brain damage which occurred at birth. His parents sued the obstetrician and several doctors testified the mother had received poor care at the time of delivery. In finding for the child, the court established a $1 million trust fund to provide for his medical and educational needs for the rest of his life.

Actress Peggy Cass received compensation when a Manhattan supreme court jury awarded her $460,000 in a suit against a surgeon at New York's Lenox Hill Hospital. He had operated on her right knee instead of her injured left knee.[30] Later, however, the amount was reduced to $260,000.

What do you have to lose from this action?

Not every suit, appeal, or other action ends the way the person making a complaint hopes it will. Frequently there are not enough witnesses, documentation, or other evidence to support the charges. Friends or family members who go to the same doctor and think he or she is a miracle worker often resent any suggestion that the doctor is incompetent, unprofessional, or impaired.

Your credibility may be challenged, your word questioned. It hurts to be called a liar, mentally unstable, disloyal, disgruntled, or even ungrateful. You may be humiliated on the witness stand. Your private life may be exposed. Being grilled by defense attorneys takes its toll—physically and emotionally. You may have second thoughts or feel guilty that you have hurt the reputation of a previously respected person in your community.

Like Peggy Cass, however, you may feel that's a risk you're willing to take to prove your case, win a settlement, or get an incompetent doctor out of practice.

Filing your complaint

When you file a complaint, give as much *specific* information as possible. Be sure your facts are correct. Be thorough but to the point. Clearly state the nature of the charges you're bringing against the doctor or nurse. It's not enough to say that a physician is "a bad doctor" or "didn't treat me properly." You must be specific. Your complaint will be more effective if you keep the following pointers in mind:

- Put your complaint in writing. Don't worry about legal or medical terms. Write in plain English and be concise.
- Include the physician's name and nature of the alleged misconduct, including date, time, and place where it occurred.

335

- Document the complaint with as much information as possible, including copies of hospital records and insurance claim forms.
- Submit the names of people who have supporting information that is specific, and if possible, include written statements from them. (Even if they have no knowledge of your case, but a similar incident happened to them involving the same doctor, this information will support your case.)
- Submit documentation of second or third opinions from other physicians about your illness and the treatment you received.
- Keep a copy of your letter and all documentation that you submit with it.

Leave your emotions out of your letter. Many valid complaints are weakened by emotional statements which bear little relevance to the facts of a complaint. "If you write a long garbled letter which includes your personal feelings about the doctor, medicine, politics, and what the disciplinary board ought to do to take that s.o.b. out of practice, you've muddied the waters," says one medical board executive secretary. "That doesn't mean you shouldn't ventilate your feelings—just do all that with someone else."

Don't forget, if your complaint is about hospital charges or physician's fees, most state boards don't handle fee disputes. In these cases, contact the administrator of the hospital, your insurance company, or the county or state medical society ethics committee which deals with unfair charges.

Whistleblowers, of course, have been called everything from heroes to self-serving traitors and publicity-seekers. But blowing the whistle may be essential to your peace of mind, your protection, and that of other innocent people.

A final word

Given the high cost of health care today and the ethical dilemmas surrounding life and death, it pays all of us to be knowledgeable and active partners in caring for our health.

Any other approach is short-changing ourselves and inviting someone else to play God for us.

"The best thing you can do," says bioethics expert Arthur Caplan, "is to inform yourself fully—reading, questioning, talking to other people with similar medical problems, and getting in touch with [self-help, support, and consumer] groups where they exist. The more input the better. It's your responsibility—the duty of the consumer. Remember, your advocate isn't going to be able to do you any good if he or she has only limited information to work with."

Simply stated, you must care enough to look out for your own best interests, and those of the people you love and are responsible for. To safeguard these interests, you may have to take on the health care system in your community, city, or state.

The whole purpose of this book is to help you understand the issues and their ethical underpinnings, how to protect yourself, and where to go for help. Remember, you don't have to sit back and passively let a doctor, nurse, or anyone else do things to you that you don't want to have done. You don't have to do what they tell you to do in the hospital—although this means you may have to change doctors, go home, or transfer to another facility.

When you are struggling with a medical dilemma, remember that help is as close as the phone. Crises don't always pull families together, but a big part of resolving any health-related moral dilemma is knowing that you are not alone and there are others who can assist you and your family.

From the relatively new specialty of biomedical ethics has emerged a whole new breed of caring and empathetic professionals who, with your doctor, can help you and your family to define the problem, sort out your values, clarify the ethical dilemma, and come up with your options for resolving it. (Appendix J contains a partial listing of bioethical centers and program directors who, if need be, can refer you to experts in your area.)

337

Consulting with an ethics committee or talking things over with an ethicist won't take away the pain of making a hard choice. But it can help you to feel the choice you do make is the right one for you.

All you have to do is ask.

Resources

Public Citizen Health Research Group
Suite 708
2000 P Street, NW
Washington, DC 20036
(202) 872-0320
Sidney M. Wolfe, M.D., director

Works on issues of health care, testifies before Congress, and monitors enforcement of health and safety legislation; publishes research and consumer action materials in reports and various publications, including a helpful booklet on obtaining your medical records titled *Medical Records: Getting Yours* ($5).

American Medical Records Association
John Hancock Center, Suite 1850
875 North Michigan Avenue
Chicago, IL 60611
(312) 787-2672
Rita Finnegan, executive director

State chapters will provide information about individual state laws pertaining to medical-record access; write for address of local chapters, attention: Legislative Affairs Department.

Federation of State Medical Boards of the United States
2630 West Freeway, Suite 138
Fort Worth, TX 76102
(817) 335-1141
Bryant L. Galusha, M.D., executive vice-president

Clearinghouse for state medical practice laws; maintains national computerized registry of physicians who have been disciplined; will refer you to your state medical licensing/disciplinary board for information about a specific doctor or your state law.

The Georgia Impaired Physicians Program
Ridgeview Institute
3985 South Cobb Drive, SE
Smyrna, GA 30080
(404) 434-4567
G. Douglas Talbott, M.D., medical director

One of the nation's oldest and most successful programs for impaired health care professionals based on a highly structured program of confrontation, intervention, treatment, and long-term follow-up; open to doctors, nurses, dentists, pharmacists, veterinarians, and others.

American Civil Liberties Union (ACLU)
132 West 43rd Street
New York, NY 10036
(212) 944-9800
Ira Glasser, executive director

Activities include test court cases, opposition to repressive legislation, public protests on every inroad of rights, and referrals to local chapters. Among publications available from the ACLU Literature Department are *The Rights of the Critically Ill*, *The Rights of Mentally Retarded Persons*, and *The Rights of Gay People*.

Suggested reading

Bowen, Ezra. "Weeding Out the Incompetents." *Time*, May 26, 1986, pp. 57–58. (Medical profession acts to discipline dangerous doctors.)

Brinkley, Joel. "U.S., Industry and Physicians Attack Medical Malpractice" and "Medical Discipline Laws: Confusion Reigns." *New York Times*, September 2–3, 1985.

Federation of State Medical Boards of the United States, Inc. *A Guide to the Essentials of a Modern Medical Practice Act*, rev. ed. Fort Worth, TX: 1985.

Feinstein, Richard J., M.D. "The Ethics of Professional Regulation

—Special Report." *New England Journal of Medicine*, vol. 312, no. 12 (March 21, 1985), p. 801.

Flaster, Donald J., M.D., LL.B. "Do You Have a Case Against Your Doctor for Negligence? Malpractice?" *New Woman*, December 1983, p. 44.

Klugman, Ellen. "Access To Your Medical Records." *Working Woman*, June 1984, pp. 57–58. (Few things seem as precious as your health or as personal as the records kept on it. You should know who has access to this information—and how to protect your privacy.)

President's Commission for the Study of Ethical Problems in Medicine and Biomedical and Behavioral Research. *Whistleblowing in Biomedical Research.* Washington, D.C.: U.S. Government Printing Office, 1981. (Proceedings of a workshop which examined the role of government, teaching hospitals, local institutions, and review boards in responding to reports of fraud and whistleblowing and protecting rights of human subjects and whistleblowers.)

Rooney, Rita. "Doctors, Patients and Sex." *Ladies' Home Journal*, June 1986, p. 107. (A report on doctors who abuse their patients; suggests where to turn for help.)

Smothers, Ronald. "Addict-Doctors Get Aid Under Georgia Program." *New York Times*, May 8, 1983, p. 16.

Stein, Andrew. "Doctors Who Get Away with Killing and Maiming Must Be Stopped." *New York Times*, February 2, 1986, p. 23-E. (Why is there no public outcry?)

Appendices

A A Patient's Bill of Rights

B A Medical Research Patient's Bill of Rights

C A Pregnant Patient's Bill of Rights

D An Institutionalized Person's Bill of Rights

E A Nursing Home Patient's Bill of Rights

F Living Will and Durable Power of Attorney for Health Care (sample forms)

G Uniform Anatomical Gift Act; Donor Card and Consent by Next of Kin for Removal of Organs (sample forms)

H Withholding or Withdrawing of Life-Prolonging Medical Treatment: AMA Statement

I Pointers on Working with the Media

J National and Regional Centers for Medical Ethics

APPENDIX A
A Patient's Bill of Rights

This policy document presents the official position of the American Hospital Association as approved by the Board of Trustees and House of Delegates.

The American Hospital Association presents a Patient's Bill of Rights with the expectation that observance of these rights will contribute to more effective patient care and greater satisfaction for the patient, his physician, and the hospital organization. Further, the Association presents these rights in the expectation that they will be supported by the hospital on behalf of its patients, as an integral part of the healing process. It is recognized that a personal relationship between the physician and the patient is essential for the provision of proper medical care. The traditional physician-patient relationship takes on a new dimension when care is rendered within an organizational structure. Legal precedent has established that the institution itself also has a responsibility to the patient. It is in recognition of these factors that these rights are affirmed.

1. The patient has the right to considerate and respectful care.

2. The patient has the right to obtain from his physician complete current information concerning his diagnosis, treatment, and prognosis in terms the patient can be reasonably expected to understand. When it is not medically advisable to give such information to the patient, the information should be made available to

an appropriate person in his behalf. He has the right to know, by name, the physician responsible for coordinating his care.

3. The patient has the right to receive from his physician information necessary to give informed consent prior to the start of any procedure and/or treatment. Except in emergencies, such information for informed consent should include but not necessarily be limited to the specific procedure and/or treatment, the medically significant risks involved, and the probable duration of incapacitation. Where medically significant alternatives for care or treatment exist, or when the patient requests information concerning medical alternatives, the patient has the right to such information. The patient also has the right to know the name of the person responsible for the procedures and/or treatment.

4. The patient has the right to refuse treatment to the extent permitted by law and to be informed of the medical consequences of his action.

5. The patient has the right to every consideration of his privacy concerning his own medical care program. Case discussion, consultation, examination, and treatment are confidential and should be conducted discreetly. Those not directly involved in his care must have the permission of the patient to be present.

6. The patient has the right to expect that all communications and records pertaining to his care should be treated as confidential.

7. The patient has the right to expect that within its capacity a hospital must make reasonable response to the request of a patient for services. The hospital must provide evaluation, service, and/or referral as indicated by the urgency of the case. When medically permissible, a patient may be transferred to another facility only after he has received complete information and explanation concerning the needs for and alternatives to such a transfer. The institution to which the patient is to be transferred must first have accepted the patient for transfer.

8. The patient has the right to obtain information as to any relationship of his hospital to other health care and educational institutions insofar as his care is concerned. The patient has the right to obtain information as to the existence of any professional relationships among individuals, by name, who are treating him.

9. The patient has the right to be advised if the hospital proposes to engage in or perform human experimentation affecting his care or treatment. The patient has the right to refuse to participate in such research projects.

10. The patient has the right to expect reasonable continuity of care. He has the right to know in advance what appointment times and physicians are available and where. The patient has the right to

expect that the hospital will provide a mechanism whereby he is informed by his physician or a delegate of the physician of the patient's continuing health care requirements following discharge.

11. The patient has the right to examine and receive an explanation of his bill regardless of source of payment.

12. The patient has the right to know what hospital rules and regulations apply to his conduct as a patient.

No catalog of rights can guarantee for the patient the kind of treatment he has a right to expect. A hospital has many functions to perform, including the prevention and treatment of disease, the education of both health professionals and patients, and the conduct of clinical research. All these activities must be conducted with an overriding concern for the patient, and, above all, the recognition of his dignity as a human being. Success in achieving this recognition assures success in the defense of the rights of the patient.

APPENDIX B
A Medical Research Patient's Bill of Rights

NORTHERN CALIFORNIA CANCER PROGRAM
PATIENT CONSENT FORM ATTACHMENT
Medical Research Patient's Bill of Rights

California law and Northern California Cancer Program (NCCP) policies require that any person asked to take part as a subject in research involving a medical experiment, or any person asked to consent to such participation on behalf of another, is entitled to receive the following list of rights written in a language in which the person is fluent. This list includes the right to:

1. Be informed of the nature and purpose of the experiment.
2. Be given an explanation of the procedures to be followed in the medical experiment, and any drug or device to be utilized.
3. Be given a description of any attendant discomforts and risks reasonably to be expected from the experiment.
4. Be given an explanation of any benefits to the subject reasonably to be expected from the experiment, if applicable.
5. Be given a disclosure of any appropriate alternative procedures, drugs, or devices that might be advantageous to the subject, and their relative risks and benefits.
6. Be informed of the avenues of medical treatment, if any, available to the subject after the experiment if complications should arise.

7. Be given an opportunity to ask any questions concerning the experiment or the procedures involved.

8. Be instructed that consent to participate in the medical experiment may be withdrawn at any time and the subject may discontinue participation in the medical experiment without prejudice.

9. Be given a copy of the signed and dated written consent form.

10. Be given the opportunity to decide to consent or not to consent to a medical experiment without the intervention of any element of force, fraud, deceit, duress, coercion, or undue influence on the subject's decision.

APPENDIX C
A Pregnant Patient's Bill of Rights

The Pregnant Patient has the right to participate in decisions involving her well-being and that of her unborn child, unless there is a clearcut medical emergency that prevents her participation. In addition to the rights set forth in the American Hospital Association's "Patient's Bill of Rights" (which has also been adopted by the New York City Department of Health), the Pregnant Patient, because she represents TWO patients rather than one, should be recognized as having the additional rights listed below.

1. *The Pregnant Patient has the right*, prior to the administration of any drug or procedure, to be informed by the health professional caring for her of any potential direct or indirect effects, risks or hazards to herself or her unborn or newborn infant which may result from the use of a drug or procedure prescribed for or administered to her during pregnancy, labor, birth or lactation.

2. *The Pregnant Patient has the right*, prior to the proposed therapy, to be informed, not only of the benefits, risks and hazards of the proposed therapy but also of known alternative therapy, such as available childbirth education classes which could help to prepare the Pregnant Patient physically and mentally to cope with the discomfort or stress of pregnancy and the experience of childbirth, thereby reducing or eliminating her need for drugs and obstetric intervention. She should be offered such information early in her pregnancy in order that she may make a reasoned decision.

3. *The Pregnant Patient has the right*, prior to the administration of any drug, to be informed by the health professional who is pre-

scribing or administering the drug to her that any drug which she receives during pregnancy, labor and birth, no matter how or when the drug is taken or administered, may adversely affect her unborn baby, directly or indirectly, and that there is no drug or chemical which has been proven safe for the unborn child.

4. *The Pregnant Patient has the right* if Cesarean birth is anticipated, to be informed prior to the administration of any drug, and preferably prior to her hospitalization, that minimizing her and, in turn, her baby's intake of nonessential pre-operative medicine will benefit her baby.

5. *The Pregnant Patient has the right*, prior to the administration of a drug or procedure, to be informed of the areas of uncertainty if there is NO properly controlled follow-up research which has established the safety of the drug or procedure with regard to its direct and/or indirect effects on the physiological, mental and neurological development of the child exposed, via the mother, to the drug or procedure during pregnancy, labor, birth or lactation—(this would apply to virtually all drugs and the vast majority of obstetric procedures).

6. *The Pregnant Patient has the right*, prior to the administration of any drug, to be informed of the brand name and generic name of the drug in order that she may advise the health professional of any past adverse reaction to the drug.

7. *The Pregnant Patient has the right* to determine for herself, without pressure from her attendant, whether she will accept the risks inherent in the proposed therapy or refuse a drug or procedure.

8. *The Pregnant Patient has the right* to know the name and qualifications of the individual administering a medication or procedure to her during labor or birth.

9. *The Pregnant Patient has the right* to be informed, prior to the administration of any procedure, whether that procedure is being administered to her for her or her baby's benefit (medically indicated) or as an elective procedure (for convenience, teaching purposes or research).

10. *The Pregnant Patient has the right* to be accompanied during the stress of labor and birth by someone she cares for, and to whom she looks for emotional comfort and encouragement.

11. *The Pregnant Patient has the right* after appropriate medical consultation to choose a position for labor and for birth which is least stressful to her baby and to herself.

12. *The Obstetric Patient has the right* to have her baby cared for at her bedside if her baby is normal, and to feed her baby according to her baby's needs rather than according to the hospital regimen.

13. *The Obstetric Patient has the right* to be informed in writing of the name of the person who actually delivered her baby and the professional qualifications of that person. This information should also be on the birth certificate.

14. *The Obstetric Patient has the right* to be informed if there is any known or indicated aspect of her or her baby's care or condition which may cause her or her baby later difficulty or problems.

15. *The Obstetric Patient has the right* to have her and her baby's hospital medical records complete, accurate and legible and to have their records, including Nurses' Notes, retained by the hospital until the child reaches at least the age of majority, or, alternatively, to have the records offered to her before they are destroyed.

16. *The Obstetric Patient,* both during and after her hospital stay, has the right to have access to her complete hospital medical records, including Nurses' Notes, and to receive a copy upon payment of a reasonable fee and without incurring the expense of retaining an attorney.

It is the obstetric patient and her baby, not the health professional, who must sustain any trauma or injury resulting from the use of a drug or obstetric procedure. The observation of the rights listed above will not only permit the obstetric patient to participate in the decisions involving her and her baby's health care, but will help to protect the health professional and the hospital against litigation arising from resentment or misunderstanding on the part of the mother.

Prepared by Doris Haire, Chair., Committee on Health Law and Regulation, National Women's Health Network

An Institutionalized Person's Bill of Rights

Rights listed below have been abstracted from Guide to Services Including Treatment Alternatives and Client Rights, *published by the Division of Mental Hygiene and Retardation, Department of Human Resources of the State of Nevada. Before you voluntarily admit yourself to an institution or commit someone else to such a facility, ask to see a copy of the guidelines for client rights and services which pertain to your state.*

Rights of the person who is institutionalized

When working with a client unable to give voluntary informed consent, special care must be taken to protect the person's best interest. Therefore, these rights have been developed for clients placed out of their normal home.... *Each client must be fully informed of these rights before or at admission, and must be informed if these rights are amended, with a third person witnessing this.* (Italics added.)

When clients receive services:

- Each adult client is considered legally competent unless there has been a court decision of incompetence.
- Each client retains all rights, benefits, and privileges guaranteed by law.

- Each client continues to have the right to vote in local, state, and federal elections; make contracts; make a will; hold or transfer property; marry; obtain a driver's license; and manage his or her own affairs.

Medical condition and treatment

Each client has the right to:

- Be fully informed by a physician of his health and medical condition, unless the physician decides that informing the patient is medically contraindicated and, if so, this is documented by the physician in the patient's record.
- Be given the opportunity to participate in planning his total care and medical treatment.
- Be given the opportunity to refuse treatment and to give or withhold consent to any and all treatment procedures to be employed.
- Give informed, written consent before participating in experimental research.
- Receive treatment in the least restrictive environment, and that environment must be safe, sanitary, and humane.
- Have an individualized plan of treatment prepared and reviewed thoroughly at least every three months.
- Receive treatment to address individual medical, psychosocial, and habilitative/rehabilitative needs.

Personal rights

Each client has the right:

- To a safe, sanitary, humane living environment.
- To privacy.
- To have his or her records, including information in an automated data bank, treated confidentially.
- To be permitted to share a room with spouse if both are residents.
- To wear his or her own clothing.
- To keep and use personal possessions unless such possessions may be used to endanger his or her or others' lives.
- To refuse to be photographed by still, motion picture, or video cameras unless written consent is given by that client or his or her guardian.

Communication

Each client has the right:

- To see visitors each day.
- To have reasonable access to the telephone.
- To have letter-writing materials, including stamps, and to receive unopened correspondence.
- To communicate, associate, and meet privately with individuals of his or her choice unless this infringes on the rights of another person.

Activities

Each client has the right to participate in social, religious, and community group activities (unless these are contraindicated for a mentally retarded resident and this determination is documented in the resident's record).

Work

No client will be required to perform services for the facility. A client shall be adequately compensated for performing labor which contributes to the operation and maintenance of the facility.

Client's finances

Each client has the right:

- To be allowed to manage his or her personal financial affairs to the fullest extent of his or her ability.
- To have money, earnings, or income deposited in an account in his or her name.

Freedom from abuse and restraint

Each resident must be free from:

- Mental, physical, and verbal abuse.
- Chemical restraint unless chemical restraints are authorized by a physician in writing for a specified period of time.

- Physical restraints unless authorized in writing by a physician or a qualified mental retardation professional (QMRP); or the parent or legal guardian of the client gives informed consent; or an emergency exists, e.g., physical restraints are necessary to protect the client from injuring himself or others.

Exercising rights

Each client is to be:

- Encouraged and assisted to exercise his or her rights as a resident of the facility and as a citizen.
- Allowed to submit complaints or recommendations concerning the policies and services of the facility to staff or to outside representatives of the client's choice or both, and to do so without restraint, interference, coercion, discrimination, or reprisal.

APPENDIX E
A Nursing Home Patient's Bill of Rights

Rights listed below are abstracted from Medicare Regulations #405.1121, Health Care Financing Administration, Department of Health and Human Services. Request a copy of the complete regulations before admission to a nursing home or extended care facility.

A NURSING HOME PATIENT'S BILL OF RIGHTS

The patient's rights policies and procedures shall insure that each patient admitted to the facility:

1. is fully informed...of these rights and of all rules and regulations governing the patient's conduct and responsibilities;
2. is fully informed...of services available in the facility, and of related charges, including any charges for services not covered by sources of third-party payments or...the facility's basic per diem rate;
3. is fully informed, by a physician, of his medical condition unless medically contraindicated...and is afforded the opportunity to participate in the planning of his medical treatment and to refuse to participate in experimental research;
4. is transferred or discharged only for medical reasons, or for his welfare or that of other patients, or for nonpayment of his stay... and is given reasonable advance notice...;

354

5. is encouraged and assisted...to exercise his rights as a patient and as a citizen, and to this end may voice grievances and recommend changes in policies and services...free from restraint, interference, coercion, discrimination, or reprisal;

6. may manage his personal financial affairs, or is given at least a quarterly accounting of financial transactions made on his behalf should the facility accept his written delegation of this responsibility...in conformance with state law;

7. is free from mental and physical abuse, and free from chemical and (except in emergencies) physical restraint except as authorized in writing by a physician for a specified and limited period of time, or when necessary to protect the patient from injury to himself or to others;

8. is assured confidential treatment of his personal and medical records...;

9. is treated with consideration, respect, and full recognition of his dignity and individuality, including privacy in treatment and in care for his personal needs;

10. is not required to perform services for the facility...;

11. may associate and communicate privately with persons of his choice, and send and receive his personal mail unopened, unless medically contraindicated (as documented by his physician in his medical record);

12. may meet with, and participate in activities of, social, religious, and community groups at his discretion, unless medically contraindicated...;

13. may retain and use his personal clothing and possessions...unless to do so would infringe upon rights of other patients, and unless medically contraindicated...and,

14. if married, is assured privacy for visits by his/her spouse; if both are inpatients in the facility, they are permitted to share a room, unless medically contraindicated (as documented by the attending physician in the medical record).

APPENDIX F

Living Will and Durable Power of Attorney for Health Care (sample forms)

LIVING WILL

TO: Family, Physician, Hospital

Should the time come when it is medically confirmed that there is no reasonable hope for my recovery, I direct that I be allowed to die naturally, receiving only the administration of comfort care. I do not wish to have my dying prolonged by artificial means or heroic measures. Should I become unable to participate in decisions regarding my medical treatment, it is my intention that these directions be honored by family and physician(s).

Signature _____

My "living will" document, signed and witnessed,
is among my personal papers.

Living Will Declaration

To My Family, Doctors, and All Those Concerned with My Care

I, _____, being of sound mind, make this statement as a directive to be followed if I become unable to participate in decisions regarding my medical care.

If I should be in an incurable or irreversible mental or physical condition with no reasonable expectation of recovery, I direct my attending physician to withhold or withdraw treatment that merely prolongs my dying. I further direct that treatment be limited to measures to keep me comfortable and to relieve pain.

These directions express my legal right to refuse treatment. Therefore I expect my family, doctors, and everyone concerned with my care to regard themselves as legally and morally bound to act in accord with my wishes, and in so doing to be free of any legal liability for having followed my directions.

I especially do not want: _____
_____
_____
_____

Society for the Right to Die

250 West 57th Street/New York, NY 10107

INSTRUCTIONS
Consult this column for help and guidance.

This declaration sets forth your directions regarding medical treatment.

You have the right to refuse treatment you do not want, and you may request the care you do want.

You may list specific treatment you do not want. For example:

Cardiac resuscitation
Mechanical respiration
Artificial feeding/fluids by tubes

Otherwise, your general statement, top right, will stand for your wishes.

358

Other instructions/comments:

_____

_____

_____

_____

You may want to add instructions for care you do want—for example, pain medication; or that you prefer to die at home if possible.

Proxy Designation Clause: Should I become unable to communicate my instructions as stated above, I designate the following person to act in my behalf:

Name _____

Address _____

If the person I have named above is unable to act in my behalf. I authorize the following person to do so:

Name _____

Address _____

If you want, you can name someone to see that your wishes are carried out, but you do not have to do this.

Signed: _____ Date: _____

Witness: _____ Witness: _____

Keep the signed original with your personal papers at home. Give signed copies to your doctors, family, and to your proxy.

Sign and date here in the presence of two adult witnesses, who should also sign.

Tear off and mail to: **Society for the Right to Die, 250 West 57th Street, New York, NY 10107.**

The Annual Report of Society for the Right to Die is available from NY State Dept. of State, Office of Charitable Contributions, 162 Washington Ave., Albany, NY 12230.

Please send me _____ additional copies of the Living Will Declaration.
Enclosed is my contribution in support of the Society's program:

☐ $15 ☐ $35 ☐ $100 ☐ $

*(Contributions are tax deductible. Contributors of $15 or more receive a Living Will/Annual Membership wallet card and Society Newsletter. Please make checks payable to **Society for the Right to Die**.)*

Name _____

Street Address _____

City _____ State _____ Zip _____

☐ I am enclosing names and addresses of others to receive information from you.

CALIFORNIA
STATUTORY FORM DURABLE POWER OF ATTORNEY FOR HEALTH CARE
(California Civil Code Section 2500)

> This document complies with California's Uniform Durable Power of Attorney Act as amended in 1983 and 1985, permitting you to designate an agent empowered to make medical treatment decisions on your behalf in the event of incompetency. If you elect to execute this document, we recommend its use in conjunction with the "Directive to Physicians" authorized by the California Natural Death Act of 1976. Forms are available from the Society for the Right to Die.

Warning to Person Executing This Document

This is an important legal document which is authorized by the Keene Health Care Agent Act. Before executing this document, you should know these important facts:

This document gives the person you designate as your agent (the attorney in fact) the power to make health care decisions for you. Your agent must act consistently with your desires as stated in this document or otherwise made known.

Except as you otherwise specify in this document, this document gives your agent the power to consent to your doctor not giving treatment or stopping treatment necessary to keep you alive.

Notwithstanding this document, you have the right to make medical and other health care decisions for yourself so long as you can give informed consent with respect to the particular decision. In addition, no treatment may be given to you over your objection at the time, and health care necessary to keep you alive may not be stopped or withheld if you object at the time.

This document gives your agent authority to consent, to refuse to consent, or to withdraw consent to any care, treatment, service, or procedure to maintain, diagnose, or treat a physical or mental condition. This power is subject to any statement of your desires and any limitations that you include in this document. You may state in this document any types of treatment that you do not desire. In addition, a court can take away the power of your agent to make health care decisions for you if your agent (1) authorizes anything that is illegal, (2) acts contrary to your known desires, or (3) where your desires are not known, does anything that is clearly contrary to your best interests.

Unless you specify a shorter period in this document, this power will exist for seven years from the date you execute this document and, if you are unable to make health care decisions for yourself at the time when this seven-year period ends, this power will continue to exist until the time when you become able to make health care decisions for yourself.

You have the right to revoke the authority of your agent by notifying your agent or your treating doctor, hospital, or other health care provider orally or in writing of the revocation.

Your agent has the right to examine your medical records and to consent to their disclosure unless you limit this right in this document.

Unless you otherwise specify in this document, this document gives your agent the power after you die to (1) authorize an autopsy, (2) donate your body or parts thereof for transplant or therapeutic or educational or scientific purposes, and (3) direct the disposition of your remains.

This document revokes any prior durable power of attorney for health care.

You should carefully read and follow the witnessing procedure described at the end of this form. This document will not be valid unless you comply with the witnessing procedure.

If there is anything in this document that you do not understand, you should ask a lawyer to explain it to you.

Your agent may need this document immediately in case of an emergency that requires a decision concerning your health care. Either keep this document where it is immediately available to your agent and alternate agents or give each of them an executed copy of this document. You may also want to give your doctor an executed copy of this document.

Do not use this form if you are a conservatee under the Lanterman-Petris-Short Act and you want to appoint your conservator as your agent. You can do that only if the appointment document includes a certificate of your attorney.

Society for the Right to Die
250 West 57 Street, New York, NY 10107 (212)246-6973

1. Designation of Health Care Agent.

I, _____

(Insert your name and address)

_____

do hereby designate and appoint _____

(Insert name, address and telephone number of one individual only as your agent to make health care decisions for you. None of the following may be designated as your agent: (1) your treating health care provider, (2) a nonrelative employee of your treating health care provider, (3) an operator of a community care facility, or (4) a nonrelative employee of an operator of a community care facility.)

as my attorney in fact (agent) to make health care decisions for me as authorized in this document. For the purposes of this document, "health care decision" means consent, refusal of consent, or withdrawal of consent to any care, treatment, service, or procedure to maintain, diagnose, or treat an individual's physical or mental condition.

2. Creation of Durable Power of Attorney for Health Care.

By this document I intend to create a durable power of attorney for health care under Sections 2430 to 2443, inclusive, of the California Civil Code. This power of attorney is authorized by the Keene Health Care Agent Act and shall be construed in accordance with the provisions of Sections 2500 to 2506, inclusive, of the California Civil Code. This power of attorney shall not be affected by my subsequent incapacity.

3. General Statement of Authority Granted.

Subject to any limitations in this document, I hereby grant to my agent full power and authority to make health care decisions for me to the same extent that I could make such decisions for myself if I had the capacity to do so. In exercising this authority, my agent shall make health care decisions that are consistent with my desires as stated in this document or otherwise made known to my agent, including, but not limited to, my desires concerning obtaining or refusing or withdrawing life-prolonging care, treatment, services, and procedures.

(If you want to limit the authority of your agent to make health care decisions for you, you can state the limitations in paragraph 4 ["Statement of Desires, Special Provisions, and Limitations"] below. You can indicate your desires by including a statement of your desires in the same paragraph.)

4. Statement of Desires, Special Provisions, and Limitations.

(Your agent must make health care decisions that are consistent with your known desires. You can, but are not required to, state your desires in the space provided below. You should consider whether you want to include a statement of your desires concerning life-prolonging care, treatment, services, and procedures. You can also include a statement of your desires concerning other matters relating to your health care. You can also make your desires known to your agent by discussing your desires with your agent or by some other means. If there are any types of treatment that you do not want to be used, you should state them in the space below. If you want to limit in any other way the authority given your agent by this document, you should state the limits in the space below. If you do not state any limits, your agent will have broad powers to make health care decisions for you, except to the extent that there are limits provided by law.)

In exercising the authority under this durable power of attorney for health care, my agent shall act consistently with my desires as stated below and is subject to the special provisions and limitations stated below:

(a) Statement of desires concerning life-prolonging care, treatment, services, and procedures:

(b) Additional statement of desires, special provisions, and limitations:

(You may attach additional pages if you need more space to complete your statement. If you attach additional pages, you must date and sign EACH of the additional pages at the same time you date and sign this document.)

5. Inspection and Disclosure of Information Relating to My Physical or Mental Health.

Subject to any limitations in this document, my agent has the power and authority to do all of the following:

(a) Request, review, and receive any information, verbal or written, regarding my physical or mental health, including, but not limited to, medical and hospital records.

(b) Execute on my behalf any releases or other documents that may be required in order to obtain this information.

(c) Consent to the disclosure of this information.

(If you want to limit the authority of your agent to receive and disclose information relating to your health, you must state the limitations in paragraph 4 ["Statement of Desires, Special Provisions, and Limitations"] above.)

6. Signing Documents, Waivers, and Releases.

Where necessary to implement the health care decisions that my agent is authorized by this document to make, my agent has the power and authority to execute on my behalf all of the following:

(a) Documents titled or purporting to be a "Refusal to Permit Treatment" and "Leaving Hospital Against Medical Advice."

(b) Any necessary waiver or release from liability required by a hospital or physician.

7. Autopsy; Anatomical Gifts; Disposition of Remains.

Subject to any limitations in this document, my agent has the power and authority to do all of the following:

(a) Authorize an autopsy under Section 7113 of the Health and Safety Code.

(b) Make a disposition of a part or parts of my body under the Uniform Anatomical Gift Act (Chapter 3.5 [commencing with Section 7150] of Part 1 of Division 7 of the Health and Safety Code).

(c) Direct the disposition of my remains under Section 7100 of the Health and Safety Code.

(If you want to limit the authority of your agent to consent to an autopsy, make an anatomical gift, or direct the disposition of your remains, you must state the limitations in paragraph 4 ["Statement of Desires, Special Provisions, and Limitations"] above.)

8. Duration.

(Unless you specify a shorter period in the space below, this power of attorney will exist for seven years from the date you execute this document and, if you are unable to make health care decisions for yourself at the time when this seven-year period ends, the power will continue to exist until the time when you become able to make health care decisions for yourself.)

This durable power of attorney for health care expires on:

_____

(Fill in this space ONLY if you want the authority of your agent to end EARLIER than the seven-year period described above.)

9. Designation of Alternate Agents.

(You are not required to designate any alternate agents but you may do so. Any alternate agent you designate will be able to make the same health care decisions as the agent you designated in paragraph 1, above, in the event that the agent is unable or ineligible to act as your agent. If the agent you designated is your spouse, he or she becomes ineligible to act as your agent if your marriage is dissolved.)

If the person designated as my agent in paragraph 1 is not available or becomes ineligible to act as my agent to make a health care decision for me or loses the mental capacity to make health care decisions for me, or if I revoke that person's appointment or authority to act as my agent to make health care decisions for me, then I designate and appoint the following persons to serve as my agent to make health care decisions for me as authorized in this document, such persons to serve in the order listed below:

A. First Alternate Agent _____

_____

(Insert name, address, and telephone number of first alternate agent)

B. Second Alternate Agent _____

_____

(Insert name, address, and telephone number of second alternate agent)

10. Nomination of Conservator of Person.

(A conservator of the person may be appointed for you if a court decides that one should be appointed. The conservator is responsible for your physical care, which under some circumstances includes making health care decisions for you. You are not required to nominate a conservator but you may do so. The court will appoint the person you nominate unless that would be contrary to your best interests. You may, but are not required to, nominate as your conservator the same person you named in paragraph 1 as your health care agent. You can nominate an individual as your conservator by completing the space below.)

If a conservator of the person is to be appointed for me, I nominate the following individual to serve as conservator of the person:

_____

(Insert name and address of person nominated as conservator of the person)

11. Prior Designations Revoked.

I revoke any prior durable power of attorney for health care.

Date and Signature of Principal
(YOU MUST DATE AND SIGN THIS POWER OF ATTORNEY)

I sign my name to this Statutory Form Durable Power of Attorney for Health Care on

_____ at _____, _____
   (Date)   (City)   State)

_____
                                    (You sign here)

(This power of attorney will not be valid unless it is signed by two qualified witnesses who are present when you sign or acknowledge your signature. If you have attached any additional pages to this form, you must date and sign each of the additional pages at the same time you date and sign this power of attorney.)

Statement of Witnesses

(This document must be witnessed by two qualified adult witnesses. None of the following may be used as a witness: (1) a person you designate as your agent or alternate agent, (2) a health care provider, (3) an employee of a health care provider, (4) the operator of a community care facility, (5) an employee of an operator of a community care facility. At least one of the witnesses must make the additional declaration set out following the place where the witnesses sign.)

(READ CAREFULLY BEFORE SIGNING. You can sign as a witness only if you personally know the principal or the identity of the principal is proved to you by convincing evidence.)

(To have convincing evidence of the identity of the principal, you must be presented with and reasonably rely on any one or more of the following:

(1) An identification card or driver's license issued by the California Department of Motor Vehicles that is current or has been issued within five years.

(2) A passport issued by the Department of State of the United States that is current or has been issued within five years.

(3) Any of the following documents if the document is current or has been issued within five years and contains a photograph and description of the person named on it, is signed by the person, and bears a serial or other identifying number:

(a) A passport issued by a foreign government that has been stamped by the United States Immigration and Naturalization Service.

(b) A driver's license issued by a state other than California or by a Canadian or Mexican public agency authorized to issue drivers' licenses.

(c) An identification card issued by a state other than California.

(d) An identification card issued by any branch of the armed forces of the United States.)

(Other kinds of proof of identity are not allowed.)

    I declare under penalty of perjury under the laws of California that the person who signed or acknowledged this document is personally known to me (or proved to me on the basis of convincing evidence) to be the principal, that the principal signed or acknowledged this durable power of attorney in my presence, that the principal appears to be of sound mind and under no duress, fraud, or undue influence, that I am not the person appointed as attorney in fact by this document, and that I am not a health care provider, an employee of a health care provider, the operator of a community care facility, nor an employee of an operator of a community care facility.

_____   _____
(Signature—Witness I)   (Signature—Witness II)

_____   _____
(Print Name)   (Print Name)

_____   _____
(Residence Address)   (Residence Address)

_____   _____

_____   _____
(Date)   (Date)

(AT LEAST ONE OF THE ABOVE WITNESSES MUST ALSO SIGN THE FOLLOWING DECLARATION.)

    I further declare under penalty of perjury under the laws of California, that I am not related to the principal by blood, marriage, or adoption, and, to the best of my knowledge, I am not entitled to any part of the estate of the principal upon the death of the principal under a will now existing or by operation of law.

Signature:_____Signature:_____

Statement of Patient Advocate or Ombudsman

(If you are a patient in a skilled nursing facility, one of the witnesses must be a patient advocate or ombudsman. The following statement is required only if you are a patient in a skilled nursing facility—a health care facility that provides the following basic services: skilled nursing care and supportive care to patients whose primary need is for availability of skilled nursing care on an extended basis. The patient advocate or ombudsman must sign both parts of the "Statement of Witnesses" above AND must also sign the following statement.)

    I further declare under penalty of perjury under the laws of California that I am a patient advocate or ombudsman as designated by the State Department of Aging and that I am serving as a witness as required by subdivision (f) of Section 2432 of the Civil Code.

Signature: _____

APPENDIX G

Uniform Anatomical Gift Act; Donor Card and Consent by Next of Kin for Removal of Organs (sample forms)

UNIFORM ANATOMICAL GIFT ACT

8 U.L.A. 22 (Master ed. 1968).

§ 2. [Persons Who May Execute an Anatomical Gift]

(a) Any individual of sound mind and 18 years of age or more may give all or any part of his body for any purpose specified in section 3, the gift to take effect upon death.

(b) Any of the following persons, in order of priority stated, when persons in prior classes are not available at the time of death, and in the absence of actual notice of contrary indications by the decedent or actual notice of opposition by a member of the same or a prior class, may give all or any part of the decedent's body for any purpose specified in section 3:

(1) the spouse,

(2) an adult son or daughter,

(3) either parent,

(4) an adult brother or sister,

(5) a guardian of the person of the decedent at the time of his death,

(6) any other person authorized or under obligation to dispose of the body.

(c) If the donee has actual notice of contrary indications by the decedent or that a gift by a member of a class is opposed by a member of the same or a prior class, the donee shall not accept the gift. The persons authorized by subsection (b) may make the gift after or immediately before death.

(d) A gift of all or part of a body authorizes any examination necessary to assure medical acceptability of the gift for the purposes intended.

(e) The rights of the donee created by the gift are paramount to the rights of others except as provided by Section 7(d).

§ 3. [Persons Who May Become Donees; Purposes for Which Anatomical Gifts May be Made]

The following persons may become donees of gifts of bodies or parts thereof for the purposes stated:

(1) any hospital, surgeon, or physician, for medical or dental education, research, advancement of medical or dental science, therapy, or transplantation; or

(2) any accredited medical or dental school, college or university for education, research, advancement of medical or dental science, or therapy; or

(3) any bank or storage facility, for medical or dental education, research, advancement of medical or dental science, therapy, or transplantation; or

(4) any specified individual for therapy or transplantation needed by him.

§ 4. [Manner of Executing Anatomical Gifts]

(a) A gift of all or part of the body under Section 2(a) may be made by will. The gift becomes effective upon the death of the testator without waiting for probate. If the will is not probated, or if it is declared invalid for testamentary purposes, the gift, to the extent that it has been acted upon in good faith, is nevertheless valid and effective.

(b) A gift of all or part of the body under Section 2(a) may also be made by document other than a will. The gift becomes effective upon the death of the donor. The document, which may be a card designed to be carried on the person, must be signed by the donor in the presence of 2 witnesses who must sign the document in his presence. If the donor cannot sign, the document may be signed for him at his direction and in his presence in the presence of 2 witnesses who must sign the document in his presence. Delivery of the document of gift during the donor's lifetime is not necessary to make the gift valid.

(c) The gift may be made to a specified donee or without specifying a donee. If the latter, the gift may be accepted by the attending physician as donee upon or following death. If the gift is made to a specified donee who is not available at the time and place of death, the attending physician upon or following death, in the absence of any expressed indication that the donor desired otherwise, may accept the gift as donee. The physician who becomes a donee under this subsection shall not participate in the procedures for removing or transplanting a part.

(d) Notwithstanding Section 7(b), the donor may designate in his will, card, or other document of gift the surgeon or physician to carry out the appropriate procedures. In the absence of a designation or if the designee is not available, the donee or other person authorized to accept the gift may employ or authorize any surgeon or physician for the purpose.

(e) Any gift by a person designated in Section 2(b) shall be made by a document signed by him or made by his telegraphic, recorded telephonic, or other recorded message.

§5. [Delivery of Document of Gift]

If the gift is made by the donor to a specified donee, the will, card, or other document, or an executed copy thereof, may be delivered to the donee to expedite the appropriate procedures immediately after death. Delivery is not necessary to the validity of the gift. The will, card, or other document, or an executed copy thereof, may be deposited in any hospital, bank or storage facility or registry office that accepts it for safekeeping or for facilitation of procedures after death. On request of any interested party upon or after the donor's death, the person in possession shall produce the document for examination.

§6. [Amendment or Revocation of the Gift]

(a) If the will, card, or other document or executed copy thereof, has been delivered to a specified donee, the donor may amend or revoke the gift by:

(1) the execution and delivery to the donee of a signed statement, or

(2) an oral statement made in the presence of 2 persons and communicated to the donee, or

(3) a statement during a terminal illness or injury addressed to an attending physician and communicated to the donee, or

(4) a signed card or document found on his person or in his effects.

(b) Any document of gift which has not been delivered to the donee may be revoked by the donor in the manner set out in subsection (a), or by destruction, cancellation, or mutilation of the document and all executed copies thereof.

(c) Any gift made by a will may also be amended or revoked in the manner provided for amendment or revocation of wills, or as provided in subsection (a).

§ 7. [Rights and Duties at Death]

(a) The donee may accept or reject the gift. If the donee accepts a gift of the entire body, he may, subject to the terms of the gift, authorize embalming and the use of the body in funeral services. If the gift is of a part of the body, the donee, upon the death of the donor and prior to embalming, shall cause the part to be removed without unnecessary mutilation. After removal of the part, custody of the remainder of the body vests in the surviving spouse, next of kin, or other persons under obligation to dispose of the body.

(b) The time of death shall be determined by a physician who tends the donor at his death, or, if none, the physician who certifies the death. The physician shall not participate in the procedures for removing or transplanting a part.

(c) A person who acts in good faith in accord with the terms of this Act or with the anatomical gift laws of another state [or a foreign country] is not liable for damages in any civil action or subject to prosecution in any criminal proceeding for his act.

(d) The provisions of this Act are subject to the laws of this state prescribing powers and duties with respect to autopsies.

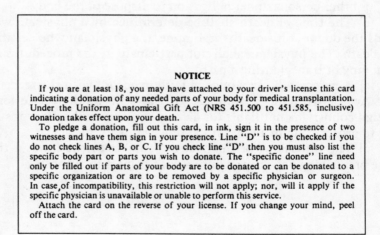

Date _____

Pursuant to the Uniform Anatomical Gift Act, I hereby give, effective upon my death:

A. Eyes: To Reno Host Lions Club Eye Bank, Inc.

B. Kidneys: _____

C. Any needed parts: _____

D. Specific parts of body as listed: _____

_____

Signature of donor in presence of witnesses

_____

Witness _____   Witness _____

NOTICE

If you are at least 18, you may have attached to your driver's license this card indicating a donation of any needed parts of your body for medical transplantation. Under the Uniform Anatomical Gift Act (NRS 451.500 to 451.585, inclusive) donation takes effect upon your death.

To pledge a donation, fill out this card, in ink, sign it in the presence of two witnesses and have them sign in your presence. Line "D" is to be checked if you do not check lines A, B, or C. If you check line "D" then you must also list the specific body part or parts you wish to donate. The "specific donee" line need only be filled out if parts of your body are to be donated or can be donated to a specific organization or are to be removed by a specific physician or surgeon. In case of incompatibility, this restriction will not apply; nor, will it apply if the specific physician is unavailable or unable to perform this service.

Attach the card on the reverse of your license. If you change your mind, peel off the card.

ADDRESSOGRAPH HERE

SAINT MARY'S HOSPITAL

CONSENT BY NEXT-OF-KIN FOR REMOVAL OF ORGANS

I, _____, next-of-kin* (_____),
         Name   Relationship

of _____, for humanitarian reasons hereby give
        Donor

consent for removal of any needed organs or tissues**, or

_____, from _____
   Specify organs or tissues   Donor

after death or declaration of irrecersible cessation of brain

function for transplantation and medical research.

_____   _____
Date   Signature of next-of-kin

_____   _____
Witness   Address

_____   _____
Witness   City, State, Zip

* Order of priority: spouse, adult son or daughter, parent, adult
  brother or sister, guardian, any other person authorized or under
  obligation for disposition of the body.

** Kidneys, liver, heart, lungs, pancreas, eyes, skin, bone, artery,
   cartilage, ear bones and membrane, pituitary gland, etc.

62236 - NURSING
3-21-84

369

APPENDIX H
Withholding or Withdrawing of Life-Prolonging Medical Treatment: AMA Statement

Opinion of the AMA Council on Ethical and Judicial Affairs
March 15, 1986

Withholding or Withdrawing
Life Prolonging Medical Treatment

The social commitment of the physician is to sustain life and relieve suffering. Where the performance of one duty conflicts with the other, the choice of the patient, or his family or legal representative if the patient is incompetent to act in his own behalf, should prevail. In the absence of the patient's choice or an authorized proxy, the physician must act in the best interest of the patient.

For humane reasons, with informed consent, a physician may do what is medically necessary to alleviate severe pain, or cease or omit treatment to permit a terminally ill patient whose death is imminent to die. However, he should not intentionally cause death. In deciding whether the administration of potentially life-prolonging medical treatment is in the best interest of the patient who is incompetent to act in his own behalf, the physician should determine what the possibility is for extending life under humane and comfortable conditions and what are the prior expressed wishes of the patient and attitudes of the family or those who have responsibility for the custody of the patient.

Even if death is not imminent but a patient's coma is beyond doubt irreversible and there are adequate safeguards to confirm the accuracy of the diagnosis and with the concurrence of those who have responsibility for the care of the patient, it is not unethical to discontinue all means of life-prolonging medical treatment.

Life-prolonging medical treatment includes medication and artificially or technologically supplied respiration, nutrition or hydration. In treating a terminally ill or irreversibly comatose patient, the physician should determine whether the benefits of treatment outweigh its burdens. At all times, the dignity of the patient should be maintained.

APPENDIX I
Pointers on Working with the Media

Here are some guidelines to help you in dealing with the media if you suddenly find yourself catapulted into the public eye because of an ethical dilemma, a "first" in medical history (or perhaps in your own community), or a desire and need to tell your story.

Select one person to be a spokesperson for the family. You may be that person. But if you're the patient, remember that each reporter may want a separate interview, photo session, or videotaping time, and at odd hours. All that can be exhausting even for someone in good health.

Be aware of the "rules" the media operate by. You can't say something to a reporter, and then say, "I didn't mean that—please don't print it" or "I meant what I said, but it's off the record." A good rule of thumb is never to say anything you don't want to see in print or hear on the air.

Be prepared for some tough questions which may seem insensitive or even cruel. Some reporters are tactless, rude, and boorish, it's true. But many others are fine journalists who know that the best story will be told only when probing questions are asked and answered. You can always say, "I prefer not to discuss that" or "I don't have an answer for that" or "I need to refer that question to my doctor (or attorney)." But if you are free to talk about a topic and it's important to you to get your point across to the public, an honest and simple reply may be your best bet.

Consider preparing a typed one-page fact sheet. Include brief information about yourself, your condition, and the problem you're addressing. Handing out photocopies to reporters will help to ensure the correct spelling of your name (or the name of the patient if you're a spokesperson) and the proper term for the medical condition or problem. (If your name is unusual, sound out the pronunciation as an aid to broadcast media. If your condition is not a common one, describe it in plain English and provide sources of additional information, e.g., books, professional articles, relevant laws or guidelines, etc.) You may want to add your doctor's name and telephone number, but get permission first.

Keep your doctor informed. Let your physician know that you have been contacted by reporters, or, if you are taking your story to the media, give your doctor permission to discuss your case. Your doctor will then be prepared if reporters call for more information or quotes. (Some physicians refuse to speak to the media because they believe they are usually misquoted. Others welcome a chance to discuss a medical problem and give their point of view about treatment, research still needed, ethical dilemmas, and the like.)

Get all the help you can from your hospital's public information or community relations department. Without advance approval, media representatives are not allowed on hospital premises. Hospitals have a duty to protect the privacy of their patients and, in general, do not release any information without your consent. However, if you want to tell your story or agree to be interviewed by the media (and if it's in the hospital's best interests, too), the public information officer will schedule interviews or set up a press conference, provide a fact sheet and/or visuals (such as charts, illustrations of procedures, etc.) if doctors are taking part, and arrange for photos of you and, possibly, your family. Says one hospital director of public relations, "With our media contacts we can help a family take its story to the public. But, frankly, the success of the appeal has a lot to do with the age of the patient—if a *child* needs help, we get much better response from the media and public." (For more on the pros and cons of seeking an organ donor through the media, see Chapter 5.)

Protect your privacy and that of your family. Consider getting an unlisted phone number or a message-answering machine which will allow you to screen calls in advance. If TV crews and reporters have camped out in front of your home, you may want to have a friend or relative answer your doorbell or take your children to another location where they won't be in the limelight.

Get an attorney to represent your interests if your story becomes a hot property.

APPENDIX J
National and Regional Centers for Medical Ethics

Here is a partial listing of centers for bioethics research and education, plus college and university programs dealing with human values and moral issues in health and medicine. Many of these centers conduct educational workshops, publish newsletters, journals, and books, and welcome membership by any interested person.

In addition, there are also many other colleges and universities with departments of philosophy and/or ethics that may be able to assist you or refer you to local hospital ethics committees or other experts in bioethics who can help you in dealing with a health-related moral dilemma.

The Hastings Center
255 Elm Road
Briarcliff Manor, NY 10510
(914) 762-8500
Joyce Bermel, director of information

Center for Bioethics
Joseph and Rose Kennedy Institute of Ethics
Georgetown University
Washington, DC 20057
(202) 255-2371
LeRoy Walters, Ph.D., director

Northeast region

American Society of Law and Medicine
520 Commonwealth Avenue
Boston, MA 02215
(617) 262-4990
A. Edward Doudera, J.D., executive director

Center for Law and Health Sciences
Boston University School of Public Health
209 Bay State Road
Boston, MA 02215
(617) 353-2910
George J. Annas, J.D., chief

Program in Medical Ethics
Dartmouth Medical School
Hanover, NH 03755
(603) 646-7505
Charles M. Culver, M.D., Ph.D., director

Department of Religious Studies
College of the Holy Cross
Worcester, MA 10706
(617) 793-2011
John J. Paris, S.J., Ph.D., professor

Center for the Study of Society and Medicine
Columbia University College of Physicians and
    Surgeons
630 West 168th Street
New York, NY 10032
(212) 305-3592
David J. Rothman, Ph.D., director

Department of Social Medicine
Albert Einstein College of Medicine of Yeshiva
    University
1300 Morris Park Avenue
Bronx, NY 10461
(212) 430-3574
Ruth Macklin, Ph.D., professor

Mid-Atlantic region

Society for Health and Human Values
1100 Witherspoon Building

Philadelphia, PA 19017
(215) 735-1551
Ronald W. McNeur, Ph.D., executive director

Department of Humanities
Milton S. Hershey Medical Center
Pennsylvania State University College of Medicine
Hershey, PA 18020
(717) 534-8778
K. Danner Clouser, Ph.D., chairman

Department of Health Sciences
George Washington University School of Medicine
1229 25th Street, NW
Washington, DC 20037
(202) 676-4269
Joanne Lynn, M.D., associate professor

Department of Philosophy
Edinboro University of Pennsylvania
Edinboro, PA 16444
(814) 732-2604
James F. Drane, Ph.D., professor

Center for Biomedical Ethics
Case Western Reserve University School of
   Medicine
2119 Abington Road
Cleveland, OH 44106
(216) 368-2828
Stephen Smookler, M.D., director

Southeast region

Department of Religious Studies
University of Virginia
Charlottesville, VA 22903
(804) 924-6709
James F. Childress, Ph.D., professor

Department of Social and Administrative Medicine
University of North Carolina at Chapel Hill School
   of Medicine
Chapel Hill, NC 27514
(919) 962-1136
Glenn Wilson, chairman

Department of Medical Humanities
East Carolina University School of Medicine

Greenville, NC 27858
(919) 551-2618
Loretta Kopelman, M.D., chairwoman

Division for the Study of Human Values in
*   Medicine*
Department of Comprehensive Medicine
University of South Florida School of Medicine
13301 N. 30th Street
Tampa, FL 33612
(813) 974-3294
David H. Smith, Ph.D., director

Great Lakes region

Humanistic Studies Program
University of Illinois Health Sciences Center
808 South Wood Street
Chicago, IL 60612
(312) 996-7216
Marc Lappé, Ph.D., chairman

University of Chicago, Section of General Internal
*   Medicine*
Pritzker School of Medicine
5841 South Maryland Avenue
Chicago, IL 60637
(312) 962-3045
Mark Siegler, M.D., professor

Medical Humanities Program
Loyola University Medical Center, Bldg. 54, Rm.
    114B
Stritch School of Medicine
2160 South First Avenue
Maywood, IL 60153
(312) 531-3433
David C. Thomasma, Ph.D., director

Program in Medical Ethics
University of Wisconsin Center for Health Sciences
470 North Charter Street
Madison, WI 53706
(608) 263-3414
Norman Fost, M.D., director

Bioethics Center
Medical College of Wisconsin

8701 Watertown Plank Road
P.O. Box 2509
Milwaukee, WI 53226
(414) 257-8498
Dennis J. Doherty, Ph.D., director

Medical Humanities Program
Michigan State University College of Human
    Medicine
East Lansing, MI 48824
(517) 355-7550
Howard Brody, M.D., Ph.D., director

Program in Public Health Nursing
University of Michigan School of Public Health
Ann Arbor, MI 48109
(313) 764-5464
Mila A. Aroskar, Ed.D., professor

*Minnesota Network for Institutional Ethics
    Committees*
2221 University Avenue, SE, Suite 425
Minneapolis, MN 55414
(612) 331-5571, ext. 73
Evelyn J. Van Allen, R.N., coordinator

Biomedical Ethics Center
University of Minnesota
Mayo Memorial Building
420 Delaware Street, SE
Minneapolis, MN 55455
(612) 625-4917
Arthur L. Caplan, Ph.D., director

Midwest region

Program on Human Values and Ethics
University of Tennessee College of Medicine
956 Court Street
Memphis, TN 38163
(901) 528-5686
Terrence F. Ackerman, Ph.D., director

Medical Humanities Program
Southern Illinois University School of Medicine
801 North Ruthledge
P.O. Box 3926
Springfield, IL 62708

(217) 782-4261
Glen Davidson, Ph.D., director

Center for Health Care Ethics
St. Louis University Medical Center
1438 S. Grand Boulevard
St. Louis, MO 63104
(314) 773-0646
Kevin O'Rourke, O.P., J.C.D., director

Midwest Bioethics Center
1200 East 104th Street
Kansas City, MO 64131
(816) 942-1992
Karen Ritchie, M.D., director

Southwest region

Ecumenical Center for Religion and Health
4507 Medical Drive
San Antonio, TX 78229
(512) 696-9966
Donald L. Anderson, Ph.D., director

Medical Humanities Program
Institute for the Medical Humanities
University of Texas Medical School at Galveston
301 University Boulevard
Galveston, TX 77550
(409) 761-2376
Ronald A. Carson, Ph.D., chairman

Center for Ethics, Medicine and Public Issues
Baylor College of Medicine
One Baylor Plaza
Houston, TX 77030
(713) 799-6290
Baruch Brody, Ph.D., director

Division of Social Perspectives in Medicine
University of Arizona College of Medicine
1505 North Campbell Avenue
Tucson, AZ 85724
(602) 626-6506
Shirley Nickols Fahey, Ph.D., chairwoman

Western region

Center for Applied Biomedical Ethics
Rose Medical Center
4567 E. 9th Avenue
Denver, CO 80220
(303) 320-2102
Frederick Abrams, M.D., director

Program in Medical Ethics
University of Nevada School of Medicine
Reno, NV 89557
(702) 784-6001
Thomas J. Scully, M.D. (Reno); Thomas Cinque,
    M.D. (Las Vegas), codirectors

Northwest Institute of Ethics and the Life Sciences
1416 E. Thomas Street
Seattle, WA 98112
(206) 322-2165
Catherine C. Morrow, Esq.

Health Policy Program in Bioethics
University of California–San Francisco School of
    Medicine
1362 Third Avenue
San Francisco, CA 94143
(415) 476-3093
Albert R. Jonsen, Ph.D., professor

Program in Medicine, Law and Human Values
University of California–Los Angeles School of
    Medicine
2859 Slichter Hall
Los Angeles, CA 90024
(213) 825-4976
Bernard Towers, M.B., Ch.B., codirector

Center for Bioethics
Sisters of St. Joseph of Orange Health System
404 South Batavia Street
Orange, CA 92668
(714) 997-7690
Sister Corrine Bayley, director

Canada

Center of Bioethics
Clinical Research Institute of Montreal
110 Pine Avenue, W.
Montreal, Quebec H2W 1R7 Canada
(514) 842-1481 ext. 256
Dr. David J. Roy, director

Medical Bioethics Program
University of Calgary Faculty of Medicine
3330 Hospital Drive, NW
Calgary, Alberta, Canada T2N 4N1
(403) 284-6541
T.D. Kinsella, M.D., director

Humanities and Social Studies in Medicine
McGill University Faculty of Medicine
3655 Drummond Street
Montreal, Quebec, Canada H3G 1Y6
(514) 392-4226
J. W. Lella, Ph.D., director

Notes and Sources

Chapter 1

1. See "Sleeping Pill Nightmare," *Time*, February 23, 1962, p. 35; and "The Thalidomide Disaster," *Time*, August 10, 1962, p. 32. Also see *The Lancet*, December 16, 1961, in which New South Wales physician W. G. McBride described multiple severe abnormalities in babies delivered of women who were given the drug Thalidomide (Distaval) during pregnancy and asked: "Have any of your readers seen similar abnormalities in babies delivered of women who have taken this drug during pregnancy?"

2. See Allen S. Goldman, M.D., "Critical Periods of Prenatal Toxic Insults," in Richard H. Schwarz, M.D., and Sumner J. Yaffe, M.D., eds., *Drug and Chemical Risks to the Fetus and Newborn* (New York: Alan R. Liss, 1980), p. 15, Table II.

3. See Sherri Finkbine as told to Joseph Stocker, "The Baby We Didn't Dare to Have," *Redbook*, January 1963, p. 50.

4. As the 1960s closed, two research centers began scholarly inquiry into a broad range of bioethical issues: the Institute of Society, Ethics and Life Science, known as the Hastings Center, in Hastings-on-Hudson, N.Y. (now located in Briarcliff, N.Y.), founded in 1969, and the Kennedy Institute of Ethics at Georgetown University, Washington, D.C., established in 1971. Both carry out research projects, train fellows in ethics, publish extensively, and provide resource materials on request. (See Appendix J.)

5. Daniel Callahan, speech at University of Nevada School of Medicine, reported in *Reno Gazette-Journal*, February 19, 1984, p. C-1.

6. Down syndrome (formerly known as mongolism or Down's syndrome) is the official nomenclature used by the President's Commission and the American Academy of Pediatrics.

7. Daniel Callahan, commentary on "The WHO Definition of Health," *Hastings Center Studies*, vol. 1, no. 3, 1973. The World Health Organization (WHO) has defined health as "a state of complete physical, mental and social well-being and not merely the absence of disease or infirmity." Many experts believe this definition is too broad and sets up expectations that cannot be met—either by doctors or by society at large.

   Callahan concludes that some minimal level of health is necessary if there is to be any possibility of human happiness. Only in exceptional circumstances can the good of self be long maintained in the absence of the good of the body—although one can be healthy without being in a state of complete mental, physical, and social well-being. That conclusion, he writes, can be justified in two ways: (a) because some degree of disease and infirmity is perfectly compatible with mental and social well-being; and (b) because it is doubtful that there ever was, or ever could be, more than a transient state of "complete physical, mental, and social well-being" for individuals or societies.

8. James F. Childress, *Who Should Decide? Paternalism in Health Care* (New York: Oxford University Press, 1982), flyleaf.

9. It's not uncommon to find a discrepancy between what people *say* they value and what their actions reveal about their values. That's why "it's important to clarify your values, making sure you understand what you believe so you can live in accordance with your beliefs," according to Barbara J. Combs, Dianne R. Hales, and Brian K. Williams, *An Invitation to Health: Your Personal Responsibility*, 2nd ed. (Menlo Park, Calif.: Benjamin-Cummings, 1983), p. 23.

10. Milton Rokeach divides thirty-six values into two categories: those which he labels *terminal* values, such as equality, happiness, and family security, and those he calls *instrumental* values, such as ambition, broadmindedness, cheerfulness, and responsibility (*Understanding Human Values*, pp. 133–34, table titled "Changes in Terminal and Instrumental Values for Entire Adult American Sample, 1968–1971"). Results of a 1984 national survey on values conducted by the National Opinion Research Center (reported in *Reno Gazette-Journal*, May 5, 1985) showed that of twenty values, family security ranked first; a world at peace, second; freedom, third; self-respect, fourth; and happiness, fifth. At the bottom of the list were social recognition and an exciting life.

11. Adapted from Kitty Kotchian Smith, "Difficult Decisions—Let Us Help You Think It Through," brochure for patients and fami-

lies, North Memorial Medical Center, Robbinsdale, Minn. Smith is the center's hospice coordinator.

12. Tom L. Beauchamp and James F. Childress, *Principles of Biomedical Ethics*, 2nd ed. (Englewood Cliffs, N.J.: Prentice-Hall, 1983), states that in a dilemma, "the reasons on each side of a problem are weighty ones, and none is in any obvious way the right set of reasons. If one acts on either set of reasons, one's actions will be desirable in some respects but undesirable in other respects. Yet one thinks that ideally one ought to act on all the reasons, for each is, considered by itself, a good reason" (p. 4).

13. Graham B. Blaine, "Ethicists in the Hospital" (letter), *New England Journal of Medicine*, January 17, 1985, p. 188. Dr. Blaine refers to R. B. Purtilo, "Ethics Consultations in the Hospital," *New England Journal of Medicine*, October 11, 1984.

14. A survey prepared by the National Institutes of Health (NIH) indicates that ethics consultants may wield considerable influence in hospitals and other health care settings. The survey, covering data from 1980 to 1984, resulted in a self-portrait of the profession. Of thirty-eight ethics consultants participating in the survey, twenty-eight say they have some jurisdiction over specific issues and eighteen maintain that hospital staffs are obliged to follow their advice in cases involving those issues. See *Hastings Center Report*, December 1985.

15. Jenny Gleich, "New America's People," *Esquire*, March 1985, p. 64.

16. The Massachusetts supreme court in *Superintendent of Belchertown State School* v. *Saikewiecz* (1977) and *In the matter of Spring* (1979) stressed the role of court review in certain cases, especially when the patient is mentally retarded or incompetent. In contrast, in *In the matter of Shirley Dinnerstein* (1978) the same court upheld a "no-code" order and ruled that such orders did not need approval by the court. (For more on no-code orders, see Chapter 4.)

Most state courts agree with this latter approach, and have taken the position that the proper place to settle such medical problems is within hospitals, and between doctor and family. For example, the New York State supreme court in *Application of Eichner (Brother Fox)* (1980) acknowledged the patient's prior wishes in decision-making.

The District of Columbia court of appeals in *Parker* v. *U.S.* (1979) acknowledged the Living Will and said there was no need for court intervention when a valid Living Will was available. The New Jersey supreme court in *In re Quinlan* (1976) laid out procedures for review by hospital ethics committees of decisions to withdraw treatment. The same court in *In re Conroy* placed responsibility for protection of elderly nursing home patients' decisions concerning removal of life support with the state ombudsman for nursing homes. The California Court of Appeals in the *Bartling* case (see Chapter 3) upheld the competent patient's right to have his life-sustaining respirator removed and noted that "requiring judicial intervention in all cases is unnecessary and may be unwise."

Chapter 2

1. As described in *Strategies for Good Health*, a booklet published by the American Association of Retired Persons, *HMOs* (health maintenance organizations) are prepaid health care plans with predetermined, fixed benefits. They operate like insurance companies and negotiate contracts with hospitals, pharmacies, doctors, and other health care providers to cut costs while providing service to patients. *IPAs* (independent practice associations) are groups of doctors who maintain private practice in addition to seeing HMO patients. *PPOs* (preferred provider organizations) are groups of physicians and hospitals who agree to hold down costs through combinations of price discounts and pattern of practice—what services will be provided and where.

   If you are an employee of a business or organization that has a contract with an HMO, IPA, or PPO, you may be assigned a primary care physician or be given a limited choice among several doctors or hospitals. If you are on your own—with or without private insurance—you will have to find your own doctor. And it may be an accident. If you go to a hospital emergency room or walk-in clinic and don't already have your own physician, whoever is on call will be your doctor.

2. Morris B. Abram, "Medical Ethics in the New Era: An Informed Patient's Perspective," speech at conference on "a new ethic for the new medicine," jointly sponsored by the American Medical Association Council on Ethical and Judicial Affairs and the Hastings Center, New Orleans, March 14–16, 1986.

3. Robert M. Veatch's "On the Other Hand" (opinion piece), *Medical World News*, May 17, 1974, p. 68. Veatch argues that the physician cannot be expected to know what will benefit the patient if he does not know the patient's values. "If the medical consumer can never understand the unique role of the medical professional in the technological era, neither can that medical professional hope to understand fully the uniqueness of the medical consumer. Not just a machine with interchangeable parts from the transplant surgeon's warehouse, the individual is a unique mix of ethnic, familial, socioeconomic, religious, and gender-related values—

values that may be radically different from those of the physician."

4. Thomasma and his colleague Edmund D. Pellegrino reject the "contract" model of doctor-patient relationships and argue for the *fiduciary* model based on beneficence—expressed through a negotiating role rather than a paternalistic one. Physicians, they argue, must share their values with patients beforehand, and patients should also share what's important to them with their doctors. See David C. Thomasma and Edmund D. Pellegrino, *For the Patient's Good: The Restoration of Beneficence in Medical Ethics* (New York: Oxford University Press, in press), section titled "The Good Patient."

5. Lloyd H. Smith, Jr., M.D., "Medicine as an Art," in James B. Wyngaarden and Lloyd H. Smith, *Cecil Textbook of Medicine,* rev. ed. (Philadelphia: Saunders, 1985), pp. 1–4, discusses what patients expect of their physicians in greater detail.

6. In a 1982 AMA public opinion survey, 63 percent of respondents said the recommendation of friends and relatives was "very important" in choosing a doctor, and 26 percent said "fairly important." See Larry J. Freshnock, Ph.D., *Physician and Public Attitudes on Health Care Issues.*

7. Isadore Rosenfeld, M.D., *Second Opinion* (New York: Simon & Schuster, 1981), p. 27.

8. Personal communication, telephone interview with Dr. Rosenfeld.

9. Robert M. Veatch, "When Should the Patient Know?" *Barrister Magazine,* American Bar Association, vol. 8, no. 1 (Winter 1981). The so-called "therapeutic privilege" was first labeled as such in Hubert Smith, "Therapeutic Privilege to Withhold Specific Prognosis from the Patient Sick with Serious or Fatal Illness," *Tennessee Law Review,* 1946. Although Smith recognized that no legal authority exists for such a privilege, hints of its legitimacy have surfaced in court cases ever since. Now, however, courts are increasingly striking it out as a valid reason to withhold medical information from patients.

10. Quoted in Martha Weinman Lear, *Heartsounds* (New York: Pocket Books, 1984), p. 57.

11. Georgia Edwards, M.D., discussion of team care for the patient in the private doctor's office, at University of Nevada School of Medicine, October 13, 1983.

12. See Ralph J. Alfidi, M.D., "Informed Consent: A Study of Patient Reaction," *Journal of the American Medical Association,* vol. 216 (1971), pp. 1325–29.

13. *Schloendorff* v. *Society of New York Hospital*, 211 N.Y. 125, 105 N.E. 92,93 (1914).

14. According to a 1982 Louis Harris and Associates poll conducted for the President's Commission on medical ethics, 56 percent of physicians and 64 percent of the public surveyed felt that increasing the patient's role in medical decision-making would improve the quality of health care. Many doctors and patients said they believed an increased patient role would give the patient a better understanding of the medical condition and treatment, would improve physician performance in terms of the honesty and scope of discussion, and would generally improve the doctor-patient relationship. However, a number of physicians claimed that greater patient involvement would improve the quality of care because it would improve compliance and would make patients more cooperative and willing to accept the doctor's judgment. See President's Commission for the Study of Ethical Problems in Medicine and Biomedical and Behavioral Research, *Making Health Care Decisions* (Washington, D.C.: U.S. Government Printing Office, 1982), vol. 1, p. 44.

   A recent study of patients undergoing coronary bypass surgery at the University of Alabama–Birmingham suggests that denial was a useful coping and adaptive mechanism for short-term adjustment following the surgery. However, the benefit of such denial in avoiding depression and anxiety was short-lived; one year later, there was no discernible difference between those patients who used denial to pretend their illness was not very serious and those who did not.

15. See Norman Cousins, *The Healing Heart* (New York: Avon, 1984), p. 13.

16. K. I. Shine, M.D., "Editor's Notes," *American Health*, November/December 1983, p. 108.

Chapter 3

1. Eugene D. Robin, M.D., *Matters of Life and Death: Risks vs. Benefits of Medical Care* (New York: Freeman, 1984), p. 19.

2. Morris B. Abram, "Ethics and the New Medicine," *New York Times Magazine*, June 5, 1983, p. 68.

3. A survey of physicians and the public conducted by the President's Commission on medical ethics revealed that 21 percent of the Americans surveyed did not know the meaning of the term "informed consent"; only 10 percent mentioned "risks" and less than 1 percent mentioned "alternatives." Of physicians responding, 47 percent mentioned "risks" but only 14 percent mentioned treatment alternatives. See President's Commission for the Study

of Ethical Problems in Medicine and Biomedical and Behavioral Research, *Making Health Care Decisions* (Washington, D.C.: U.S. Government Printing Office, 1982), vol. 1, Report, p. 18.

4. Ibid., p. 2. According to the commission, a person's capacity to make decisions requires, to a greater or lesser degree, (1) a set of values and goals that are reasonably stable and consistent; (2) the ability to communicate and understand information; and (3) the ability to reason and to deliberate about one's choices.

5. *A Patient's Bill of Rights* is not a legal document, but rather a public statement of intent that sets a standard of care. (See Appendix A.)

6. George J. Annas, *The Rights of Hospital Patients: An American Civil Liberties Union Handbook* (New York: Avon/Discus Books, 1975), p. 60.

7. *Canterbury* v. *Spence*, 464 F 2d 722, D.C. Cir. (1972).

8. *Cooper* v. *Roberts*, 220 Pa. Super. 260, 286 A.2d 647 (Super. Ct. 1971) allocatur refused, 221 Pa. Super. xviii (1972).

9. Chart titled "Why You Need a Second Medical Opinion" in *Glamour*, September 1985, p. 400.

10. Victor R. Fuchs, "What Is Cost-Benefit Analysis?" *New England Journal of Medicine*, vol. 303, no. 16 (October 16, 1980), pp. 937–38.

11. Associated Press, "Cummings Almost Quit Playing Ball," October 27, 1983.

12. *Bouvia* v. *Superior Court of the State of California for the County of Los Angeles*, no. B019134 (Cal. Ct. App. 2d Dist., April 16, 1986). Bouvia, who won the right to have her force-feeding apparatus removed, has filed a $10 million malpractice suit against the Los Angeles County–High Desert Hospital, Lancaster, California, and against its ethics committee for having violated her constitutional rights by forcing her to continue nasogastric tube feedings without her consent; see *Hospital Ethics*, January/February 1987, p. 13.

13. See Andrew H. Malcolm, "Right to Die Dispute Focuses on Californian," *New York Times*, October 21, 1984, p. 10.

14. Quality of life judgments are subjective evaluations based on the mental, physical, and emotional health of the patient and his or her ability to interact with other people. When there appears to be severe physical debilitation, total loss of intellectual activity, and no evidence of sensory feeling, most people judge this quality of life to be below any acceptable minimum. This is known as the "reasonable person" standard. But reasonable people often view quality of life issues differently. Some believe life should be sustained at all costs; others believe the quality of that life should be

the deciding factor in whether or not to sustain it.

And until recently, many doctors and even family members of patients with cancer or other debilitating or painful conditions seemed to lump quality of life discussions into the "soft" or "touch-feely" areas of medicine. Now, however, cancer researchers can measure quality of life in their patients through use of a test which may also play an important role in their survival. Created by Dr. Harvey Schipper and reported in the *Journal of Clinical Oncology*, vol. 2, no. 5 (May 1984), the quality of life test is thought to be the first scientifically designed index of that elusive element, and may even help doctors determine which patients will do best under treatment.

15. Margaret Schroeder, "An Affair of the Heart," *People*, December 16, 1985, p. 60. An Associated Press article, "Heart Patients' Wives Under Special Strain," quotes Dr. Allan M. Lansing, medical director of Humana Heart Institute International at Humana Hospital Audubon, as saying that wives of artificial heart patients experience more pressure and strain than the recipients themselves.

16. Robin, *Matters of Life and Death*, p. 168.

17. Associated Press, "Spleen Donor Wants Share of Research Profits," August 18, 1985; Associated Press and United Press, "Arguments Over Who Owns the Profits from Patients' Cells," October 30, 1985.

18. See David Perlman, "Why a Baby's Death Was in Vain," *San Francisco Chronicle*, May 5, 1986, p. 1. See also "Why Transplant Offers Have to be Refused," same issue, p. 4.

Chapter 4

1. Rex Julian Beaber, "Facing, Making the Choice of How We Will Die," *Reno Gazette-Journal*, October 14, 1984, p. 6-C.

2. David C. Thomasma and Edmund D. Pellegrino, *For the Patient's Good: The Restoration of Beneficence in Medical Ethics* (New York: Oxford University Press, in press).

3. UPI News, Washington News Section, "Deaths," File 261, DIALOG Database, March 12, 1986.

4. Quoted in "Spock's Sendoff," *Reno Gazette-Journal*, March 10, 1985, p. 11-E.

5. Quoted in Judith Horstman, "Javits Supports Right to Die," *Standard Star-Gannett Westchester Newspapers*, July 10, 1985, and in "Javits Wants Living Wills," *Reno Gazette-Journal*, July 10, 1985, p. 2.

6. "Nurses Speak Out: Does a Terminal Patient Have the Right to Die?" *NursingLife*, March/April 1984, p. 81.

7. In a 1985 Media General–Associated Press nationwide poll, 68 percent of the 1,532 respondents said that people dying of incurable diseases should be allowed to end their lives, 22 percent said they should not be allowed to do so, and 10 percent didn't know or didn't answer. (See "Survey Finds People Favor Right to Die," *Standard-Star/Gannett Westchester Newspapers*, April 1, 1985, p. 6-A.) A 1985 Harris survey indicated 85 percent of Americans think a patient with a terminal disease ought to be able to tell his doctor to let him die rather than to extend his life when no cure is in sight (see "Support Increases For Euthanasia," in *The Harris Survey*, no. 18, March 4, 1985, p. 1), and a 1986 nationwide Roper Organization poll revealed that 76 percent of 2,000 adults surveyed said that doctors should be bound by law to obey patient's living wills and ought to help the terminally ill to die (Associated Press, "Americans Back Right to Die," *Reno Gazette-Journal*, June 10, 1986, p. 2-D).

8. Courtesy of the Society for the Right to Die.

9. Robert G. Twycross, "Euthanasia," in A. S. Duncan, G. R. Dunstan, and R. B. Welbourn, eds., *Dictionary of Medical Ethics* (New York: Crossroad, 1981), pp. 164–67.

10. See "Dutch Physicians and Euthanasia Availability," *Hemlock Quarterly*, issue 22 (January 1986), p. 2.

11. Twycross, "Euthanasia."

12. Sacred Congregation for the Doctrine of the Faith, *Declaration on Euthanasia* (June 26, 1980), Section IV, "Due Proportion in the Use of Remedies," available from The United States Catholic Conference, 1312 Massachusetts Ave. N.W., Washington, D.C. 20005 or the Society for the Right to Die, 250 West 57th St., New York, New York 10107.

13. See President's Commission for the Study of Ethical Problems in Medicine and Biomedical and Behavioral Research, *Deciding to Forego Life-Sustaining Treatment* (Washington, D.C.: U.S. Government Printing Office, 1983), Chapter 1, "Setting of the Report," pp. 28–30 ("'Slippery Slope' Arguments").

14. See George T. Annas, "Patients' Rights" (letter), *New York Times*, March 15, 1983.

15. For further discussion of family members as surrogates for an incapacitated relative, see President's Commission, *Deciding to Forego Life-Sustaining Treatment*, Chapter 4, "Patients Who Lack Decisionmaking Capacity," pp. 126–29.

16. Eugene D. Robin, M.D., *Matters of Life and Death: Risks vs. Benefits of Medical Care* (New York: Freeman, 1984), suggests that patients and/or family who feel insecure about decision-making and interpreting doctors' opinions and recommendations

for treatment might look to an intermediary, whom Dr. Robin calls an *ombudsdoctor*, "to advise you and represent you in health care encounters so that you can make the most rational and informed choices possible" (p. 118). Basically, this doctor would serve as patient representative and advocate.

Chapter 5

1. "This Is What You Thought About...Donating (or Selling) Human Body Organs" (report of results from an earlier readership survey), *Glamour*, July 1984. In a 1986 *Redbook* readership survey, 80 percent of respondents indicated they would be willing to donate their organs to help someone else live, but only 50 percent agreed with the recommendation that laws be changed to *presume* organ donation consent unless the deceased had expressed his or her objection beforehand.

2. Quoted in Polly Ross Hughes and William Cooney, "Boy Gives His Heart to Save Dying Girl," *San Francisco Chronicle*, January 7, 1986.

3. Quoted in Polly Ross Hughes, "Sad Farewell to Boy Who Gave His Heart," *San Francisco Chronicle*, January 9, 1986.

4. Initially the artificial heart held out hope to terminally ill heart patients, but poor survival rates and major complications following surgery have raised serious questions about the value of the current permanent implant. Although research continues on long-term use, the immediate focus has shifted to use of the artificial heart as a temporary "bridge" until a human donor heart becomes available. See Arnold S. Relman, M.D., "Artificial Hearts—Permanent and Temporary" (editorial), *New England Journal of Medicine*, March 6, 1986, p. 644. Of all kidney transplants in 1985, approximately 25 percent were from living related donors; 75 percent were cadaveric organs. See "Top 10 U.S. Transplant Centers for 1985," *Contemporary Dialysis & Nephrology*, October 1986, p. 17.

5. Associated Press, February 23, 1986.

6. See Ronald Sullivan, "New York's Shortage of Organ Donors Grows Acute," *New York Times*, September 8, 1985.

7. Figure, quote, and statistics which follow from "Organ Transplantation: Will Success Spoil the Stock Hunter?" *Hospital Ethics*, November/December 1985. According to a survey conducted by the Batelle Human Affairs Research Centers in Seattle and published in the June 7 issue of the *Journal of the American Medical Association*, 94 percent of respondents had heard of organ transplantation, but only 19 percent carried donor cards. Fifty-three percent said they would donate organs of a relative, while 50 per-

cent said they would donate their own. Significantly, less than 7 percent of the population supported the concept of presumed, or implied, consent. Under that concept, organ donation compliance is assumed unless otherwise noted by the potential donor.

8. Associated Press, "Gary Coleman Is Treated for 2nd Kidney Rejection," December 21, 1985.

9. Nationwide, there are about fifty independent organ procurement agencies and eighty that are hospital-based. These organizations coordinate activities related to retrieval of donated organs, including preserving them, making arrangements to transport organs, and arranging for tissue-typing. Initially, costs of organ donation are picked up by the transplant facility that recovers the donated organs and tissues.

10. Consent may be either written or oral, e.g., a telegram or recorded telephone consent which is kept on file at a transplant center. In addition, many hospital autopsy permits include a next-of-kin consent for removal of organs.

11. Cristine Russell, "Last March: Leukemia Patient Sues for Name of Possible Donor," *Washington Post*, March 4, 1983.

12. Quoted in Charles Marwick, "Pondering Past, Future of Implantable Heart," *Journal of the American Medical Association*, December 20, 1985, "Medical News" section.

13. From Renee C. Fox, "Organ Transplantation—Sociocultural Aspects," in Reich, Warren T., ed., *Encyclopedia of Bioethics* (New York: Free Press/Macmillan, 1978), vol. 3, p. 1166.

14. See Andrew S. Levey, Susan Hou, and Harry Bush, Jr., "Kidney Transplantation from Unrelated Living Donors: Time to Reclaim a Discarded Opportunity," *New England Journal of Medicine*, vol. 314, no. 14 (April 3, 1986), p. 914.

15. Quoted in Ellen Goodman, "The Business of Buying and Selling Spare Body Parts Erodes Morality" (column), *Reno Gazette-Journal*, September 30, 1983.

16. Ibid.

17. See "Organ Transplantation—Will Success Spoil the Stock Hunter?"

18. Daniel Q. Haney, "Jamie, Parents Beat the Odds," *Reno Gazette-Journal*, October 30, 1983. Also, Associated Press, "Fiske Doing Fine 2 Years After Transplant" (follow-up article), *Reno Evening Gazette*, November 7, 1984.

19. See Joyce Bermel, "Is the Media the Last Resort in Donor Cases?" *Medica*, Fall 1983. Fight to get a liver? Be more aggressive? Ethicists question what kind of society imposes such a burden on patients and their families that they must *compete* publicly for the next available liver or kidney. They are also critical of media cam-

paigns that enable some people to circumvent established procedures for choosing candidates for transplants and suggested criteria aimed at achieving fair allocation procedures.

20. Quoted in Beverly Merz, "The Organ Procurement Problem: Many Causes, No Easy Solutions," *Journal of the American Medical Association*, December 20, 1985, "Medical News" section.

21. Arthur L. Caplan, "Fix the Legal Ground for Organ Transplants" (letter), *New York Times*, October 7, 1983.

Chapter 6

1. Statistic from John Naisbitt, "More Reproductive Technologies Available to Infertile Couples: Trendnotes," *San Francisco Chronicle*, June 25, 1986, p. 2. See also Victor Fuchs and Leslie Perreault, "Expenditures for Reproduction-Related Health Care," *Journal of the American Medical Association*, January 3, 1986, pp. 7–81.

2. Australian In Vitro Fertilisation Collaborative Group, "High Incidence of Pre-term Births and Early Losses in Pregnancy After in Vitro Fertilisation," *British Medical Journal*, October 26, 1985, pp. 1160–63. See also Sue Downie, "Most Test-tube Babies Are Normal," *San Francisco Chronicle*, July 8, 1987, p. 6-A.

3. Quoted in David Perlman, " 'Test Tube' Triplets," *San Francisco Chronicle*, December 28, 1984, p. 1.

4. Quoted in Sandra Blakeslee, "New Issue in Embryo Case Raised over Use of Donor," *New York Times*, June 21, 1984, p. 16–A. Although present Australian legislation allows the Minister of Health to make the Rios's embryos available for implantation, the Victoria state government is seeking legal advice on what should be done with the two frozen embryos still in their possession. See "The Australian Frozen Embryos," *Hastings Center Report*, vol. 17, no. 2, April 1987, p. 51.

5. There are many ways of looking at the concept of personhood and self. Most scientists and philosophers believe that "man" is not only human (in a genetic and biologic sense) but is also a *person* possessing many characteristics which distinguish him or her from other living beings. These characteristics include self-awareness; minimal intelligence; a sense of past, present, and future; and the ability to feel, communicate, relate to others, reason, imagine, make decisions, and exercise judgment. For a fuller discussion, see Joseph Fletcher, *Humanhood: Essays in Biomedical Ethics* (Buffalo, N.Y.: Prometheus, 1979); and Clifford Grobstein, *From Chance to Purpose: An Appraisal of External Human Fertilization* (Reading, Mass.: Addison-Wesley, 1981), Chapter 5, "Becoming a Person."

6. Thomas Aquinas, *Summa Contra Gentiles*, 2:89.

7. See Ravi Taj Singh Khalsa, "When the Soul Enters" (letter), *New York Times,* September 30, 1984.

8. Quote from Sherman Elias, M.D., and George J. Annas, J.D., M.P.H., "Social Policy Considerations in Noncoital Reproduction," *Journal of the American Medical Association,* January 3, 1986, p. 63.

9. See American Fertility Society, "Ethical Statement on *in Vitro* Fertilization" and "Minimal Standards for Programs of *in Vitro* Fertilization," *Fertility and Sterility,* vol. 41, no. 1 (January 1984, p. 12). See also "Ethical Considerations of the New Reproductive Technologies," *Fertility and Sterility,* Supplement 1, September 1986.

10. See Claudia Wallis, "Quickening Debate over Life on Ice," *Time,* July 2, 1984, p. 68. See also David T. Ozar, "The Case Against Thawing Unused Frozen Embryos," *Hastings Center Report,* August 1985, p. 7; and Peter Singer, "Making Laws on Making Babies," same issue, p. 5.

11. Quoted in Lenita Power, "Reno Doctors Consider Freezing Embryos," *Reno Gazette-Journal,* June 21, 1984, p. 1.

12. See Gena Corea and Susan Ince, "IVF a Game for Losers at Half of U.S. Clinics," *Medical Tribune,* vol. 26, no. 19 (July 3, 1985), p. 1.

13. Statistic from "People, People, People," *Time,* August 6, 1984, p. 25.

14. Naisbitt, "More Reproductive Technologies Available."

15. Even Pope Pius XII acknowledged the legitimacy of "certain artificial methods intended simply either to facilitate the natural act, or enable the natural act, effected in a normal manner to attain its end"—pregnancy. Such methods include collecting a husband's semen from his wife's vagina following natural intercourse and concentrating the sperm density for later insemination. But the Roman Catholic hierarchy remains opposed to masturbation, the usual method of obtaining semen. See Pope Pius XII's *Allocution to the Second World Congress on Fertility and Sterility,* HB nn. 650–66, May 19, 1956, in *The Human Body: Papal Teachings* (Boston: St. Paul Editions, 1960).

    In a major Vatican document issued in March 1987 and titled "Instruction on Respect for Human Life and the Dignity of Procreation: Replies to Certain Questions of the Day," the Congregation for the Doctrine of the Faith asserted that "test-tube" fertilization, surrogate motherhood, sex-selection and other recent medical practices associated with procreation are immoral. It restates the church's total opposition to abortion and reaffirms the teaching in Pope Paul VI's encyclical "Humanae Vitae," which banned contraception, and stated that conjugal sex and procreation morally cannot be separated.

Some Roman Catholic theologians, however, believe that even standard methods of artificial insemination can be justified when a loving couple cannot achieve pregnancy through regular intercourse. Artificial insemination by donor is still not permitted. See Benedict M. Ashley and Kevin D. O'Rourke, in *Health Care Ethics: A Theological Analysis*, 2nd ed. (St. Louis: Catholic Health, 1982), Chapter 10, "Sexuality and Reproduction," p. 288.

According to Immanuel Jakobovits, *Jewish Medical Ethics* (New York: Bloch, 1975), "if Jewish law nevertheless opposes AID [artificial insemination by donor] without reservation as utterly evil, it is mainly for moral reasons.... the revulsion against the practice is the fear of abuses to which its legalization would lead, however great the benefits may be in individual cases. By reducing human generation to stud-farming methods, AID severs the link between the procreation of children and marriage, indispensable to the maintenance of the family...

"On AIH [artificial insemination by husband], however, rabbinic opinions are rather more favorable.... the argument hinges largely around the controversy on whether a man who begot a child *sine concubito* has therefore fulfilled his duty of procreation." The argument deals with the morality of masturbation, since Jewish law condemns "the bringing forth of semen for no purpose" (pp. 248–49).

16. Statistic from Elias and Annas, "Social Policy Considerations in Noncoital Reproduction," p. 63.

17. Quoted in "'Artificial' Human Reproduction Poses Medical, Social Concerns," *Journal of the American Medical Association*, January 3, 1986, pp. 13–15.

18. See "Some Sperm Donors Can Be Legal Fathers," *Reno Gazette-Journal*, March 29, 1986, p. A-2. In the first known ruling of its kind in California, the 1st District court of appeal said the donor can claim paternity unless the woman has followed a state law which permits her to exclude the donor as the child's father.

19. See 1985 Nevada Revised Statutes 126.061, 126.071, and 126.081, p. 4951.

20. Elias and Annas, "Social Policy Considerations in Noncoital Reproduction," p. 63.

21. Quoted in "'Artificial' Human Reproduction Poses Medical, Social Concerns."

22. Associated Press, June 27, 1986.

23. Ellen Goodman, "Today's bizarre parenthood options unnerving," *Reno Gazette-Journal*, April 4, 1986, p. 21-A.

24. Quoted in Courtney Brenn, "Surrogate Mothers Tough Issue," *Reno Gazette-Journal*, June 18, 1986, p. 2-C.

25. Quote attributed to the Sterns' attorney, Gary N. Skoloff, from Robert Hanley, "Plea by Baby M's Mother is Recalled," *New York Times*, January 7, 1987, p. 2-B.

26. The Surrogacy Arrangements Act, which became law in Great Britain on July 16, 1985, attempts to prevent third parties from deriving financial benefit from surrogacy. To date, however, voluntary surrogacy is not illegal in Britain, and no attempt has been made to define the status of babies born under such circumstances. See Diana Brahams, "The Hasty British Ban on Commercial Surrogacy," *Hastings Center Report*, February 1987, pp. 16–19.

27. George J. Annas, "The Baby Broker Boom," *Hastings Center Report*, June 1986, pp. 30–31.

28. For a fuller discussion of the Boff case (*Smith and Smith* v. *Jones and Jones*, 85-532014 DZ, Detroit, MI, 3d Jud. Dist., March 14, 1986, Battani, J.), see Annas, "The Baby Broker Boom."

29. Burton Sokoloff, M.D., "Surrogate Motherhood Should Be Abolished in U.S." (opinion piece), *AMA Medical News*, November 8, 1985, p. 35.

30. Quoted in "Choice vs. Life," *People*, August 8, 1985, p. 70.

31. See George Gallup, Jr., "U.S. Evenly Divided on Legalized Abortion," *San Francisco Chronicle*, February 20, 1986, p. 62.

32. According to the Alan Guttmacher Institute, a nonprofit research organization associated with Planned Parenthood, about 30 percent of all pregnancies in the United States were ended by abortion in 1983, with the largest proportion of abortions (35 percent) found in the 20-to-24 age category. About 51 percent of abortions were performed within eight weeks of conception, and 91 percent within three months of conception. See "Characteristics of U.S. Women Having Abortions, 1982–1983," Stanley K. Henschaw, *Family Planning Perspectives*, vol. 19, no. 1, January/February 1987, pp. 5–9.

33. For ruling on spousal consent and parental consent for a minor, see *Bellotti* v. *Baird*, Supreme Court of the United States, 1979, 443 U.S. 622, 99S.Ct. 3035, 61 L.Ed.2d 797.

34. Thomas A. Shannon and Jo Ann Manfra, *Law and Bioethics: Texts with Commentary on Major U.S. Court Decisions* (Ramsey, N.J.: Paulist Press, 1982), discussing spousal consent and parental consent for minors, states that "an important ethical dimension of abortion involves the relations of second and third parties to a pregnant woman. What rights, if any, does the husband of a pregnant woman have with respect to an abortion decision? And what rights, if any, do parents have with respect to a minor daughter who desires an abortion?" (p. 3).

Discussing *Bellotti* v. *Baird,* Shannon and Manfra point out that the U.S. Supreme Court said that "because of their vulnerability and need for parental attention, children's rights cannot be equated with those of adults and the state is 'entitled to adjust its legal system to account for' these special needs. The Court further stated that an abortion decision is of a 'unique nature' and requires a state 'to act with particular sensitivity when it legislates to foster parental involvement in this matter'" (p. 5).

The justices conclude that if a state requires parental consent, then it must also provide an alternative procedure. This alternative must allow the pregnant minor to obtain an independent judgment that either she is mature and capable enough to make the abortion decision on her own or else that the abortion is in her best interests.

35. See "*Roe* v. *Wade* Came Too Late for the Real Jane Roe," *People,* August 5, 1985, p. 72.

36. See Bill Wallace, "S.F. 'Birth-Control Agency' Probed as Anti-Abortion Unit," *San Francisco Chronicle,* June 23, 1986, p. 1.

37. Quoted in Randy Shilts, " 'Free Pregnancy Test' Offer Leads to Suit Against Agency," *San Francisco Chronicle,* June 23, 1986, p. 14. On August 26, 1986, Superior Court Judge Lucy McCabe ordered the anti-abortion clinic known as the Free Pregnancy Center to state in its advertising that it urges alternatives to abortion. She said that the center engaged in misleading advertising when it claimed in the phone book that it was a free pregnancy-testing and birth-control information center without making its anti-abortion position clear. (See "S.F. Judge's Order to Anti-Abortion Clinic," *San Francisco Chronicle,* August 27, 1986, p. 22.)

38. See Thomas G. Keane, "Father Sues for Fetus in 'Dead' Woman," *San Francisco Chronicle,* June 13, 1986, p. 1. Fifty-three days after Michele Odette Henderson was declared brain-dead, a four-pound, five-ounce girl in excellent health was delivered by cesarean section. Minutes later, doctors disconnected the life-support system which had sustained the 34-year-old mother's life since the twenty-sixth week of pregnancy, when she lapsed into irreversible coma because of a brain tumor. Henderson's parents had asked doctors to allow their daughter to die, but Derrick Poole, the baby's father, won a last-minute court order preventing doctors from removing life supports and was appointed the legal guardian of the fetus—an action which attorneys said set a legal precedent, since the couple were not married. (See Thomas Keane, "Brain-Dead Mother Has Her Baby," *San Francisco Chronicle,* July 31, 1986, p. 1.) See also, Jerry Carroll, "Another First for Little Michele: 'Miracle baby' has a birthday," *San Francisco Chronicle,* July 31, 1987, p. 36.

Chapter 7

1. See Claudia Wallis, "The Stormy Legacy of Baby Doe," *Time*, September 26, 1983; and E. Salholz, "Baby Doe's Legal Fate," *Newsweek*, November 14, 1983, p. 58.

2. Bonnie Steinbock, "Baby Jane Doe in the Courts," *Hastings Center Report*, February 1984, pp. 13–15.

3. Associated Press, January 15, 1986.

4. See Lisa Krieger, "Baby Doe Rule's Successes Told: Three Lives Reported Saved," *American Medical News*, August 19, 1983, p. 1.

5. *Otis R. Bowen, Secretary of Health and Human Services, Petitioner* v. *American Medical Association et al.*, Supreme Court of the United States, No. 84-1529 (B2750-B2804), June 9, 1986.

6. Richard A. McCormick, "To Save or Let Die: The Dilemma of Modern Medicine," *Journal of the American Medical Association*, July 8, 1974, p. 174.

7. Quoted in Dr. "N" as told to David R. Zimmerman, "Should This Baby Be Kept Alive...Who Can Best Decide?" *Woman's Day*, April 24, 1984, p. 70. See also Kathleen Kerr, "Reporting the Case of Baby Jane Doe," *Hastings Center Report*, August 1984, pp. 7–9.

8. Carson Strong, "The Neonatologist's Duty to Patient and Parents," *Hastings Center Report*, August 1984, pp. 10–16.

9. Peggy and Robert Stinson, *The Long Dying of Baby Andrew* (Boston: Little, Brown, 1983). See also Robert and Peggy Stinson, "On the Death of a Baby," *Atlantic Monthly*, July 1979, pp. 64–72.

10. Pope Pius XII, "Prolongation of Life: Allocution to an International Congress of Anesthesiologists," November 24, 1957, in *The Pope Speaks: The Church Documents Quarterly*, 4:393–98.

11. Norman Fost, "How Decisions Are Made: A Physician's View," in Chester A. Swinyard, *Decision Making and the Defective Newborn* (C. C. Thomas, 1978), p. 224.

12. Dr. "N," "Should This Baby Be Kept Alive?"

13. Paul Bridge and Marlys Bridge, "The Brief Life and Death of Christopher Bridge," *Hastings Center Report*, December 1981, pp. 17–19.

14. Robert Weir, *Selective Nontreatment of Handicapped Newborns* (New York: Oxford University Press, 1984), Chapter 9, "Procedure: Criteria, Options and Recommendations," pp. 261–62.

15. More than half of 426 hospitals responding to a 1984 American Academy of Pediatrics survey reported having set up infant bioethics committees (IBCs), and most of those which did not yet have such panels were considering establishing them. As reported

in the October 9, 1984, issue of the academy's publication *News & Comment*, survey results were compiled shortly before President Reagan signed child abuse prevention legislation encouraging formation of IBCs.

16. For a useful guide to resolving conflicts, see President's Commission for the Study of Ethical Problems in Medicine and Biomedical and Behavioral Research, *Deciding to Forego Life-Sustaining Treatment* (Washington, D.C.: U.S. Government Printing Office, 1983), p. 218.

17. Edward Walwork, A.C.S.W., and Patricia H. Ellison, M.D., "Follow-up of Families of Neonates in Whom Life Support Was Withdrawn," *Clinical Pediatrics*, vol. 24, no. 1 (January 1985), pp. 14–20.

18. See Mark Rust, "Scientists Ponder Ethics of Genetic Era," *American Medical News*, April 20, 1984, p. 3.

Chapter 8

1. Many articles about the Karen Ziegler case appeared in the *Reno Gazette-Journal* in 1984, among them Kate Santich, "Legal fight over Young Sparks Cancer Victim," February 18; Lenita Powers, "Cancer Victim Has Brief, Tearful Reunion," February 22; Kate Santich, "County Says It's Trying to Protect Cancer Victim," February 24; Kate Santich, "District Attorney: Ziegler Case 'Ripe for Misunderstanding,'" February 26; and Kate Santich, "Cancer Victim's Mom: Karen 'Wanted Peace,'" December 28. See also Wayne Melton, "Controversial Cancer Patient Dead at 13," December 27; and two editorials: "Officials Must Review Handling of Ziegler Case," February 29, and "Zieglers Had Right to Pick Wrong Path," December 30.

2. Washoe County Social Services officials acted under a state child abuse law that allows emergency removal of a child whose health or welfare is believed to be in jeopardy.

3. Originally, Washoe County District Attorney Mills Lane's office had filed the petition in court seeking to remove Karen from her parents' home and place her in the county's custody. Later, Lane was quoted as saying he was not "competent" to say what kind of treatment should be prescribed for Karen. See Kate Santich, "District Attorney: Return Cancer Victim to Parents," *Reno Gazette-Journal*, February 25, 1984. See also April Mayville, "Should a child die?" (letter), *Reno Gazette-Journal*, March 5, 1984; the writer asks: "Why did the district attorney, Mr. Lane, choose to remove Karen from her parents 'in her best interest' and then when the public opinion was clearly against his position, reverse his thing? Was the law more clear to him on Friday morning than

on Wednesday or did the political ramifications become more clear to him?"

4. Quoted in Kate Santich, "Karen Goes Home—Court: Daughter's Cancer Treatment up to Parents," *Reno Gazette-Journal*, February 25, 1984.

5. Willard Gaylin and Ruth Macklin, eds., *Who Speaks for the Child: The Problems of Proxy Consent* (New York: Plenum, 1982), p. 26.

6. See discussion of Joseph Hofbauer case in Bonnie Steinbock, "Baby Jane Doe in the Courts," *Hastings Center Report*, February 1984, pp. 13–19.

7. Irving Dickman and Dr. Sol Gordon, *One Miracle at a Time: How to Get Help for Your Disabled Child* (New York: Simon & Schuster, 1985), makes the distinction between a disability and a handicap: "The deficit with which a child is born (or that results from a later trauma or illness) is termed a *disability; handicaps* are the secondary problems that occur later, sometimes from society's discrimination or mistreatments but more often from help delayed or denied. It is a sad fact that most disabled children are also handicapped" (p. 137).

8. Quote from ibid., p. 146.

9. Ibid., p. 136.

10. See Matt Clark *et al.*, "A Breakthrough Transplant?" *Newsweek*, November 12, 1984; and "The Subject Is Baby Fae" (six articles by experts), *Hastings Center Report*, February 15, 1985, pp. 8–17.

11. See Dennis L. Breo, "Interview with Baby Fae's Surgeon: Therapeutic Intent Was Topmost," *American Medical News*, November 16, 1984, p. 1.

12. "Informed Consent Procedure Adequate for Baby Fae: NIH," *American Medical News*, March 29, 1985. See also "NIH Approves the Consent for Baby Fae, or Does It?" *Hastings Center Report*, April 1985, p. 2.

13. Olga Honasson, M.D., and Mark A. Hardy, M.D., "The Case of Baby Fae: Editorial," *Journal of the American Medical Association*, vol. 254, no. 23 (December 20, 1985), p. 3358–59.

14. Ellen Goodman, "Don't Experiment on Patients Who Have No Say" (column), *Reno Evening-Gazette*, November 11, 1984, p. 19-A.

15. In 1963 the Food and Drug Administration reviewed the world scientific literature regarding the controversial product laetrile (synthesized amygdalin, a derivative of peach pits) and concluded that there was no acceptable evidence that laetrile is effective in the treatment of cancer. See Dr. Arnold S. Relman, "Closing the Books on Laetrile" (editorial), *New England Journal of Medicine*, vol. 306, no. 4 (January 28, 1982), p. 236.

16. See J. C. Holland, "Why Patients Seek Unproven Cancer Remedies: A Psychological Perspective," *CA—a Cancer Journal for Clinicians*, vol. 32 (1982), p. 10.

17. *Prince* v. *Massachusetts* (1944) is discussed in Arnold J. Rosoff, *Informed Consent* (Rockville, Md.: Aspen Systems Corp., 1981), p. 199.

18. For analysis of *In re Pogue*, see Joseph Goldstein, "Medical Care for the Child at Risk," in Gaylin and Macklin, *Who Speaks for the Child*, p. 163.

19. For discussion of criteria for state intervention, see ibid., pp. 153–88.

20. See George Annas, "'A Wonderful Case and an Irrational Tragedy': The Phillip Becker Case Continues," *Hastings Center Report*, February 1982, p. 25; "The Phillip Becker Case: Was 'My Turn' Out of Turn?" *Hastings Center Report*, October 1983, p. 2; and Mark Rust, "Down's Child Gets New Family, Surgery," *American Medical News*, January 6, 1984, p. 31. For discussion of the Chad Green case, *In Custody of a Minor*, 375, 379 N.E.2d 1053 (1978), see Michael H. Shapiro and Roy G. Spece, Jr., *Bioethics and Law: Cases, Materials and Problems* (St. Paul: West, 1981), pp. 654–56.

21. Quoted in Kate Santich, "Karen Goes Home," *Reno Evening Gazette*, February 24, 1984.

22. Quoted in Kate Santich, "Cancer Victim's Mom: Karen 'Wanted Peace,'" *Reno Gazette-Journal*, December 28, 1984.

23. Quoted in Kate Santich, "Unorthodox Doctors: Quacks or Saviors?" *Reno Evening Gazette*, January 19, 1986.

24. See Susan Cunningham, "Prevention Studies May Clash with Ethics," *APA Monitor*, April 1984, p. 19.

25. See Ruprecht Nitschke *et al.*, "Therapeutic Choices Made by Patients with End-Stage Cancer," *Journal of Pediatrics*, vol. 101, no. 3 (September 1982), pp. 471–76; and Olle Jane Z. Sahler, commentary, *1984 Year Book of Pediatrics*, pp. 263–64.

26. For fuller discussion of the development of competence in children, see Sanford L. Leiken, M.D., "Minors' Assent or Dissent to Medical Treatment," *Journal of Pediatrics*, vol. 102, no. 2 (February 1983).

27. Ibid., p. 173

28. Willard Gaylin and Ruth Macklin, eds. *Who Speaks for the Child: The Problems of Proxy Consent*, p. 14

29. Leiken, "Minors' Assent or Dissent to Medical Treatment," p. 173.

30. The average stay of patients in the hospice program is from thirty-one to ninety days, as most children referred to hospice programs

are close to death, and, in fact, many hospice programs have set as an admission criterion a life expectancy of six months or less, according to Children's Hospice International, *1985 Pediatric Hospice Conference Report,* ed. Mary M. Hunter (Alexandria, VA: Children's Hospice International).

31. Elisabeth Kübler-Ross, M.D., "Challenges for Those Who Work with Dying Children," *1985 Pediatric Hospice Conference Report,* pp. 13–14. Dr. Kübler-Ross commented on nonverbal communication of dying children and explained three expressions of this universal symbolic language which children use. One type is spontaneous drawings, another spontaneous poems, and a third the collage. In discussing the drawings, she stressed that it's important in interpreting them to have the assistance of someone who knows how to read such pictures, for "otherwise, you can end up doing more harm than good."

    Dying children and young teenagers frequently write poems that they claim "just came to me" and that Kübler-Ross said reflect their awareness of impending death. "It's an incredible gift to parents whose child has died to find a poem afterward and realize that their child was in effect saying goodbye to them," she said. However, she placed most significance on the collage, in which words are added to pictures in an attempt to communicate the children's "inner language of what is happening to them. If you have children in remission or on the verge of relapse, you always know in which direction they will go from their collages and other nonverbal communication."

32. Ann Landers, "Be honest with the terminally ill," *The Standard Star-Gannett Westchester Newspapers,* May 2, 1985, p. 8-D.

33. J. J. Spinetta and L. J. Maloney, "The Child with Cancer: Patterns of Communication and Denial," *Journal of Consulting Clinical Psychology,* vol. 46, no. 6 (December 1978), pp. 1540–41. This widely quoted study of communication patterns in school-age children with terminal cancer showed children cope best when there is open communication among family members. Coping was defined as successful attempts by the child to master troublesome situations relative to the illness, a nondefensive personal posture, closeness to parental figures, happiness with oneself and the freedom to express negative feelings within the family. The researchers concluded that choosing silence (noncommunication) can lead to denial and a feeling of rejection and isolation in the child. See Eugenia H. Waechter, "Dying Children: Patterns of Coping," in Hannelore Wass and Charles A. Corr, eds., *Childhood and Death* (New York: Hemisphere, 1984), p. 63.

34. Controversy surrounds so-called "new" techniques currently being used by some physicians to hasten recovery of brain functions in patients in coma. Such methods include biofeedback to

reinforce neural pathways to the brain, feeding patients with twice as many calories as usual, drugs to minimize swelling and supply more oxygen to damaged parts of the brain, behavior modification of comatose patients to reinforce spontaneous movements so they will become voluntary, and promoting muscle tone through electrical stimulation of the patient's muscles. Many experts believe, however, that in cases where such unproven methods seem to have worked "miracles," the patient's level of coma had been incorrectly assessed to begin with. Thus, the diagnosis of "persistent vegetative state" (an irreversible condition) was incorrect, and some improvement would have been expected whether or not new methods of treating comatose patients were used.

35. Contrary to the prediction of a high divorce rate among these families, Shirley B. Lansky, M.D., together with other University of Kansas Medical Center researchers, found a person-year divorce rate of 1.19 percent—slightly lower than the 2.03 percent person-year divorce rate among married couples with children in Kansas and Missouri. Reported in Shirley B. Lansky *et al.*, "Childhood Cancer: Parental Discord and Divorce," *Pediatrics*, Vol. 62, No. 2 (August 1978), pp. 184–88. See also Ida M. Martinson, R.N., *et al.*, "Home Care for Children Dying of Cancer," *Pediatrics*, vol. 62, no. 1 (July 1978), pp. 106–13. Of fifty-eight families in four states Dr. Martinson studied from 1976 to 1978, 88 percent remained together; she is still researching the long-term effects of the death of a child on these families.

Chapter 9

1. See *In re Eichner* (1980, 2d Dept.) 73 App Civ 2d 431, 426 NYS2d 517 modified 1981.

2. Among additional reasons outlined in the commission report are (1) that the family deserves recognition as an important social unit that ought to be treated, within limits, as a responsible decision-maker in matters that intimately affect its members, and (2) that since a protected sphere of privacy and autonomy is required for the flourishing of this interpersonal union, institutions and the state should be reluctant to intrude, particularly regarding matters that are personal and on which there is a wide range of opinion in society. See the President's Commission for the Study of Ethical Problems in Medicine and Biomedical and Behavioral Research, *Deciding to Forego Life-Sustaining Treatment* (Washington, D.C.: U.S. Government Printing Office, 1983), pp. 127–28.

3. George J. Annas, "Do Feeding Tubes Have More Rights Than Patients?" *Hastings Center Report*, February 1986, p. 26.

4. Although testimony revealed that Karen had discussed her feelings with friends, the court wrote that "we cannot discern her supposed choice based on the testimony of her previous conversations with friends" since such testimony appeared remote and impersonal and lacked significant weight. Thus the substituted judgment standard could not be used in this case. See *In re Quinlan* (Supreme Court of New Jersey, 1976 70 N.J. 10, 355 A.2d 647). However, in 1985, the same court reversed itself in the Claire Conroy case, described later in this chapter.

5. See President's Commission, *Deciding to Forego Life-Sustaining Treatment*, pp. 132–36.

6. The seven cases are *Barber and Nejdl* in California; *Conroy, Jobes,* and *Peters* in New Jersey; *Brophy* and *Hyer* in Massachusetts; and *Corbett* in Florida.

7. Nancy Dickey, M.D., presentation on withdrawing of life supports at AMA–Hastings Center conference "A New Ethic for the New Medicine," New Orleans, March 14–16, 1986. (See Appendix H.)

8. According to the California court of appeal in *Barber* v. *Superior Court* (147 Cal. App. 3d 186, 195 (1984), "even if a proposed course of treatment might be extremely painful or intrusive, it would still be proportionate treatment if the prognosis was for complete cure or significant improvement in the patient's condition. . . . a treatment course which is only minimally painful or intrusive may nonetheless be considered disproportionate to the potential benefits if the prognosis is virtually hopeless for any significant improvement in the patient's condition." A discussion of this case, John J. Paris, S.J., "When Burdens of Feeding Outweigh Benefits," *Hastings Center Report*, February 1986, comments: "Thus the determination as to whether the burdens of treatment are worth enduring for any individual patient depends on facts unique to each case, namely, how long the treatment is likely to extend life under what conditions" (pp. 30–32).

9. John J. Paris, S.J., "Withholding Life Support" (presentation), AMA–Hastings Center conference, New Orleans, March 14–16, 1986. John Paris's testimony in the Brophy case appears in Paris, "When Burdens of Feeding Outweigh Benefits."

10. Quoted in Annas, "Do Feeding Tubes Have More Rights than Patients?" p. 26.

11. Quoted in Claudia Wallis, "To Feed or Not to Feed?" *Time*, March 31, 1986, p. 60.

12. "Judge OKs Removal of Tube That Has Kept Woman Alive," *San Francisco Chronicle*, April 24, 1986, p. 7. See also Joseph F. Sullivan, "Jersey Court Wrestles Again with Death and Civil Rights," *New York Times*, October 20, 1986. See also "Nancy Ellen Jobes" (obituary), *San Francisco Chronicle*, August 8, 1987, p. 5.

13. John J. Paris, S.J., "Withholding Life Support." A 1987 study by the Office of Technology Assessment, "Life Sustaining Technologies and the Elderly," found that most U.S. hospitals lack guidelines on when to extend or withdraw life-sustaining treatments for the elderly and often ignore the patient's wishes. Researchers emphasized the importance of advance directives, such as living wills, in ensuring the patient's wishes regarding treatment will be known when he or she is terminally ill. See "Hospitals Criticized for Ignoring Patient Wishes," San Francisco Chronicle, August 1, 1987, p. 1.

14. Story and following quotes from "Excerpts from Jersey Ruling on Withholding of Life Support," New York Times, January 18, 1985.

15. In 1985, a Louis Harris and Associates survey of 1,254 adults found that 85 percent thought a terminally ill patient "ought to be able to tell his doctor to let him die," and 82 percent supported the idea of withdrawing feeding tubes if that was the patient's wish. See "Support Increases For Euthanasia," The Harris Survey, no. 18, March 4, 1985, pp. 1–3.

16. Statistics from American Association of Retired Persons, "A Profile of Older Americans 1985" (brochure); and Robert Katzman, M.D., "Alzheimer's Disease," New England Journal of Medicine, vol. 314, no. 15 (April 10, 1986), pp. 964–72.

17. Daniel Callahan, "What Do Children Owe Elderly Parents?" Hastings Center Report, April 1985, pp. 32–37.

18. "Grim Report on Nursing Homes," San Francisco Chronicle, May 22, 1986, p. 18.

19. In her seminar presentation "Family Caregivers: Their Perspective On Institutional Decisions" (University of Tennessee seminar, "Informed Consent and Elderly Patients with Limited Decision-Making Capacity," April 3, 1986), Aloen Townsend, Ph.D., of the Rose Institute in Cleveland, Ohio, indicated that although less than 25 percent of families studied preferred nursing homes as a solution to their elders' problems, 92 percent said they had no alternative, and 75 percent said they had few choices. Of forty-nine families studied, six of the elders had made the final decisions to enter the home, ten were consulted, and thirty-three were considered too impaired to participate in the decision-making.

20. See "Nursing-Home Residents Seek Freedom of Choice," Reno Gazette-Journal, May 5, 1985, p. D-6.

21. David C. Thomasma, Jurrit Bergsma, and Gerard Daggelders, "Doctors and Patients on Autonomy and Decision Making," submitted to Archives of Internal Medicine.

Chapter 10

1. See the following articles in *New York Times:* Dena Kleiman, "Twin Brothers, Both East Side Gynecologists, Apparent Suicides," July 20, 1975, p. 38; Mary Breasted, "Death of Twin Doctors Linked to Despondency," July 21, p. 25; Boyce Rensberger, "Death of 2 Doctors Poses a Fitness Issue," August 15, p. 1; and Boyce Rensberger, "New York Hospital Defends Its Actions on Marcus Twins," August 19, p. 1.

2. According to the St. Paul Fire and Marine Insurance Company, one of the major medical malpractice insurers in the United States, the ten leading allegations in medical malpractice claims against doctors and hospitals in 1983 were bad treatment results, such as post-surgical care; falling out of bed; delay or omission of needed treatment; injury of body adjacent to the treatment site; wrong diagnosis; incorrect treatment and other miscellaneous treatment problems; exposure to infection; falling while walking; and falling in bathroom. See Joel Brinkley, "Physicians Have an Image Problem—It's Too Good," *New York Times*, February 10, 1985.

3. According to Brinkley, "Physicians Have an Image Problem," in 1983 there were sixteen malpractice claims for every hundred doctors, 20 percent more than in 1982 and three times more than in 1975. In 1982, more than 250 exceeded $1 million, a tenfold increase in just four years. See also John Naisbitt, "Trendnotes: Record Malpractice Claims," *San Francisco Chronicle*, August 7, 1985, p. 16; and "Medical Malpractice," *Medical Tribune*, January 23, 1985, p. 19.

4. Interview with Alexander Capron, "Internal Policing Called Best Malpractice Solution," *American Medical News*, March 15, 1985, p. 30.

5. Statistic from Charlotte L. Rosenberg, "Why Doctor-Policing Laws Don't Work," *Medical Economics*, March 4, 1984, pp. 84–96.

6. Statistics and Dr. Arnold Relman's estimate of grossly incompetent or negligent doctors from Andrew Stein, "Doctors Who Get Away With Killing and Maiming Must Be Stopped," *New York Times*, February 2, 1986, p. 23-E.

7. Arnold S. Relman, M.D., "Professional Regulation and the State Medical Boards," *New England Journal of Medicine*, vol. 312, no. 12 (March 21, 1985), pp. 784–85.

8. Nevada State Medical Association Meeting, May 1986.

9. See Appendix A, the American Hospital Association's "A Patient's

Bill of Rights," items 5 and 6, regarding privacy and confidentiality of patient records and communications.

10. Associated Press, "AMA president says confidentiality ethic a hindrance in war on AIDS," April 14, 1987.

11. *Tarasoff* v. *Regents of University of California*, Supreme Court of California, 1976. In 1967, University of California–Berkeley student Prosenjit Poddar fell in love with fellow student Tatiana Tarasoff, who did not share his feelings and told him so. Poddar became depressed, neglected his studies, and showed signs of poor health. After six months, he sought psychiatric help as a voluntary outpatient at the university's hospital, where he revealed to Dr. Lawrence Moore his intent to kill Tatiana upon her return from summer vacation. Moore and two other doctors agreed that Poddar was "at this point a danger to the welfare of other people and himself."

In a letter of diagnosis, Dr. Moore asked campus police to detain Poddar for a seventy-two-hour emergency psychiatric treatment, but Poddar was released when he appeared sane and promised to stay away from Tatiana. Moore's superior, Dr. Powelson, then closed the case and ordered Poddar's records destroyed. Two months later, Poddar murdered Tatiana. No one had warned the girl or her parents of Poddar's threat, and the Tarasoffs brought a wrongful-death action against the regents, campus police, and hospital doctors.

In its ruling, the California supreme court stated that "the protective privilege ends where the public peril begins" and that psychotherapists, who have reason to believe a patient may harm someone, have a duty to warn the potential victim and confine dangerous patients.

12. See Claudia Wallis, "Weeding Out the Incompetents," *Time*, May 26, 1986, pp. 57–58; and Karen Dandrick, "Illinois Physicians Work to Weed Out Bad Apples," *Private Practice*, August 1983, pp. 17–20.

13. See Joel Brinkley, "U.S., Industry and Physicians Attack Medical Malpractice" and "Medical Discipline Laws: Confusion Reigns," *New York Times*, September 2–3, 1985. See also Carole Horn, "When Doctors Go Shockingly Wrong," *Washington Post*, June 9, 1985, p. 1-D.

14. As of October 1986, states permitting patients unrestricted access to their medical records include Alaska, California, Colorado, Connecticut, Florida, Georgia, Hawaii, Illinois, Michigan, Minnesota, Nevada, Oklahoma, Virginia, West Virginia, and Wisconsin. Source: "Where Patients Can See Medical Records," *Good Housekeeping*, October 1986. In January 1987, New York passed a law allowing most interested patients to have unrestricted access to

their medical records, according to Arthur A. Levin, M.P.H., director, Center for Medical Consumers in New York City. See also, Ronald Sullivan, "New York Patients to Have More Access to Their Records," *New York Times*, July 14, 1986, p. 30, and Allan H. Bruckheim, "Family Doctor: Medical Records" (column), *Reno Gazette-Journal*, April 2, 1987, p. 7-D.

15. The Federation of State Medical Boards in its *Guide to the Essentials of a Modern Medical Practice Act* (revised 1985) lists thirty-three grounds for which a state licensing board should be authorized to take disciplinary action against physicians. Not every state act includes all thirty-three, but the list is representative of most state laws.

16. Robert C. Derbyshire, M.D., "Medical Discipline in Disarray" (series), *Hospital Practice*, November 1983–June 1984.

17. Donald J. Flaster, M.D., LL.B., "Do You Have a Case Against Your Doctor for Negligence? Malpractice?" *New Woman*, December 1983, p. 44. See also Dr. James Sammons, executive vice president of the American Medical Association, letter headed "The People Support Curbs on Malpractice Awards," *New York Times*, March 24, 1985. See also comments in *Medical World News*, March 11, 1985, p. 27, which read in part: "Medicine is a complex, rapidly changing, inexact science, and patients' needs, histories, and responses vary greatly. Many claims involve no negligence at all— only unfulfilled expectations.... Make no mistake about it, society is paying these costs.... Physicians and hospitals are merely conduits, passing these costs on to their patients."

18. See Marcia Chambers, "Parents of Septuplets Sue in Desperation," *San Francisco Chronicle*, December 12, 1985, p. 26.

19. Associated Press, *Reno Gazette-Journal*, August 23, 1986. See also J.H. Eichhorn, M.D., *et al.*, "Standards for Patient Monitoring During Anesthesia at Harvard Medical School," *Journal of the American Medical Association*, vol. 256, no. 8 (August 22–29, 1986), p. 1017.

20. See "Malpractice Foes Enter Computer Age," *Medical World News*, December 9, 1985, p. 22; also, Associated Press, "Doctors, Lawyers Square Off Over Lawsuit Hot Lines," *San Francisco Chronicle*, December 26, 1985, p. 6.

21. See American Medical Association Special Task Force on Professional Liability and Insurance, "Report 2: Professional Liability in the '80s" (November 1984), p. 6, chart (Claims filed, closed, with and without indemnity: 1979–1983).

22. See Robert Lindsey, "2 Doctors Cleared in Death of Patient in California," *New York Times*, March 10, 1983, p. 18-A; Dennis L. Breo, Doug Lefton, and Mark Rust, "MDs Face Unprecedented

Murder Charge," *American Medical News*, September 16, 1983; and Mark Rust, "Appellate Ruling Breaks New Legal Ground," *American Medical News*, October 28, 1983. (For more information on withholding food and nutrition from terminally ill patients, see Chapter 9.)

23. Statistics from Ronald Smothers, "Addict-Doctors Get Aid Under Georgia Program," *New York Times*, May 8, 1983, p. 16.

24. Personal communication from executive director, Nevada State Nurses Association.

25. G. Douglas Talbott, "Impaired Physicians Program," address given at annual meeting of Nevada State Medical Association, May 1985.

26. See Carl R. Robinson, M.D., J.D., "Why the Conspiracy of Silence Won't Die," *Medical Economics*, February 20, 1984, pp. 180–86.

27. "The Marcus Tragedy" (editorial), *New York Times*, August 16, 1975, p. 18.

28. "Malpractice Crisis: Public Aware but Confused on Details," *Medical World News*, December 9, 1985, p. 22.

29. According to Rita Rooney, "Sexual Exploitation Is Shockingly Prevalent in the Medical Community," *Ladies' Home Journal*, June 1986, "There is no accurate count of the number of physicians around the country who sexually exploit their patients, but lawyers and medical experts assert that the problem is far more commonplace than people realize" (p. 109). Each month, the Federation of State Medical Boards of the United States receives about three reports of such abuse, and for every one investigated, it's estimated that fifteen to twenty-five more go unreported.

30. See N.Y. Supreme Court Index 834 (1981).

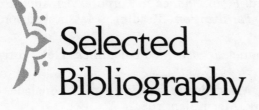

Selected Bibliography

The following list of books, articles, and reports includes those which we believe will be most helpful to patients and their families, and most readily found in hospital, medical center and major public libraries. Suggested readings at the end of each chapter contain specific references related to topics covered in the chapter.

Books

Ashley, Benedict M., O.P., and Kevin D. O'Rourke, O.P., *Health Care Ethics: A Theological Analysis*, 2nd ed. St. Louis: Catholic Health Association of the United States, 1982.

Bachelor, Edward, Jr. *Abortion: The Moral Issues.* New York: Pilgrim, 1982.

Beauchamp, Tom L., and Leroy Walters. *Contemporary Issues in Bioethics*, 2nd ed. Belmont, Calif.: Wadsworth, 1982.

Bloch, Sidney, and Paul Chodoff. *Psychiatric Ethics.* New York: Oxford University Press, 1981.

Callahan, Sidney, and Daniel Callahan. *Abortion: Understanding Differences.* New York: Plenum, 1984.

Childress, James F. *Who Should Decide? Paternalism in Health Care.* New York: Oxford University Press, 1982.

Doudera, A. Edward, and Douglas J. Peters. *Legal and Ethical Aspects of Treating Critically and Terminally Ill Patients.* Ann Arbor: AUPHA Press, 1982.

Fletcher, Joseph. *Humanhood: Essays in Biomedical Ethics.* Buffalo, N.Y.: Prometheus, 1979.

Gaylin, Willard, and Ruth Macklin, eds. *Who Speaks for the Child: The Problems of Proxy Consent.* New York: Plenum, 1982.

Grobstein, Clifford. *From Chance to Purpose: An Appraisal of External Human Fertilization.* Reading, Mass.: Addison-Wesley, 1981.

Jakobovits, Immanuel. *Jewish Medical Ethics.* New York: Bloch, 1959; New Matter, 1975.

Jonsen, Albert R., Mark Siegler, and William J. Winslade. *Clinical Ethics.* New York: Macmillan, 1982.

Katz, Jay. *The Silent World of Doctor and Patient.* New York: Free Press, 1984.

Kopelman, L., and J.C. Moskop, eds. *Ethics and Mental Retardation.* Boston: D. Reidel, 1984.

Kushner, Harold S. *When Bad Things Happen to Good People.* New York: Shocken, 1981.

Lyon, Jeff. *Playing God in the Nursery.* New York: Norton, 1985.

Robertson, John A. *The Rights of the Critically Ill,* rev. ed. New York: American Civil Liberties Union, 1983.

Robin, Eugene D., M.D. *Matters of Life and Death: Risks vs. Benefits of Medical Care.* New York: Freeman, 1984.

Rosoff, A.J. *Informed Consent.* Rockville, Md.: Aspen Systems Corp., 1981.

Shannon, Thomas A., and JoAnn Manfra. *Law and Bioethics: Texts with Commentary on Major U.S. Court Decisions.* Ramsey, N.J.: Paulist Press, 1982.

Shaw, Margery W., M.D., J.D., and A. Edward Doudera, J.D. *Defining Human Life: Medical, Legal, and Ethical Implications.* Ann Arbor: AUPHA Press, 1983.

Siegel, Bernie S., M.D. *Love, Medicine and Miracles.* New York: Harper & Row, 1986.

Veatch, Robert M. *A Theory of Medical Ethics.* New York: Basic Books, 1981.

Weir, Robert. *Selective Nontreatment of Handicapped Newborns.* New York: Oxford University Press, 1984.

Articles

Abram, Morris B. "Ethics and the New Medicine." *New York Times Magazine*, June 5, 1983.

"America's Abortion Dilemma." *Newsweek*, January 14, 1985.

Andrews, Lori B. "When Baby's Mother Is Also Grandma—and Sister: Commentary." *Hastings Center Report*, vol. 15, no. 5 (October 1985).

Annas, George J. "Baby Fae: The 'Anything Goes' School of Human Experimentation." *Hastings Center Report*, vol. 15, no. 1 (February 1985).

———. "Do Feeding Tubes Have More Rights Than Patients?" *Hastings Center Report*, vol. 16, no. 1 (February 1986).

———. "Elizabeth Bouvia: Whose Space Is This Anyway?" *Hastings Center Report*, April 1986.

———. "The Baby Broker Boom." *Hastings Center Report*, vol. 16, no. 3 (June 1986).

Becker, Warren, and Patricia Becker. "My Turn: Mourning the Loss of a Son." *Newsweek*, May 30, 1984.

Binkley, Deana, as told to Edwin Black. "Young Mother's Story: 'We Weren't Going to Let Jesse Die.'" *Redbook*, November 1986.

Blair, Beatrice. "The Right-to-Life Debate." *New York Times Magazine*, January 27, 1985.

Caplan, Arthur. "Toward Greater Donor Organ Availability for Transplantation." *New England Journal of Medicine*, vol. 312, no. 5 (January 3, 1985).

Cousins, Norman. "How Patients Appraise Physicians." *New England Journal ofMedicine*, vol. 313, no. 22 (November 28, 1985).

Derr, Patrick G. "Why Food and Fluids Can Never Be Denied." *Hastings Center Report*, vol. 16, no. 1 (February 1986).

Elias, Sherman, M.D., and George J. Annas, J.D., M.P.H. "Social Policy Considerations in Noncoital Reproduction." *Journal of the American Medical Association*, vol. 255, no. 1 (January 3, 1986).

"Excerpts from Jersey Ruling on Withholding of Life Support." *New York Times*, January 18, 1985.

Fost, N.E. "Parental Control over Children." *Journal of Pediatrics*, vol. 103, no. 4 (October 1983).

Holder, A.R. "Parents, Courts and Refusal of Treatment." *Journal of Pediatrics*, vol. 103, no. 4 (October 1983).

"Hospices: Not to Cure but to Help." *Consumer Reports*, 1986.

Huttmann, Barbara. "My Turn: A Crime of Compassion." *Newsweek*, August 8, 1983.

Kleiman, Dena. "Hospital Care of the Dying: Each Day, Painful Choices." *New York Times*, January 14, 1985.

Knoll, Elizabeth, M.Phil., and George D. Lundberg, M.D. "Informed Consent and Baby Fae." *Journal of the American Medical Association*, vol. 254, no. 23 (December 20, 1985).

Lawrence, Raymond J. "David the 'Bubble Boy' and the Boundaries of the Human." *Journal of the American Medical Association*, vol. 253, no. 1 (January 4, 1985).

Lawson, Carol. "Surrogate Mothers Grow in Number Despite Questions." *New York Times*, October 1, 1986.

Lynn, Joanne, and James F. Childress. "Must Patients Always Be Given Food and Water?" *Hastings Center Report*, October 1983.

"Making a 'Living Will.'" *New York Times*, November 23, 1985.

Malcolm, Andrew H. "The Dialysis Dilemma: Extending Life or Prolonging Death?" *New York Times*, March 23, 1986.

Manney, James. "The Right-to-Life Debate." *New York Times Magazine*, January 27, 1985.

Marwick, Charles. "Pondering Past, Future of Implantable Heart." *Journal of the American Medical Association*, vol. 254, no. 23 (December 20, 1985).

May, William F. "Religious Justifications for Donating Body Parts." *Hastings Center Report*, vol. 15, no. 1 (February 1985).

Moskop, John C., and Rita L. Saldanha. "The Baby Doe Rule: Still a Threat." *Hastings Center Report*, April 1986.

Murray, Thomas H., Ph.D. "Ethical Issues in Fetal Surgery." *American College of Surgeons Bulletin*, vol. 70, no. 6 (June 1985).

Otten, Alan L. "New 'Wills' Allow People to Reject Prolonging of Life in Fatal Illness." *Wall Street Journal*, July 2, 1985.

Paris, John J., S.J., Ph.D. "When Burdens of Feeding Outweigh Benefits." *Hastings Center Report*, vol. 16, no. 1 (February 1986).

———, and Frank E. Reardon, J.D. "Court Responses to Withholding or Withdrawing Artificial Nutrition and Fluids." *Journal of the American Medical Association*, vol. 253, no. 15 (April 19, 1985).

Relman, Arnold S., M.D. "Artificial Hearts—Permanent and Temporary." *New England Journal of Medicine*, vol. 314, no. 10 (March 6, 1986).

Singer, Peter. "Making Laws on Making Babies." *Hastings Center Report*, August 1985.

Stein, Andrew. "Doctors Who Get Away with Killing and Maiming Must Be Stopped." *New York Times*, February 21, 1986.

———. "Picking a Doctor in an Information Vacuum." *New York Times*, August 18, 1986.

Steinbrook, Robert, M.D., and Bernard Lo, M.D. "Decision Making for Incompetent Patients by Designated Proxy." *New England Journal of Medicine*, vol. 310, no. 24 (June 14, 1984).

Sullivan, Joseph F. "Jersey Court Wrestles Again with Death and Civil Rights." *New York Times*, October 20, 1986.

Wallis, Claudia. "To Feed or Not to Feed?" *Time*, March 31, 1986.

Wanger, Sidney H., *et al.* "The Physician's Responsibility Toward Hopelessly Ill Patients." *New England Journal of Medicine*, vol. 310, no. 15 (April 12, 1984).

Wilde, Richard. "Parenting our Parents." *New Woman*, May 1986.

Younger, Stuart J., M.D., *et al.* "Psychosocial and Ethical Implications of Organ Retrieval." *New England Journal of Medicine*, vol. 313, no. 5 (August 1, 1985).

Reports

The President's Commission for the Study of Ethical Problems in Medicine and Biomedical and Behavioral Research. Reports. 10 reports. Washington, D.C.: U.S. Government Printing Office, 1983. For copies, contact the Superintendent of Documents, U.S. Government Printing Office, Washington, D.C. 20402.

Willoughby, Deborah, ed. *Organ Transplantation: Issues and Recommendations*. Rockville, Md.: Task Force on Organ Transplantation, Health Resources and Services Administration, U.S. Department of Health & Human Resources, April 1986.

General Reference

Callahan, Daniel, and H. Tristram Engelhardt, Jr. *The Roots of Ethics: Science, Religion and Values*. New York: Plenum, 1981.

Duncan, A.S., G.R. Dunstan, and R.B. Welbourn, eds. *Dictionary of Medical Ethics*. New York: Crossroad, 1981.

Reich, Warren T., ed. *Encyclopedia of Bioethics*, 4 vols. New York: Free Press/Macmillan, 1978.

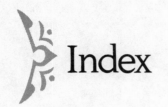 Index

Abbotts, Carla, 186
abortion, 48, 155, 158, 179, 180–90,
   191
  case-by-case view on, 188–89
  laws regarding, 182–83
  minors and, 182
  options and, 184–85
  pro-choice view on, 187–88
  pro-life view on, 186–87
  questions to ask about, 189–90
  rape and, 183–84, 189
  rights and, 182–86
  therapeutic, 16
Abram, Morris B., 37–38, 61–62
achondroplasia, 226
active euthanasia, 111, 327
acupuncture, 250
Admiraal, Pieter, 111
adoption, 175, 184, 190–91
AIDS (acquired immune deficiency
  syndrome), 136, 165, 167, 312–
  315
Albert Einstein College of Medicine,
  30
Alcoholics Anonymous, 330
Alfidi, Ralph J., 54
alpha fetoprotein (AFP) tests, 178

Alternatives to Abortion
  International, 185, 191
Alzheimer's disease, 293
Alzheimer's Disease and Related
  Disorders Association, 303
American Academy of Family
  Physicians, 39
American Academy of Pediatrics,
  147, 215
American Association for the
  Advancement of Science, 252
American Association of Retired
  Persons (AARP), 57
American Board of Family Practice,
  40
American Cancer Society, 72
American Civil Liberties Union
  (ACLU), 65, 68, 339
American College of Obstetrics and
  Gynecology, 65
American Council on
  Transplantation (ACT), 150
American Fertility Society, 159, 161,
  167–68, 190
American Health, 55
American Health Care Association,
  296, 302

American Heart Association, 72
American Hospital Association, 67, 136, 342
American Kidney Fund, 267
American Medical Association (AMA), 37, 42, 286, 322, 328, 333
  Council on Ethical and Judicial Affairs, 285, 370
  Family Medical Guide, 72
  Medical News, 176
  on withholding treatment, 370–71
American Medical Directory, 41–42, 322
American Medical News, 240
American Medical Records Association, 338
American Red Cross, 149, 150
amniocentesis, 21, 48, 175, 177, 185, 188, 225, 228
amputations, 253–54
amyotrophic lateral sclerosis, 98
M. D. Anderson Cancer Center, 246
Andrews, Lori, 167–68
anencephaly, 89
anesthesia, 326
aneurysms, 107, 287
angiograms, 54
animal-heart transplants, 239–42
Annas, George J., 68, 114, 167, 172, 281
aplastic anemia, 135
apnea, 196
Aquinas, Thomas, 158
artificial hearts, 83
artificial insemination, 164–68, 176
  see also surrogate motherhood
Ashlock, Donna, 125–26, 130
Assisted Suicide: The Compassionate Crime, 122
Associated Press, 169, 314
Australia, 159
autonomy, 18, 20, 25, 37–38, 54–55, 247, 293, 294

Baby Andrew, 204–5
Baby Bryan, 195–98, 207, 222
Baby Doe, 198
Baby Doe cases, 194–229
  bioethics committees for, 214–21
  child's best interests in, 203–4
  costs in, 207–8
  death in, 222–23
  doctor's duties in, 204–5, 208–12
  federal regulations on, 200–202
  heroic treatment in, 205–6, 216
  medical records and, 213–14
  parents' and family's interests in, 204
  parents as primary decision-makers in, 202
  quality of life in, 206–7
  questions to ask about, 210–11
Baby Fae, 239–42
Baby Jane Doe, 199–200, 203–4
Baby M, 170–71
Baby Moses, 242–43
Baby Stiver, 173–74
Bailey, Leonard, 240
Barber, Neil L., 285–86, 327
Barnard, Christiaan, 138
Barrister Magazine, 49
Bartling, William, 81–82, 88
Beaber, Rex Julian, 93
Becker, Phillip, 250
Bellon, Laird and LeAnn, 147–48
beneficence, 18, 38, 239
Benson, Earl B., 329
Better Business Bureau, 185
biliary atresia, 135
Bills of Rights:
  Institutionalized Person's, 350–53
  Medical Research Patient's, 345–346
  Nursing Home Patient's, 298, 354–55
  Patient's, 67–68, 342–44
bioethics committees, 30–31, 283–284
  infant, 214–21
biopsies, 75
birth defects, 15–16, 21
  causes of, 225–27
  prenatal testing for, 177–80
  surrogate motherhood and, 173–174
  see also Baby Doe cases
Birth Defects: Tragedy and Hope, 227

Bischoff, Ernest, 269
Blaine, Graham B., 29
Blom, Randy, 302
blood plasma, 142
blood transfusions, 208, 247, 257
Blue Cross/Blue Shield, 307, 323
   Second Opinion Referral Center,
   46
Boff, Shannon, 175
bone cancer, 253–54
bone marrow transplants, 135, 166
Bouvia, Elizabeth, 78–80, 82, 88
brain death, 265, 277
   organ transplants and, 126, 133–
   134
   pregnancy and, 187
Brazil, organ sales in, 142
Breaden, Dale, 316
breast cancer, 59–60, 74–75
Bridge, Paul and Marlys, 212–13
British Medical Journal, 155
Brophy, Paul, 287–88
Brown, Louise, 152
Broznick, Brian, 135
Burlington County (N.J.) *Times*,
   147

Caduceus Clubs, 330
Callahan, Daniel, 16, 24, 142, 294
cancer, 49, 139
   bone, 253–54
   breast, 59–60, 74–75
   children with, 230–33, 237–38,
   245, 249–52, 253–54, 259–60,
   262
   colon, 80
   Hodgkin's disease, 21, 230–33,
   249–52
   leukemia, 61, 80, 135, 137,
   165–166
   lung, 51, 81
   pancreas, 52
Cancer Information Service, 267
Candlelighters Childhood Cancer
   Foundation, 267
Can Genetic Counseling Help You?,
   228
Canterbury v. *Spence*, 69
Caplan, Arthur, 19, 53, 54, 117, 142,
   150, 337
cardiopulmonary resuscitation,

108–9, 119, 196
Cardozo, Benjamin, 54
Cass, Peggy, 334, 335
Catholics for a Free Choice, 185,
   191
CAT scans, 208
Center for Medical Consumers, 57
cerebral palsy, 78, 334
cesarean sections, 64–65, 153
chemotherapy, 165–66, 251, 254,
   313
Chicago Bears, 25
child abuse, 201, 214, 247
Child Abuse Amendments, 201–2
childbirth, 63–65, 153
child neglect, 230–31, 249–50
Children's Hospice International
   (CHI), 258, 268
children's illnesses, 230–71
   alternative treatments for,
   245–256
   cancer, 230–33, 237–38, 245,
   249–52, 253–54, 259–60, 262
   child's competency and, 254–56
   child's rights and, 253–56
   conventional therapy for, 237–39
   death from, 256–66
   development and, 234–35, 236,
   254–55
   experimental treatment for,
   239–44, 249–52
   hospices and, 257–59, 268
   informed consent and, 240–42,
   243–44
   questions to ask about, 235–37,
   265
   rights and, 246–49, 253–56
   waiting and, 234–35
   withholding treatment for,
   256–66
   see also Baby Doe cases
chorionic villus sampling (CVS),
   178
Christian Scientists, 257
Claire Conroy pattern, 288–91
Clark, Barney, 83
Cleveland Clinic, 54
cocaine, 331
Coleman, Gary, 130
coma, 277–78
communication, 48–56, 317–19

Compassionate Friends, 268
*Complete Guide to Prescription
    and Non-Prescription Drugs*
    (Griffith), 72
Concern for Dying, 102, 121
confidentiality, 36–37, 87, 137,
    312–15, 331
Conroy, Claire, 288–89
consumerism, 37–38
*Consumer's Guide to Improved
    Nursing Home Care*, 303
*Consumer's Guide to Nursing
    Home Care, A*, 303
Consumers Union, 121
Cooke, Terence Cardinal, 78
Cooper v. *Roberts*, 69
corneal transplants, 128, 141
costs, medical:
    in Baby Doe cases, 207–8
    billing fraud and, 323–24
    high, 306–7, 318, 336
    of organ donations, 134–36
    second opinions and, 46
Cotes, Susan and Roland, 262–63
Coury, John J., Jr., 314
Cousins, Norman, 55–56
cryopreservation, 153
Cummings, Terry, 77–78
cyclosporin, 125, 140
cystic fibrosis, 266
Cystic Fibrosis Foundation, 267

Dailey, Ann, 258, 268
Day, Carol and Dennis, 156
death:
    in Baby Doe cases, 222–23
    brain, 126, 133–34, 187, 265, 277
    of children, 256–66
    definitions of, 277
    informed consent and, 68–69
    right to, 23, 60, 78–80, 99,
        282–83, 287–90; *see also* Baby
        Doe cases; treatment,
        withholding
    risk of, 68–69
Declaration of Independence, 24
Declaration on Euthanasia, 112
Deering, Warren, 79
denial, 27, 51
depression, 80–81
Derbyshire, Robert C., 320

diabetes, 139, 140, 141, 223, 267
diaphragmatic hernias, 179
Dickey, Nancy, 285
Dickman, Irving, 234
Dictionary of Medical Ethics
    (Twycross), 111
dilatation and curettage (D & C),
    189
Directory of Medical Specialists,
    41–42, 322
dissociation, 51
doctors, 34–58
    authority of, 25
    communication and, 48–56,
        317–19
    complaints against, 317–24,
        335–36
    confidentiality and, 36–37,
        312–15, 331
    criminal charges against, 327–28
    drug and alcohol abuse among,
        308, 321, 327–31
    duties of, in Baby Doe cases,
        204–5, 208–12
    glut of, 17, 316
    hospital privileges of, 319–20
    incompetent, 306–39
    limited paternalism of, 81
    malpractice suits against, 309–10,
        324–26
    patient's relationship with,
        34–58, 217, 314–15
    primary care, 40
    qualifications of, 41–42
    secondary care, 40
    second opinions and, 44–46
    selection of, 39–44, 47–48,
        95–96
    truth-telling dodges of, 49–56
    unacceptable, warning signs for,
        43–44
    values of, 24–25, 47–48
Donahue, 82, 173
"Do not resuscitate" code, 108–9,
    118, 119, 274–75, 299
Down syndrome, 21–22, 198, 216,
    226, 267
Dozeretz, Linda, 269
Drug Enforcement Administration,
    U.S., 324
drugs:

antirejection, 125, 140
cocaine, 331
cyclosporin, 125, 140
doctors' abuse of, 308, 327–31
laetril, 232, 249–50, 252
Pergonal, 152, 325
RU 486, 183
side effects of, 69–70, 81, 144
Thalidomide, 15–16
Dudding, Burton, 260–61
Dudding, Georgia, 32
Durable Powers of Attorney for
    Health Care Decisions, 29, 85,
    105–7, 137, 273, 276
    insurance and, 106
    "no code" and, 108–9
    pregnancy and, 187–88
    sample of, 360–63
    suicide and, 106
dwarfism, 226

Edwards, Georgia, 53
EEG (electroencephalogram), 208
Eichhorn, John H., 326
Eichner, Father, 279
Albert Einstein College of Medicine,
    30
Elias, Sherman, 167, 172
Ellison, Patricia, 223
embryos:
    experimental use of, 153–54,
        159–61
    freezing of, 153, 155, 159, 160
    orphan, 157
    rights of, 157
emergencies:
    informed consent and, 68
    Living Wills and, 100
    rights during, 61
Encyclopedia of Bioethics (Fox),
    139
England, 19, 159
Epilepsy Information Hotline, 267
Esposito, Elaine, 287
Esquire, 30
ethicists, defined, 29–30
ethics committees, 30–31, 283–84
    infant, 214–21
eugenics, 166
euthanasia, 111–13, 207, 283, 327
experimental research:

animal-heart transplants, 239–42
children's illnesses and, 239–44,
    249–52
on embryos, 153–54, 159–61
genetic engineering, 87–88
participation in, 83, 84–88
Patient's Bill of Rights for,
    345–46
placebos in, 86
extraordinary treatment, 205–6,
    278

Facts in Brief on Long-Term Care,
    296, 302
Family Health History Scan, 228
Federation of State Medical Boards,
    320–21, 328
feeding tubes, 285–88
Ferguson, Tom, 72
fetoscopy, 178
Finkbine, Sherri, 16
Finnegan, Rita, 338
Fiske, Jamie, 147–48
Flaster, Donald J., 324
*For the Concerned Couple Planning
    a Family*, 228
*For the Patient's Good: The
    Restoration of Beneficence in
    Medical Ethics* (Thomasma and
    Pellegrino), 95–96
Fost, Norman, 207
Fox, Brother, 278–79
Fox, Renee C., 139–40
Framingham Group Study, 50
fraud:
    billing, 323–24
    health, 252–53
    insurance, 321
Freeman, Beverly, 190
Friends and Relatives of
    Institutionalized Aged, Inc.,
    302
Frustaci, Patti and Sam, 325
Fuchs, Victor R., 77
funerals, 97, 222, 261

Gallup poll, 24
Galusha, Bryant L., 338
Garn, Jake, 140
Garza, Felipe, Jr., 125–26, 130
Gaylin, Willard, 232, 248n, 255

Lou Gehrig's disease, 98
generalizations, 51–52
genetic counseling, 179, 223–27
Genetic Counseling, 227
genetic diseases, 223–25, 228
genetic engineering, profits from,
    87–88
Genna, John, 127–28
Georgia Impaired Physicians
    Program, 339
German measles, 188, 225
Glamour, 125
Glasser, Ira, 339
Glendale Adventist Medical Center,
    82
Gohlke, Mary, 83
Goldstein, Joseph, 247–48
Goodman, Ellen, 143, 169, 243
Goodrich, Therese, 268
Government Printing Office, U.S.,
    17
Gray, Laura Beryl, 129–30, 132
Greene, Chad, 250
Griffith, H. Winter, 72
Guidelines on Human
    Experimentation, U.S., 84
Guiler, Gerri, 155, 163
Woody Guthrie's disease, 223

Haas, Toni, 267
Haire, Doris, 349
Hanafin, Hilary, 192
harassment, 80–81
Harvard Medical School, 325
*Harvard Medical School Health
    Newsletter*, 72
Hastings Center Report, 172, 213,
    293–94
Head, William, 137–38
Healing Heart, The (Cousins), 55
Health and Human Services, U.S.
    Department of, 46, 96, 159, 201
    Administration on Aging, 302
Health Care Finance
    Administration, 46
Healthfacts, 57
Health Insurance Association, 46
health maintenance organizations
    (HMOs), 37
Health Resources and Services
    Administration, 151

heart attacks, 50, 55–56
HeartLife, 267
heart-lung transplants, 129, 135
hearts, artificial, 83
Heartsounds (Lear), 50
heart transplants, 125–26, 127–28,
    138, 239–44
    animal-to-human, 239–42
Heinz, John, 295
Helsinki Declaration, 84
Hemlock Society, 102, 111, 121–22
hemophilia, 179
Henderson, Morrice and Marilyn,
    107–9
hepatitis, 107, 139, 165, 167
Herbert, Clarence, 286
hernias, diaphragmatic, 179
heroic treatment, 278
    in Baby Doe cases, 205–6, 216
Hicks, Linda, 259–60
Hippocratic Oath, 16
Hodgkin's disease, 21, 230–33,
    249–52
Hofbauer, Joseph, 232, 250
homicide, 134
hormonal tests, 178
hospices, children's, 257–59, 268
hospitals, 96–97
    emergency rooms of, 39–40
*How Genetic Disease Can Affect
    Your Family*, 228
How Safe Is Safe?, 56
Hoxsey treatment, 239, 250
Humane and Dignified Death Act,
    111–12
Huntington's chorea, 223
Huxley, Thomas, 53
hydrocephalus, 179, 209
hydronephrosis, 179
Hyman, Helen Kandel, 296
hyperparathyroidism, 35–36
hypertension (high blood pressure),
    35–36, 69–70, 139
hypoplastic left heart syndrome,
    239–40

impotence, 69–70
incest, 183–84
independent practice associations
    (IPAs), 37
India, organ sales in, 142

infant bioethics committees,
214–21
informed consent, 50, 65–73, 321
on abortion, 184
of child, 255–56
children's illnesses and, 240–42,
243–44, 255–56
elements of, 66
information sources for, 71–73
questions for, 70–71
risks and, 68–71
informed refusal, 56–57
In re John Storar, 281
In re Pogue, 247, 257
Inskip, Richard, 39
Institute for Consumer Policy
Research, 121
Institutionalized Person's Bill of
Rights, 350–53
Institutional Review Boards (IRBs),
85
insurance, health, 32
billing fraud and, 323–24
fees and, 306–7
Living Wills and, 106
organ transplants and, 134–35
records of, 117–18
withholding treatment and, 110
insurance, malpractice, 316
intermediate care homes, 296
*In the Matter of Karen Ann
Quinlan*, 282
in vitro fertilization (IVF), 152–64,
165–66
chances of, 154–57
embryo experimentation and,
153–54, 159–61
multiple births from, 156
orphan embryos from, 157
privacy and, 154
selection of program for, 161–63
Iowa, University of, 137–38

jargon, truthful, 50–51
Javits, Jacob and Marion, 98
Jean's Way: A Love Story, 122
Jehovah's Witnesses, 77, 247, 257
Jobes, Nancy and John, 288
John Paul II, Pope, 112
*Journal of the American Medical
Association*, 73, 167, 242, 326

justice, 18–19
Justice Department, U.S., 199
Juvenile Diabetes Foundation, 267

Kaiser Hospital, 285
Karen Ann, 282
Katz, Sanford, 169–70
kidney dialysis, 19, 284
kidney disease, 35, 139
kidney transplants, 125, 128,
131–32, 140
Kissling, Frances, 191
Koop, C. Everett, 180
Kübler-Ross, Elisabeth, 52, 261

laetrile, 232, 249–50, 252
Landers, Ann, 261
Lear, Hal, 50
Lear, Martha Weinman, 50
Leiken, Sanford, 255–56
Lenox Hill Hospital, 280, 334
Let Me Die Before I Wake, 122
leukemia, 61, 80, 135, 137, 165–66
life:
beginning of, 158–59
quality of, *see* quality of life
sanctity of, 30
*Life Support: Families Speak About
Hospitals, Hospice and Home
Care for the Fatally Ill*, 121
life-support systems, 97–98, 99,
120, 134, 265
DNR code and, 108–9, 118, 119
feeding tubes, 79, 285–88
Living Will and, 103
patient's wishes about, 278–81
substituted judgment standard
and, 279–81
see also Baby Doe cases;
treatment, withholding
limited paternalism, 81
liver transplants, 127–28, 135, 262
Living Wills, 29, 48, 98–104, 124,
137, 273–74, 276, 289
doctors and, 104
insurance and, 106
laws, by state, 101–2
on life-sustaining procedures, 103
limitations on, 104
"no code" and, 108–9

Living Wills *(cont.)*
  pregnancy and, 104, 187
  sample of, 357–59
  suicide and, 106
Long Dying of Baby Andrew, The
    (Stinson and Stinson), 204–5
Los Angeles Medical Center, 88
Los Angeles Times, 147
Los Angeles Trial Lawyers
    Association, 326
Lou Gehrig's disease, 98
lumpectomies, 74–75
lung cancer, 51, 81

McCormick, Richard, 203
Macklin, Ruth, 30, 232, 248*n*
McMahon, Jim, 27
Make-a-Wish Foundation, 259, 269
Malahoff, Alexander, 173–74
malpractice, 64–65, 309–10, 324–
    326
mammogram, 59
March of Dimes Birth Defects
    Foundation, 224–25, 226, 227
Marcus, Cyril C., 307–9, 329–30
Marcus, Stewart Lee, 307–8,
    329–30
Marik, Jaroslav, 325
Markle, Gerald E., 252
Marriage, Virginia, 154, 161
mastectomies, 74–75
Matters of Life and Death (Robin),
    61
M. D. Anderson Cancer Center, 246
media, 88–90
  incompetent doctors and, 331–32
  organ donations and, 147–48, 262
  pointers on working with,
    372–74
Medicaid, 297, 323
  organ transplants and, 134–35
medical ethics:
  centers for, 375–82
  decision-making and, 19–33
  defined, 19
  experts in, 29–31
  new technology and, 16, 37–38
  personal values and, 24–25
  principles of, 18–19
  see also specific topics
medical neglect, 201, 238

Medical Records: Getting Yours,
    338
Medical Research Patient's Bill of
    Rights, 345–46
Medicare, 297, 323
  organ transplants and, 135
Mehling, Alice V., 120
mental retardation, 22, 334
  in Baby Doe cases, 206–7
microcephaly, 173
Millman, Jeffrey, 45
Minor, Richard, 232, 250
miscarriage, 178
*Modern Prevention: The New
    Medicine* (Rosenfeld), 72
Monaco, Grace Powers, 267
Moore, John, 88
Mormons, 156
multiple sclerosis, 87, 170
Murphy, Judge, 247
muscular dystrophy, 179, 223
myelomeningocele, 216

N, Dr., 209
Nader, Ralph, 310
Narcotics Anonymous, 330
National Abortion Federation, 191
National Association of Surrogate
    Mothers, 192
National Center for Education in
    Maternal and Child Health, 228
National Center for Health
    Statistics, 152
National Center for Organ
    Transplantation, 131
National Citizen's Coalition for
    Nursing Home Reform, 301
National College of Juvenile Justice,
    170
National Conference of
    Commissioners on Uniform
    State Laws, 102
National Council on Aging, Inc.,
    293, 302
National Down Syndrome Society,
    267
National Genetics Foundation, Inc.,
    228
National Hospice Organization, 121
National Institutes of Health (NIH),
    88, 241

National Kidney Foundation, 143, 149, 150
National Organ Transplant Act, 131
National Self-Help Clearinghouse (NSHC), 268
National Task Force on Organ Transplantation, 131, 150
National Women's Health Network (NWHN), 56, 349
naturopathy, 230–31, 233, 249–50
Nejdl, Robert J., 285–86
Netherlands, 111, 159
Nevada State Board of Medical Examiners, 17, 310
New England Journal of Medicine, 29, 73, 77, 311
"new" medicine, 16–18, 37–38
Newsweek, 198
New Woman, 324
New York County Medical Society, 329
New York Disciplinary Board, 310
New York Hospital, 307
New York Times, 157, 311, 329
New York Times Magazine, 62
"Nobel sperm bank," 166
nonmaleficence, 18
nonverbal communication, 52
North American Transplant Coordinators Organization (NATCO), 132, 146
Northern California Transplant Bank, 129, 138–39
Northern Nevada Fertility Clinic, 153, 154, 160–61
North Memorial Medical Center, 27
Nuremberg Code, 84
Nursing Home Patient's Bill of Rights, 298, 354–55
nursing homes, 290–303
  ethics of, 299–300
  guilt about, 300–301
  ombudsmen in, 299, 303
  patient choices and, 301
  pros and cons of, 295–96
  selection of, 296–301

Office of Organ Transplantation, 129, 134, 151
Oklahoma Children's Memorial Hospital, 254

ombudsmen, 62–63, 299, 303
One Miracle at a Time (Dickman), 234
Operation Liftoff, 269
Organ donations, 21, 89, 124–51, 262, 364–67
  AIDS and, 136
  black market for, 142–43
  brain death and, 126, 133–34
  consent for, 136–37
  consent form for, 369
  criteria for, 138–39
  emotional bonds from, 139–41
  fund-raising for, 148
  living donors and, 140
  media appeals for, 147–48
  motivations for, 126–27
  networks for, 131–32
  payment for, 134–36
  privacy in, 137–38
  questions to ask about, 143–46
  required request laws for, 131, 132–33
  shortage of, 127–31
  waiting lists for, 146–47
Organ Donor Card, 130, 137, 149, 368
orphan embryos, 157

palliative care, 238
pancreas transplants, 127–28, 135, 141
Parade, 97
Paris, John, 286, 288
passive euthanasia, 112, 207
paternalism, limited, 81
patients:
  advocates and ombudsmen for, 62–63, 299, 303
  autonomy of, 18, 20, 25, 37–38, 54–55, 247, 293, 294
  benefit to, 16–17
  denial by, 27, 51
  doctor's relationship with, 34–58, 217, 314–15
  media and, 88–90
  nursing homes for, 290–303
  privacy of, 36–37, 38, 65, 87, 247, 279, 282
  proxies for, 99, 103, 105, 114–18
  responsibility of, 37

patients *(cont.)*
  rights of, *see* rights, patient
  selective hearing by, 51
  values of, 24–26, 47–48
Patient's Bill of Rights, 67–68,
  342–44
Peacock, John, 83
Pellegrino, Edmund D., 25, 94
People, 84, 262
People's Book of Medical Tests, The
  (Sobel and Ferguson), 72
People's Medical Society (PMS), 57
Pergonal, 152, 325
peritonitis, 212
Permanent Families for Children,
  190–91
persistent vegetative states, 277–78,
  287, 288
Peter F., 253–54
Peterson, James C., 252
physician's aid committees, 330–31
Physician's Alert Screening Service,
  326
Physician's Recognition Award, 42
Piaget, Jean, 254–55
Pittsburgh Press, 146
Pius XII, Pope, 205
placebos, 86
Plaintext Doctor-Patient Checklist,
  56
Planned Parenthood Federation of
  America, Inc. (PPFA), 185, 191–
  92
Plater, Dan, 25–27
*Politics, Science and Cancer: The
  Laetrile Phenomenon* (Markle
  and Peterson, eds.), 252
polydactyly, 226
Postgraduate Medicine, 329
Potter, Laurie, 73
Poulsen, Mike and Shauna, 153–54,
  163, 165–66
preferred provider organizations
  (PPOs), 3
pregnancy, 48
  Living Will and, 104
  see also surrogate motherhood
Pregnant Patient's Bill of Rights,
  347–49
prenatal testing, 177–80

questions to ask about, 179–80
  risks of, 178–79
President's Commission for the
  Study of Ethical Problems in
  Medicine and Biomedical and
  Behavioral Research, 17, 37, 38,
  283
  on Baby Doe cases, 202, 214
  on embryo experimentation, 189
  on informed consent, 66
  on withholding treatment, 113
primary care physicians, 40
Prince v. *Massachusetts*, 247, 257
privacy, 36–37, 38, 65, 87, 247, 279,
  282
  Baby Doe cases and, 202–3
  in vitro fertilization and, 154
professional review organizations
  (PROs), 324
Prottas, Jeffrey, 149
proxies, 99, 103, 105, 114–18
  assertiveness of, 115–16
  health of, 116–17
  selection of, 115–17
  values of, 115–16
Public Citizen Health Research
  Group, 310, 338
Purke, Don, 174

quackery, 252–53
quality of life, 30, 81–84
  in Baby Doe cases, 206–7
*Questions and Answers on Organ
  Transplantation*, 151
Quinlan, Karen Ann, 279, 282–83,
  287

Radford, Barbara, 191
rape, 183–84, 189
rationality, 19
records, medical, 307–9, 318–19,
  333
  in Baby Doe cases, 213–14
Rehabilitation Act, 200, 202
religion, 20, 77–78, 156, 185, 191,
  247, 257, 282
Relman, Arnold S., 311
remission, 238
Repository for Germinal Choice,
  166

Reproductive Council of the American Association of Tissue Banks, 167
required request laws, 131, 132–33
research, *see* experimental research
Resolve, Inc., 190
resuscitation, 99, 108–9, 119
  DNR code and, 108–9, 118, 119, 299
  Living Will and, 108–9
Riessman, Frank, 268
rights, embryo, 157
rights, patient, 18–19, 59–91
  abortion and, 182–86
  autonomy, 18, 20, 25, 37–38, 247, 293, 294
  in Baby Doe cases, 202–8
  beneficence, 18, 38, 239
  Bills of, 67–68, 342–55
  of children, 246–49, 253–56
  confidentiality, 36–37, 87, 137, 312–15, 331
  to die, 23, 60, 78–80, 99, 282–83, 287–90; *see also* Baby Doe cases; treatment, withholding
  in emergencies, 61
  in experimental research programs, 83, 84–85
  informed consent, *see* informed consent
  nonmaleficence, 18
  parents and, 246–49
  privacy, 36–37, 38, 65, 87, 154, 202–3, 247, 279, 282
  self-determination, 54, 80–81
  violations of, 306–39
Rights of Gay People, The, 339
Rights of Hospital Patients, The (Annas), 68
Rights of the Critically Ill, The, 65–66, 339
Rights of the Mentally Retarded, The, 339
Rios, Mario and Elsa, 157, 160
risk-benefit analysis, 18, 77, 248
Robin, Eugene D., 61, 87
Roe, Jane, 183–84
Roe v. *Wade*, 158, 180, 183
Rokeach, Milton, 26*n*
Ronald McDonald House, 258, 268

Rosenfeld, Isadore, 46, 48, 72
RU 486, 183
Rutherford, Pat, 262–63
Ryser, Janet, 266

Sacred Congregation for the Doctrine of the Faith, 112
Sandburg, Carl, 33
San Diego Clippers, 77
San Diego Tribune, 78
San Francisco Chronicle, 89, 156, 186
Sapadin, Lois, 269
Schloendorff v. *Society of New York Hospital*, 54
Schroeder, William and Margaret, 84
seat belt laws, 129
secondary care physicians, 40
Second Opinion, 46
second opinions, 35–36, 44–46, 75–76, 144
selective hearing, 51
self-determination, right to, 54, 80–81
self-fulfilling prophecies, 53
Senate Select Committee on Aging, 295
senile dementia, 289
sexually transmitted diseases, 314
Shankel, Stewart, 69
Sher, Geoffrey, 160–61
Sherman, Jerome K., 167
Shine, K. I., 55–56
Should You Consider Amniocentesis?, 228
sickle-cell disease, 179, 226
side effects of drugs, 69–70, 81, 144
Silverstone, Barbara, 296
60 Minutes, 82, 111
skilled nursing facilities (SNFs), 296
Smith, Lloyd H., 36
Smith, Sylvia, 300–301
Sobel, David, 72
Society for the Right to Die, 102, 105, 120–21, 358, 360–63
Sokoloff, Burton, 176
sonograms, 177
Sorkow, Harvey R., 171
sperm, 142

sperm *(cont.)*
  banks for, 166–68
  freezing of, 165–66
spina bifida, 199, 209
Spina Bifida Association Hotline, 267
Spinal Cord Injury Hotline, 267
Spock, Benjamin, 97–98
Springer, Charles E., 31
Starlight Foundation, 269
state boards of medical examiners, 320
sterilization, 156
Stern, William and Elizabeth, 170–171
Stinson, Robert and Peggy, 204–5
Stiver, Judy, 173
Stiver, Ray, 174
strep infections, 173
strokes, 109
Strong, Carson, 204
substituted judgment standard, 279–81
suicide, 79, 106, 112, 121–22, 127, 134, 138, 308, 327
surgery, 36, 59–60
  cesarean sections, 64–65, 153
  fetal, 179
  second opinions on, 44–45, 75–76
surrogate motherhood, 22, 168–76, 192
  altruistic, 168–69, 176
  Baby M case of, 170–71
  birth defects and, 173–74
  ethics and legality of, 176
  laws regarding, 172–73, 176

Talbott, G. Douglas, 328, 329, 339
Tannenbaum, Melvyn, 199
Tay-Sachs disease, 179, 226
test-tube babies, *see in vitro fertilization*
Thalidomide, 15–16
therapeutic abortion, 16
Thinking About a Nursing Home, 296, 302
Thinking of Having Surgery?, 90
Thomas, Herbert H., 190
Thomasma, David, 38, 94, 301
Thoreau, Henry David, 49

Thornton, Barbara, 115
Time, 15, 198, 288
Townsend, Aloen, 295
tracheostomy, 196
transplants, *see* organ donations; *specific organs*
treatment, heroic, 205–6, 216, 278
treatment, withholding, 23, 78–81, 94, 105, 109–11, 173, 201–2
  AMA on, 370–71
  best interests and, 283–85, 289
  for children, 256–66
  euthanasia and, 111–13
  feeding tubes and, 79, 285–88
  insurance and, 110
  patient's wishes about, 278–79
  for relative or friend, 272–90
  substituted judgment standard for, 279–81
  unlawful, 327
  see also Baby Doe cases
Trisomy 18, 224, 226
Trisomy 21 (Down Syndrome), 21–22, 198, 216, 226, 267
truthful jargon, 50–51
Turk, Virginia, 109–11
Twycross, Robert G., 111, 112
Tyler Medical Clinic, 325

ultrasound testing, 177, 325
Understanding Human Values (Rokeach), 26n
Uniform Anatomical Gift Act, 364–67
Uniform Determination of Death Act, 277
United Network for Organ Sharing (UNOS), 131, 146
universalizability, 19
University of California, Berkeley, Wellness Letter, 72
Utilization Review Boards, 110

values, 24–27, 47–48
  changes in, 25–27
  list of, 26
  of proxies, 115–16
  spiritual, 77–78
Van Woert, Cathie and Brad, 224–25
Van Woert, Chrissy, 224–25

Veatch, Robert M., 38, 49
viral encephalitis, 212

Walsh, Ellen, 191
Walwork, Edward, 223
Washburn, A. Lawrence, 199
Wattleton, Faye, 191
Weir, Robert, 214
Weithorn, Lois, 253
*What You Should Know About
    Durable Power of Attorney*, 121
Whitehead, Mary Beth, 170–71
Who Speaks for the Child? (Gaylin
    and Macklin, eds.), 232, 248*n*
Wilborn, Sandra, 23
Wilks, Jeanette, 168–69, 176
Wilks, Martin, 169
wills, 92

see also Living Wills
withholding treatment, *see*
    treatment, withholding
Wolfe, Sidney M., 338
Woman's Day, 209
Woody Guthrie's disease, 223
World Medical Association, 84
Wright, Frank Lloyd, 51

x-rays, 177–78, 208

You and Your Aging Parent
    (Silverstone and Hyman), 296
You and Your Living Will, 121
Young, James Harvey, 252

Ziegler, Karen, 230–33, 249–52